ENDURING MEMORIES:
A PAEDIATRIC GASTROENTEROLOGIST REMEMBERS

A TALE OF LONDON AND SYDNEY

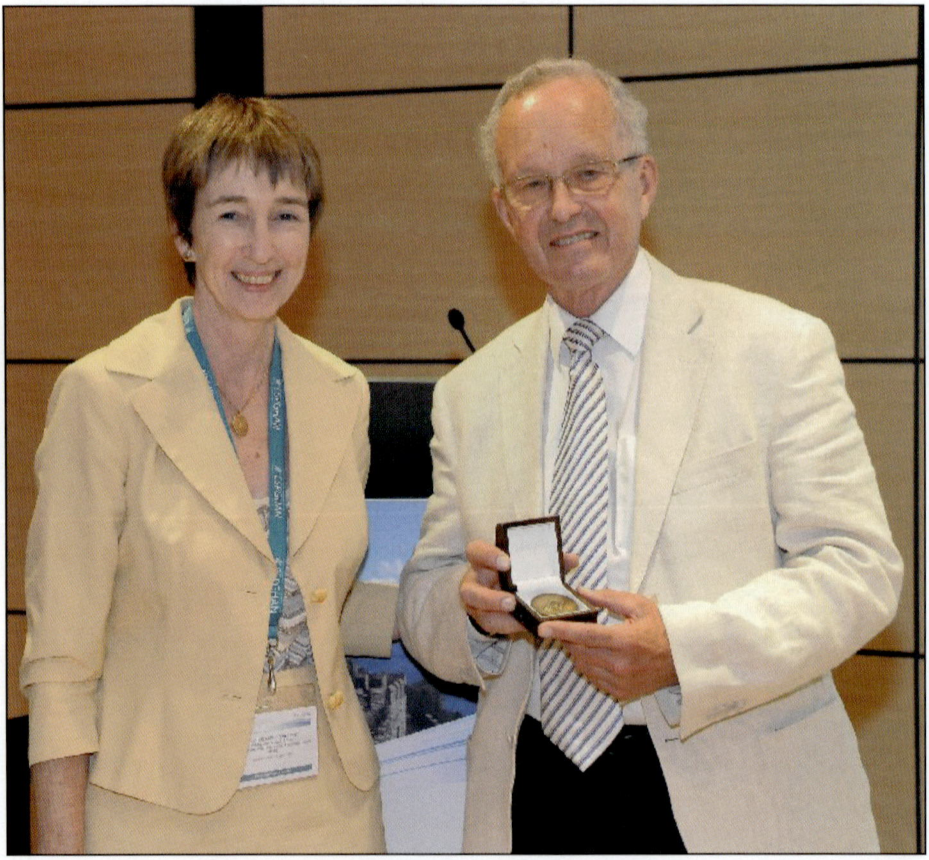

Professor Deidre Kelly President of ESPGHAN, presents Author with a distinguished service award, Istanbul 2010

ENDURING MEMORIES: A PAEDIATRIC GASTROENTEROLOGIST REMEMBERS

A TALE OF LONDON AND SYDNEY

by

John Walker-Smith

To David
with best wishes
John Walker-Smith
Jan 2014

The Memoir Club

First published in 2003 by
The Memoir Club
Reprinted in 2012 by
The Memoir Club
Arya House
Langley Park
Durham
DH7 9XE
Tel: 0191 373 5660
Email: memoirclub@msn.com

British Library Cataloguing in
Publication Data.
A catalogue record for this book
is available from the
British Library

ISBN: 978-1-84104-538-2

Printed by Xpresslitho, Washington

This book is dedicated to all my patients, both children and adult, and to my long-suffering family.

Contents

List of Illustrations ix
Preface xi
Author's Note First Edition xiii
Author's Note Second Edition xvii
Chapter 1 Growing-up in Australia; Early Childhood Influences 1
Chapter 2 School Days; Privileged Education 7
Chapter 3 University of Sydney and its Medical School 35
Chapter 4 Junior Doctor in Sydney 46
Chapter 5 Ship's Surgeon 54
Chapter 6 Physician Trainee in London 64
Chapter 7 Gastroenterology Trainee in Sydney 83
Chapter 8 Paediatric Trainee in Sydney and Zurich 91
Chapter 9 Specialist Paediatrician in Sydney, Planning the Future 110
Chapter 10 Young Academic in London, Fighting the Corner 129
Chapter 11 Recognition for Paediatric Gastroenterology, Specialism in Medicine 156
Chapter 12 A Chair in London, Perpetual Change 167
Chapter 13 Paediatric Gastroenterology, International Connections and World Travel 183
Chapter 14 The Tomlinson Report 195
Chapter 15 MMR, Crohn's Disease and Regressive Autism 207
Chapter 16 The Trial 219
Chapter 17 Time for the Family: Aspects of the Personal Life 236
Chapter 18 Reflections on Anglo-Australia, the Empire and the Monarchy 244

Chapter 19 Ecclesiastical Reflections 266
Chapter 20 Medico-Historical Postscript 273
Index 279

List of Illustrations

Between page 45-46

1. Alexandra (Alix) Buckingham Walker-Smith (née Trindall) BA (Sydney), (1901-1970)
2. Angus Buchanan Walker-Smith MB ChM (Sydney) FRCS (Edinburgh), (1900-1975)
3. Author aged five years with mother, sister Judith and grandmother (nana) in George St, Sydney 1941
4. Author in Mowbray House School uniform, photographed in back garden of 6 Milner Crescent, aged seven years, January 1943
5. Gran, auntie Ethel, Judith and Author with 1935 Vauxhall at the back of Allowah
6. Shore School with the boarding house known as School House on the left, with the chapel on the right and Sydney Harbour Bridge and harbour in the background
7. Shore boys as the '*Ladies and Gentlemen*' of Pinafore, 1953
8. University friends at 68 Shirley Rd, 1955
9. Author as fifth year medical student bathing a baby he had just delivered at King George V Memorial Hospital, 1958
10. The front of the Old Medical School, with the dissecting room on the first floor on the left, 1955
11. Author assisted by nurse performs an exchange blood transfusion on a newborn baby at King George V Memorial Hospital, 1961
12. Author on MV *Aramaic* in the Red Sea, 1962
13. Dr John Samuel Yu, general medical superintendent of the Royal Alexandra Hospital for Children, with the bust of Queen Alexandra, 1990
14. Author visiting Victoria Falls, December 1966
15. Prince Philip being shown the gastroenterology laboratory in the Institute of Child Health, Sydney 1968

Between page 109-110

16. The tomb of Rahere in the church of St Bartholomew the Great
17. View day at Barts, Author's sister Judith Peak, Howard Peak, his son James, wife Liz, niece Christine, daughter Laura, nephew Malcolm, daughter Louise and nephew Stephen, 1985
18. View day, Author with wife Liz and daughter Louise at Barts, 1973
19. View day at Barts, Author, 1995
20. Ad hoc editorial office meeting for Journal of Pediatric Gastroenterology and Nutrition in Author's office at the Royal Free School of Medicine, 1998
21. Author with child patient in outpatient clinic at the Royal Free Hospital, Septembercv 1995
22. ESPGAN working group for coeliac disease, in Paris in home of Jacques and Françoise Schmitz, 1989
23. Author signing copy of fourth edition of book in Taipei for a research fellow working with Dr Me-Hwei Chang on left, March 2000
24. Author on 65th birthday, in back garden at home with wife Liz, Chloe, Joseph, Morgan and William, 2001
25. Visit of Queen Elizabeth the Queen Mother to Queen Elizabeth Hospital for Children for 125th anniversary of the hospital, 1992
26. Family group at home of Author, Christmas Eve, 1992
27. Visit of Queen Elizabeth II and Prince Philip to entrance of Queen Elizabeth Hospital for Children on the occasion of the Queen's Silver Jubilee, 1977

Preface

AS A CLOSE personal friend and colleague, I am pleased to write the preface to John Walker-Smith's autobiography. John and I first met in London in the mid-seventies when I was visiting Chris Booth at Hammersmith Hospital and John kindly invited me to his home in Woodford Green for dinner. It was there that I initially realized our common heritage (e.g., our families had both emigrated from Scotland to Australia and to America respectively). Since then, we have had parallel career trajectories and shared many happy times together at meetings throughout the world. We have also worked together as editors of a textbook in our field (1980-1999) and as co-editors of *The Journal of Pediatric Gastroenterology and Nutrition* (1996-2000). In addition, we also co-jointly supervised a Fellowship Exchange Program (1984-2000). During this time, we have shared countless hours discussing our field, politics, cultures and values. As a participant in John's *'Festschrift'* in September, 2000, I learned about his early life in Australia and the influence that his family and educational background had on him becoming one of the pioneers in our subspecialty. Our common bond is highlighted in a review of *The History of Paediatric Gastroenterology* and *Paediatric Research* (2003:53:706-715).

However, this close association in a shared professional field has been the catalyst for a much deeper and more meaningful relationship. John and I have shared those values and aspirations on enjoyable moments encountered in life that are most meaningful (e.g., painting of a religious scene in Jerusalem; time in Silver Lake, New Hampshire; convincing my youngest son, Andrew, of the value of the monarchy) and have gotten to know each other's families through time spent together. One always wonders how someone like John Walker-Smith has achieved so many accomplishments in his field and become such a pioneer of our subspecialty. Insights into his capacity to influence this subspecialty came from reading of his early life in Australia, the influences of interaction with mentors (Chris Booth and Tony Dawson in the UK and Andrea Prader in Switzerland) in the UK and elsewhere, and his high personal standard for interactions with young paediatric gastroenterologists worldwide. It is a pleasure to attend meetings with John throughout the world, particularly in Commonwealth countries, because he is always surrounded by adoring former trainees showing their appreciation for his guidance.

Since the last edition of his memoirs was published, several tragic events have occurred in John's life including the death of his middle daughter Laura and the GMC Hearing into his evaluation of autistic children. Despite the heartache that these events have caused, John has weathered the "storm" and has recently been exonerated from the ill-conceived GMC Hearing determinations by his successful Appeal to the High Court.

My fondest regards.

Allan Walker

Harvard Medical School
Boston, MA,
2012

Author's Note First Edition

THE PROFESSIONAL HISTORIAN of medicine may find little of interest in this autobiography of one academic doctor, a minor player in the medical world, struggling to develop one small specialty within paediatrics. There are no great names, nor great discoveries here. However the general reader may perhaps be interested to read one doctor's account 'from the inside' of a profession coming under increasing scrutiny in recent years.

'The biographer is free to roam wherever his instinct takes him.' So stated Michael Holroyd in his acclaimed *Works on Paper, the Craft of Biography and Autobiography* (2002). As I have roamed across my life I have become aware of the impact of unexpected events. So I have sought to highlight these moments with the comment 'Little did I realize that . . .' at strategic moments in this account of my life. Looking back, perhaps the most unanticipated thing I ever did was to settle permanently in England having grown up in Australia. However as my early life is related, perhaps the reader will not be as surprised as I was at the time.

Virgil, in the Aeneid, described how the goddess Venus gave Aeneas the unique opportunity to see into the future, and in particular to see the deeds of his descendents. Venus brought to him the armour wrought by the hands of her husband, the god Vulcan. 'What words can tell of all the wonders of the shield and the pictured history wrought on its surface by the fire god?' Here Aeneas saw displayed the future with all the deeds of his posterity. This is not given to us, but as one looks back reflectively at oneself at an earlier given moment in life, one can then analyse and reflect on how things were seen at the time and what the ultimate reality proved to be.

An autobiography can reveal things that friends, colleagues and oneself might prefer to be buried. I hope none of my family, friends and colleagues, or indeed even my professional rivals, will feel, after reading this book, that this is so. Yet I have felt the need to record some of the conflicts in my own life and career, but not all. Some have been left out, especially in relation to more recent events, as many colleagues are still in the midst of an active career. I have not mentioned any junior doctors by name from 1995 onwards; I would not wish to do anything to embarrass or damage anyone's career. Yet I have not avoided completely the possibility of causing dissent by some of those about whom I have written, but these are my memories, not theirs. I certainly hope I do not cause any pain to those who have been my mentors, friends and colleagues. I have endeavoured throughout to try to answer the two questions - 'What was it like at the time?' and 'Why did things happen the way they did?'

So I have roamed around my life, trying to be as honest as possible, but I have been selective. Most of what I shall record concerns my own recollections and response to events. Others recalling the same events may have different memories, but this is a record of how I acted and reacted. Queen Victoria remarked that history was not an account of what actually happened but what people generally thought had happened. This book provides an account, by one doctor, of what happened to him in the latter part of the twentieth century, in two countries, Australia and Britain. With apologies to Charles Dickens, it is a tale of two cities, Sydney and London, and in part a tale of each of their universities. There are no sensations or scandals but there will be accounts of some conflicts. Medical politics can be as bitter as national politics.

I have sought to avoid the prison of chronology as described by Holroyd, although at the beginning a chronological approach is used, but this becomes thematic as the book advances.

The greatest challenge of my career was to contribute to the development of the new child specialty of paediatric gastroenterology and to help secure its recognition internationally. Paediatric generalists and adult gastroenterology specialists alike resisted this, but it is the children with gastrointestinal disorders who have been the real beneficiaries of the development of special skills to diagnose and treat their maladies. Much more could have been done and much more remains to be done to defeat these scourges of children.

My life has occurred in a world full of alarms and excursions. The Second World War over-shadowed my early childhood, but since then, at first in Australia, and then latterly in Britain, I have lived in a civil society largely at peace, apart from acts of Irish Republican terrorism in London, in 1973 and 1974. To live personally in peace has been an extraordinary privilege. However, great geopolitical events have impacted upon the societies in which I have lived. Pivotal for my life has been Britain's retreat from Empire and how that impacted upon our life in Australia and how it may have contributed to my decision to settle in England. This event has continued to shape our family life in Britain, with the ever increasing engagement with Europe. I shall attempt to describe my own experience of these changes as well as the way in which society itself and the Church particularly have changed.

Surprisingly, perhaps, increasing good health, highlighted by dramatic falls in infant mortality and general affluence in the developed world has not produced the great advances in human happiness and contentment that the reformers of the Victorian Age had anticipated. Nevertheless, for me and my family the past fifty years have been a wonderful time in which to live, at first in Australia and then in Britain, a period of calm and stability, a veritable golden age. Yet the life led by so many in the developing world provides a sad contrast, and I have tried in a small way not to be indifferent to this reality. During this time I have been privileged to be a member of what remains for me a noble profession. My autobiography gives an account of this.

John Angus Walker-Smith
MD (*Sydney*)
FRCP (*Edinburgh & London*)
FRACP
FRCPCH (*Honorary*)
Emeritus Professor of Paediatric Gastroenterology, University Of London

Woodford Green
Essex, England
September 2002

Author's Note Second Edition

NINE YEARS ON, professional historians may now indeed be interested in me, in view of the General Medical Council (GMC) Hearing, which involved Dr. Andrew Wakefield, myself and Professor Simon Murch. It was held from 16 July 2007 till 24 May 2010. I gave evidence for a total of 27 days but that was 17 months before the GMC Panel gave their determination of facts. Finally on 7th March 2012 my appeal against their decision to erase me from GMC register was upheld. The findings of the GMC panel were quashed. This was eight years after a journalist had first made allegations against me. My personal response to the Hearing, is reported in this second edition in a new chapter, entitled The Trial. In view of the immense complexity and the duration of the Hearing, I have preferred this personal response to a detailed factual account. It was the longest Hearing ever held by the GMC. Little did I realize when the first edition of this book was published in 2003 that the worst years of my professional life were still to come.

Elsewhere I have undertaken a limited revision of the text. In the latter chapters I have added more recent events. The account of MMR, Crohn's disease and Regressive Autism etc has been updated in light of documents not available at the time of the first edition. In large measure the first edition was based upon memory of past events, sometimes without supporting documentation.

In 2002 my mood was in general optimistic. Now it is more pessimistic. This pessimism is in large measure related to the GMC Hearing. It has had a profound effect upon me, my family, friends and colleagues. To some extent, it did sour my outlook on life, for a time.

This pessimism is also related to my perception of the decline of "Britishness", within the United Kingdom and the acceleration of political correctness in so many areas of life, including medicine and especially the National Health Service. This pessimism also relates to my disappointment, concerning my expectations for academic paediatric gastroenterology at the

Royal Free Hospital as expressed in 2003. Sadly these have not been fulfilled. The laboratory has closed and the colleagues who supported me at the time of my retirement, have moved on elsewhere. Then there is the sadness following the decision to close the Wellcome Trust Centre for the History of Medicine in 2012. Many of my hopes and expectations for the future expressed in the first edition have been dashed.

This pessimism is also related in some measure, to a self awareness of my own naïve expectations over many years. In the first edition I was aware to some extent. For example I referred to my hope to preserve sentiment and to avoid cynicism by moving to London. This was a very naïve hope. In the United Kingdom cynicism appears to rule the media today, perhaps more than ever. This spreads out, to society more generally.

I have always had great respect for the British Establishment and the medical establishment in particular. My experience with the General Medical Council has blunted this respect. I was treated very harshly. Apart from anything else the duration was very hard for me and my family to bear. Looking back, I may also have been at times, somewhat unrealistic in my defence of Britain and her former Empire, but only in part. I do retain my own defence of the many good qualities of the British Empire such as I experienced myself, growing up in Australia in 1930's to 1950's. My admiration for men such as Sir Robert Menzies and Lord Slim stands quite undimmed. I also have enjoyed visiting so many Commonwealth countries where their British heritage is still very real, as I have outlined in this book. Yet my expectations for the "Britishness" experienced in my youth, have proved to be unrealistic in modern Britain. I was indeed surprised on arrival in England to find in 1962 that so many people were less than respectful concerning the mother country and her institutions. This was so unlike me and my friends in Sydney, as I have described in Chapter 17. However there is room for a return of some optimism for "Britishness" in this year of the Queen's Diamond Jubilee and the London Olympics. Perhaps the Royal Wedding of Prince William and Kate Middleton was a real turning point to a restoration of pride in things British.

I have resisted the temptation to swing from naivety to cynicism . I believe I am now moving towards a new sense of reality. Two of my friends have encouraged me to take stock and to move in this direction.

Two great personal tragedies have befallen my family since the first edition was published. These have affected me profoundly and are mentioned in Chapter 17.

Yet in the long term I do remain an optimist. This is especially so in view of the justice I received eventually from the High Court. My experience of wife and family, especially grandchildren as well as young medical colleagues and my friends too, permit me to retain a positive outlook on life. Looking back now, my own golden age professionally was the period of time I spent in 1980's and 1990's at Queen Elizabeth Hospital for Children and at St. Bartholomew's Hospital in London. During this time we were able to advance knowledge concerning gastroenterological disease in childhood by means of technological advances. Tissue diagnosis, based upon biopsy of the gastrointestinal tract was at the centre of our diagnostic approach. This was innovative at the time. Important advances were made concerning the management of a range of disorders especially inflammatory bowel disease in children. The care of sick children with gastroenterological disorders was measurably improved. An international personal network in paediatric gastroenterology was established.

So even now battered though I be, by the GMC events of recent years, but restored by the receipt of justice, I retain my faith in medicine as a noble profession. It is a worthwhile life and I am proud to live in this United Kingdom where justice prevails in the Royal Courts of Justice.

John Angus Walker-Smith
MD (*Sydney*)
FRCP (*Edinburgh & London*)
FRACP
FRCPCH (*Honorary*)
Emeritus Professor of Paediatric Gastroenterology, University Of London

Woodford Green
Essex, England
June 2012

CHAPTER ONE

Growing-up in Australia; Early Childhood Influences

WE ARE ALL IN BONDAGE to our own genes, to our own parents and grandparents as well as to our forebears, lost in time. However the way our parents brought us up, together with the sum of our past experiences modifies and influences the expression of our genes. Although we may have the illusion of complete freedom of choice, yet we are not free to do exactly what we desire.

In this autobiography I shall endeavour to sketch out the professional life of one doctor, engaged in a branch of the specialty of paediatrics (the care of sick children). I shall endeavour to describe how my parents influenced me in my decision to study medicine and much more. I shall mention how I was aware of the 'medical genes' inherited from my father and both grandfathers. I shall also describe some of the rather mundane experiences which have shaped the life of one doctor, and hope that the detail provided will be of interest.

I shall also outline how my own upbringing gave me a sense of a world-wide British inspired community, a view which flourished in Australia at the time of my birth and continued whilst I was growing up, but which has now largely vanished there. This shaped my own life more than it did many of my contemporaries and continues to influence my thoughts today. In one way I am writing, in part, a kind of requiem for a Britannic Australia, long gone, but with powerful echoes and surprisingly loud resonances even today in both Australia and Britain.

More conventionally in a medical autobiography, I shall describe my own experience of the complicated world of medical practice in both Australia and the United Kingdom as well as internationally. I shall highlight the long battle for the recognition of my own particular specialty, paediatric gastroenterology, within child care. I also hope to give some insights as to how things looked from within the British National Health Service, from an Academic or University perspective for nigh on thirty years.

I was born on 1 December 1936, in Charlemount private hospital in Potts Point, Sydney. My mother was Alexandra Buckingham Walker-Smith (née Trindall). She was always known in the family as Alix, having been named after Queen Alexandra, whose name within her own family had been Alix. My mother recalled that she had heard the wireless broadcast made by King Edward VIII, announcing his abdication, while she was still nursing me in hospital. This occurred when I was 10 days old on December 11th. Clearly mothers of newborn babies remained longer in hospital at that time than they do today, as I am quite unaware of any medical problems with either mother or baby!

1936 was indeed the year of the three kings with the death of George V on 20 January and the accession of Edward VIII followed by his abdication after his brief reign. George VI succeeded him to the throne of Britain and her Empire. From my earliest moments, my mother brought me up as a royalist and loyal son of Empire, although we lived in one of its farthest outposts. She herself was third generation Australian, descended largely from English forebears with one Irish ancestor.

My father Angus Buchanan Walker-Smith was first generation Australian born, with all his ancestors from Scotland, chiefly from the Highlands. His father, also John, had constructed a double barrelled name from his mother Mary Walker of Campbeltown and father Alexander Smith of Cardross. I have often been asked over the years whether I am related to the conservative politician Sir Derek Walker-Smith. The answer is no. At the time of my birth, my father was an honorary urological surgeon (consultant equivalent) at the Royal Prince Alfred Hospital in Sydney. An urologist is a surgical specialist in the genito-urinary tract of the body.

From my earliest days I was brought up in a medical atmosphere. Both my grandfathers, who had died years before I was born, had been general practitioners, as indeed were both my paternal and maternal uncles. So there always seemed to be a tacit assumption within the family, perhaps from my birth, that I would in due course follow the family tradition into medicine.

One of my earliest memories was being ordered out of my father's study in no uncertain terms. Amidst my tears I told my mother that I 'only spitted on his scope.' The 'scope' in question, upon which I had apparently spat, was a cystoscope, an instrument used by my father to examine the inside of the urinary bladder in his urological practice. My father's study did in fact contain mysterious instruments, long cylinders containing fine tubes (catheters) and packages of strange partly black images, which I later learned, were X-ray films. I would often glimpse my father examining these closely by holding them up to the electric light bulb. I used to wonder what on earth these strange pictures revealed to him that held him so spellbound. His study also had a curious ill-defined smell, which I later came to understand to be related, in some way, to being a doctor.

I also realized early on that my father's profession meant he was away from home a great deal. In my earliest memories I only recall him appearing at breakfast time and sometimes at the weekend.

For breakfast he always had porridge in the winter, (with salt and no sugar, in the Scots manner) or cornflakes in the summer, followed by a soft boiled egg and toast. He always cut his toast into four parts before he buttered each piece individually. He was a very particular man. He insisted on referring to his table napkin whereas my mother always spoke of his serviette and she said jokingly that napkins were only for babies.

In my earliest days I lived with my parents in an upstairs flat of a large house known as Allowah in Manly. The name Manly was given to this area when Governor Arthur Phillip first arrived on 22 January 1788. He wrote concerning the local aboriginal men he encountered:

> 'Their confidence and manly bearing made me give the name of Manly Cove to this place.'

The suburb of Manly includes Manly Beach and is seven miles north from central Sydney, whence it is reached most conveniently by ferry across Sydney Harbour. Allowah was later to feature much in my childhood memories, but by my second birthday we had moved to a flat in the adjacent suburb of Balgowlah. Allowah was owned by my maiden Aunt Ethel Andrews (Auntie Ethel) whose home it was. Ethel had been a child of my grandmother's first marriage in Glasgow. Like her mother she had been a nurse. She then shared her home with her mother, my widowed Grandmother, Elizabeth Walker-Smith (1883-1947), who I was later always to know as gran. Both of them had been born in Scotland and a very Scottish household it was. Gran was a formidable, strong minded woman with very definite opinions. Gran did not approve of married couples kissing in public! My mother related that she had been informed by her mother-in-law, after enthusiastically kissing my father 'Goodbye' on several mornings, as a newly wed, that this really was not the done thing in 'public'! My mother's resulting deflation and hurt can well be imagined when my father tacitly signalled his agreement.

I was baptized John Angus at the age of a month in the Presbyterian

Church at Manly by Rev. Stevenson. My father's religious position could best be described as a Presbyterian agnostic, but my mother was an enthusiastic and active believer and member of the Church of England. The fact that I was christened as a Presbyterian was I think a ploy on my mother's behalf, to encourage my father to attend church, but as the years went by this clearly did not happen. I myself liked the Church of England and my own attendance at a Presbyterian church faded out once I went to Shore School.

Our flat in Balgowlah was situated in a new brick building two storeys high and we had a ground floor flat. There was a sitting room, a dining room, study, main bedroom and a nursery for me and later my sister. A domestic maid, Maisie, who did not live in, assisted my mother. She was a refugee from German-occupied Austria and she seemed to do a lot of weeping about her family's circumstances back in Europe. In fact my sister was born on September 20th shortly after the outbreak of the Second World War. I can vividly remember my mother crying when she heard the news on the wireless of the outbreak of war and bemoaning the terrible state of the world for a newborn baby.

My sister's birth had been quite traumatic for me, aged 2 years 9 months, with the sudden and unexpected pain of separation from my mother. One morning early, to my great surprise, my mother had disappeared without saying goodbye and there was my maternal Grandmother (Rosina Trindall, nana, 1864-1958) sitting by my bed telling me not to worry and that mummy would be back soon with a new baby. I remember it was raining at the time and she had me playing the interesting game of determining which of two raindrops landing on the window glass would reach the bottom of the pane first. Nana, like my other grandmother, was also a quite formidable woman. However she was well covered and cuddly, not fearsome and remote. Indeed she both gave and received kisses and hugs, unlike gran, who liked only the lightest peck on her cheek from a dutiful grandson. Nana however was a dedicated charity worker and was a tough member and sometimes chair of committees. One of her favourite committees was the Fresh Air League which was a charity arranging country holidays for poor city families with children. She was also on the Visiting Committee of Marrickville District Hospital where her husband and son had been on the staff. Like her husband before her, she had been a member of the synod of the Church of England, Diocese of Sydney. She was on terms of friendship with the Archbishops of Sydney up to Dr Howard Mowll. She was the pivot of her large family and centre of the annual Christmas reunion. She, like her brother Uncle Tom Warren, had been born on Christmas Day, making the festive season a very special family event.

I remember on one occasion, her arriving breathless at Balgowlah, carrying an enormous parcel which turned out to be a large wooden farmyard with associated lead toys. She had lugged this heavy load from Walther and Stephenson's store in town, across the harbour via the Manly Ferry, and then taken the tram to the end of our road in Balgowlah. When she pulled up the coarse veil surrounding her hat and sat down in the front hall to recover, I noticed her face was flushed. There is little that she would not do for her adored grandchildren.

My father's half sister Florence Borthwick (née Andrews and called Auntie Flo) lived nearby in a new bungalow with her husband Tom Borthwick (Uncle Tom) and adopted Daughter Elizabeth. He was a great gardener and had a wonderful greenhouse containing beautiful orchids which he had built himself. Tragically he died suddenly and unexpectedly, to my Father's great loss, as they had become rather close. For me his death led to the surprising arrival of a beautiful large wooden child's wheelbarrow, with a remarkable tank track instead of a wheel. He had just completed this, as a gift for me, shortly before his death. This led my dad to make contact with Tom's brother Brian living in England, in Welwyn Garden City with his wife Ethel and Daughter Jean. This contact was to become a lifetime bond for me in the years ahead. My family in fact sent regular 'Food for Britain' parcels to them. When we moved to Wollstonecraft, our parish church St Giles, Greenwich, also sent such parcels to the sister parish of St Alphege's in Greenwich, England. My family, and indeed most Australians at that time, may have exaggerated the food shortages in England. In a letter some years later, dated 30 June 1946, Uncle Brian Borthwick writing from Welwyn Garden City in Hertfordshire, wrote in a letter to me and my sister. 'I think it was extremely kind of you to send us such a very acceptable and welcome food parcel as we have recently received - we are not by any means starving here!' I can imagine his smile as he wrote those words.

Life in Balgowlah was happy. I can remember local friends, both boys and girls. There were occasional visits with dad to nearby Fairlight Beach and its beautiful rock pool at the weekend. I can remember untoward events such as repeatedly swinging on the iron front gate against parental advice, until the brick gate post collapsed, missing me by inches, and then against maternal advice eating chillies from a neighbour's garden with dire effects on my oral mucosa. I enjoyed digging in the garden and being fascinated to hear of a neighbour's garden where plants would not grow because of the dreadful cutworm which devoured their roots!

In 1940, we moved to the suburb of Wollstonecraft, as my parents wanted to move to the lower North Shore district of Sydney and to leave flat-life. We were then closer to the city which was reached conveniently by fast and regular suburban electrified trains crossing the Harbour Bridge. Our home was 'Rathcallan', 6 Milner Crescent, a modest bungalow set below the street level on a slope to the railway track. This was hidden from our view by the backs of huge advertising hoardings and a virtual forest of overgrown privet trees at the rear of our quite large back garden. The bungalow was of brick but largely covered by stucco which had been painted white. It had a large front veranda in the Australian fashion, which made the house look rather dark from the road. There was a sitting room, dining room, master bedroom, nursery for my sister and me, a study, a room for a domestic maid, a large kitchen, a playroom and a small bathroom containing the toilet with a gas fired bath heater which on occasions blew-up! It was our sole source of hot water needed for shower or bath. We had no running hot water and no central heating. Air conditioning was quite unknown. We had no refrigerator when we first arrived. My mother relied on visits of the iceman to fill the top of our ice chest. He delivered regularly, sometimes almost bent double by a large rectangular block of ice on his back inside a canvas sack. Bread was also delivered locally by the baker in his horse-drawn cart as was our daily milk. A drive ran down beside the house to a moderate sized garage and tool room for dad. We had a Vauxhall car which had been given to dad and mum by their best man John Hall as a wedding present in 1935. It lasted many years.

These pre-school years were happy calm times with mum as the central figure in my life.

CHAPTER TWO

School Days; Privileged Education

I DID NOT GO TO SCHOOL till the age of six years as my mother felt that she could do a better job in teaching me the basics of writing and reading etc. I believe she was right and it did mean that we were very close. So I never attended a pre-school. I started at Mowbray House School in 1943 at first in the 'Kindergarten' or sub-primary section led by Miss Boardman. I found it very tedious as we had to 'sleep' for an hour between 1 and 2 p.m. This I was not able to do. I could also read and spell better than the other boys. So it was not long before I moved up to Form I.

Mowbray House was a small Church of England private Boarding and Day school, which extended only to the Intermediate Certificate. It had been founded in 1906 and was situated in Mowbray Road, Chatswood. The nearest railway station was Artarmon, two rail stops from Wollstonecraft, further north along the North Shore Railway Line. So at first my mother took me to school each day by train. We had to walk up the hill from the station to the school, together. This was a great time for me as mum used to tell me stories from the Bible, Greek and Roman Legends etc. in an exciting and interesting way. However after a few weeks in Form I it transpired that my schoolmistress, Miss Griffiths, also travelled to school each day by train. So my mother would take me to Wollstonecraft station each morning. Then she made sure I got in to the correct train carriage to join Miss Griffiths for the remainder of the journey to school.

Each morning, the school day began with a short service in the beautiful school chapel conducted by the Headmaster Mr L. Bavin. Every morning we sang the hymn beginning-

> 'Holy, holy, holy, Lord God Almighty!
> Early in the morning our song shall rise to thee ... '

The hymn is in fact perhaps one of the greatest affirmations of the Triune

God, a core doctrine of Christianity, but little did we realize that, as we sang it lustily each day.

Over the next two years there were very sad occasions when the Headmaster would read out the name or names of old boys of the school recently killed in the War. I have a vivid memory of the bright Australian sun streaming through the multi-coloured stained glass of the chapel and falling upon the black-gowned white haired figure of the Headmaster reading the names, with evident holding back of emotion. There was the long silence, as an act of remembrance. Some boys sometimes shed tears, either because they knew the named old boys or perhaps as a result of the emotion of the occasion.

The War was like a constant background to life, distant but never very far away. Our maid had a brother in the army and he used to loll round the kitchen talking to her. I remember during 1943, my mother leading my sister and me in prayer during our evening prayers before going to sleep, for our brave soldiers who were about to land in France. The year before my parents had been gravely concerned when they heard that the great battleships, the *Prince of Wales* and the *Renown* had been sunk off Malaya by the Japanese, and then later the terrible fall of Singapore. I was of course not aware at the time why my parents had been so upset about the war. However I do remember the awful time when we heard the news that the Japanese Fleet was advancing on Australia and there was 'only' the American Navy and the Royal Australian Navy between them and us, 'What will become of us all?' This hand-wringing question was widely posed at that time. In the event, there followed the first great celebration of the war that I can remember, namely the great victory of what came to be called the Coral Sea Battle in May 1942.

Often at night we could hear noise above our heads of what were said to be Japanese reconnaissance planes. There were occasional air raid warnings with the awful noise of the siren and then the wait for the all clear. In the event Sydney was only once directly affected by the War. This was when a Japanese suicide midget submarine came into the Sydney Harbour in June 1942. There were casualties and gunfire. Sadly the casualties were largely due to an American Battleship firing in all directions and hitting a small ship where naval ratings were sleeping. The newspapers of the time said nothing of this. In any event the strength of the explosions was enough to crack, but not break, a large pane of opaque glass in our bathroom window. This crack remained as a dreadful reminder of what might happen until the end of the war when it was repaired. I have to say that there was a good deal of panic in Sydney next day and many people moved out west to the Blue Mountains.

Both at school and at home trenches were dug for refuge during possible air raids. However Sydney has very hard clayey soil. This meant that they were very hard to dig and tended to fill with water when it rained. I remember at home a very red-faced dad labouring away at digging a deep trench. It never could be used in fact, as it filled with water and mud whenever it rained. Of course water and mud were a schoolboy's dream and so one day at school a group of us got involved in a reasonably friendly fight, throwing mud at each other from water-filled trenches at school. My mum was collecting me on that day and she was appalled to find my school uniform soaked and covered with mud! She was very angry but did not smack me, as in my family any form of corporal punishment was taboo.

At home as an alternative to a trench, in anticipation of air raids, a huge pile of sand bags was placed in front of the front door to protect us from blast effect. The family took refuge under the dining room table which had been moved into the entrance hall, on the few occasions when the air raid siren did sound. For a child, it was all quite hilarious, as my by then rather overweight grandmother, nana, found it rather hard to both get under the table and get out again. Nana had moved in with us in 1944 and we had lost our maid, whose room nana occupied. For my sister and me, it was all good fun. All the glass panes at home became criss-crossed with black tape to prevent glass shattering in an explosion and there was a very strict blackout at night when there were air raids. These were supervised by the ARP (air-raid precaution) people, who once called on us to point out a crack of light! At Allowah, my Auntie Ethel had allowed the ARP to construct a station in her garage. Most street direction signs were removed. Children were given pieces of cork to chew on, so that when an actual air raid did occur, biting of the tongue would be avoided. This often caused great hilarity. My Cousin Richard Buswell was delighted to have been walking home from school in suburban Killara (upper North Shore), when an air raid siren sounded. He thus was able to lie in a ditch biting his cork till the all clear went.

It was in 1944 that the battleship *King George V* was dry-docked in Sydney for repairs. One of dad's oldest friends was surgeon rear admiral Dermot Walsh of the Royal Navy, who was part of her ship's company. He treated the family to an escorted visit around this amazing ship. Whilst on the admiral's bridge I smelt some smoke and raised the alert, or so I believed. A small electric fire had caused some signal flags to smoulder. I was thrilled at having 'saved the ship' as the flatteringly kind Admiral Walsh remarked. Judith and I were to visit him years later at his home in Dublin, where he spent his last years in retirement. It was interesting that he was a Roman Catholic Irishman who regarded himself also as British. He remained loyal to the crown to the end of his life.

Another great maritime moment came in 1944. As dad was driving Judith and me home after a visit to Manly along the shores of the harbour above the Spit, we were amazed to see the *Queen Mary* and the *Aquitania* coming through Sydney Harbour Heads. It was an unforgettable sight, to see these great liners especially the *Aquitania* with her massive four funnels. The ships were in fact acting as troop carriers, bringing back the Australian troops from the middle east for the war in the Pacific. This had been ordered by the Australian Prime Minister John Curtin, against the wishes of Winston Churchill.

A sad, albeit indirect casualty of the war for us, was the death from tick-bite of our little mongrel black dog, known as Puppy Smut, in 1945. Ticks in NSW are a real threat to dogs and indeed on occasion to humans. They bite into the skin and literally suck the blood at the same time secreting an anti-coagulant and neurotoxin into the unfortunate animal or person. Tragically this neurotoxin can cause paraplegia, as in Puppy Smut's case. As the ticks drink the blood so they swell and can be recognized by feeling the dog's coat or examining the skin carefully for a greyish lump. If alcohol is applied sometimes they drop off, otherwise a Spencer Wells forceps skilfully applied to the head enables it to be withdrawn completely. However once neurological damage has occurred the only treatment is an anti-serum. During the war no sera were available for pets as they were required for the troops in New Guinea and elsewhere. So he was buried wrapped in the Union Jack as dad said he had died for his country.

However the wider family had suffered a direct casualty of the war, revealing its terrible reality to me, in 1944 when my second Cousin Ted Warren, a RAAF pilot, was shot down by the Japanese. I remember having visited his home in Northbridge and seeing his impressive pilot's helmet and I even had tried it on! He was young and handsome. I regarded him with awe. Apparently the Japanese planes unseen by him came out of the sunset and shot down his plane. I remember my grandmother placing a simple wooden cross in the field of remembrance at Sydney's St Andrew's Cathedral, each subsequent year, in his memory. His name is recorded in the National War Memorial in Canberra.

It was in St Andrew's Cathedral again with nana after the war, that I saw Field Marshall Viscount Montgomery on 13 July 1947 when he made a post-war visit to Sydney. I remember he read the lesson from 2 Samuel 3,4 with the boy Samuel's words 'Here am I.'

I can still recall the unusual timbre of his voice. My grandmother also took my sister and me to services when pastor Neimoller of the German Resistance and then Archbishop Fisher of Canterbury visited the cathedral. Archbishop Geoffrey Fisher's visit was on 19 November 1950. He endeared himself to my family by placing his hand on my sister's head and saying, 'Hello darling'. She has never forgotten that moment.

For my first year at Mowbray House our classroom was situated in the main school building and where the boarders had their dormitory. For the second year we were in a purpose built classroom with a corrugated iron roof and verandah, in the Australian mode. I remember the roof well, because during 1944 there was a severe drought. This was so severe that we were limited by the amount of bath water we could use at home. Then the precious water was taken in jugs to water the garden to try and keep some of the plants, especially the roses, alive. When the drought broke with torrential rain at school, the noise of the rain drumming on our corrugated iron roof was dramatic and exciting. Uncharacteristically Miss Griffiths was carried away with the excitement of the occasion. She allowed the class to rush outside and stand and jump about in the refreshing and cooling rain, despite becoming drenched.

She was a good teacher and for some reason I had her teach me for two years in a row. Her emphasis was on the classical three Rs, 'reading writing and arithmetic'. The latter was often a problem for me, but she slowly drummed the basic multiplication tables into my head. Reading was my forte, both listening to her read us stories and reading myself. I remember her reading aloud to us *The Story of Dr Dolittle* by Hugh Lofting. It and its sequelae became amongst my favourite books as a boy. I also remember reading famous stories of history, such as how King Alfred burnt the cakes and the victory of Lord Nelson at Trafalgar. However my writing was not great. We used pens dipped into inkwells on our individual desks. Our fingers became very ink stained, as were the desks, much carved with the initials of former and current pupils. I used to sit next to Jorgenson, who was a boarder, as his family lived on Goat Island in Sydney Harbour. My friends were Lemon (Graham) and Stevens (Hugh). The latter was my best friend. We always used surnames at school but when invited to each other homes we then used Christian names. I lost touch with Hugh, although he lived in Wollstonecraft too, but he went on to boarding school at the King's School Parramatta. I did meet up with his older brother Sam at cadet camp in Singleton some years later. I wonder what happened to Hugh?

At school, a year ahead of me was a boy I knew a little, Howard Peak, who was to stay on at Mowbray House School till he passed the Intermediate

Certificate. He then went on to secondary school at Shore. As for me, I was only to stay for two years at Mowbray House and then in 1945 I went on to Shore. Years later I met up with Howard again, when he came to Shore to complete his education for two years before passing the Leaving Certificate examination. He was to become a medical colleague at Prince Alfred Hospital and I introduced him to my sister Judith, who in time he was to marry. He ultimately became a distinguished cardiologist in Canberra.

The most memorable time for me at Mowbray House School was my last Speech Day held in Chatswood Town Hall, just before Christmas 1944. I had the immense honour to be presented with the prize (*I'll Tell You a Story* by Enid Blyton) for being 'Dux' of Form II by none other than William Morris Hughes, the famous former Prime Minister of Australia in World War I (1916-22). Billy Hughes was affectionately known as 'the little digger' (a popular term for the Australian soldier of the First War and afterwards). He was the local member of the federal parliament. The speech day was presided over by Bishop De Witt Batty, Bishop of Newcastle (NSW), chairman of the school council. The Headmaster in his speech amused my father by criticizing politicians (a popular theme with dad) but then apparently suddenly realizing that Billy Hughes was a politician, he went on to praise by contrast, 'Statesmen'. Of course by inference the little digger was a statesman! He certainly was a statesman. In the National Portrait Gallery in London there is a painting by Sir James Guthrie entitled 'Statesmen of World War I' which includes Billy Hughes sitting next to the British Prime Minister Lloyd George.

Curiously, years later, I was to have another connection with Billy Hughes, albeit a sad one after his death, when I was an Army Cadet at Shore School. I was one of a group of three Shore schoolboy cadets rostered to stand completely still with reversed arms and head bowed, for four periods of half an hour, by his coffin which was lying in state in the chancel of St Andrew's Cathedral Sydney in November 1952. They were the four longest half hours I can remember in my entire life. The worst fear was to bring disgrace upon the school, and even worse upon myself, by fainting.

It was when I commenced school that my father began to take me with him on some of his hospital rounds on a Saturday morning. As a urological surgeon he was an honorary surgeon at three hospitals. These were first the great teaching hospital, the Royal Prince Alfred Hospital, then the Mater Misericordae Hospital and finally the Manly District Hospital. Later on my sister Judith was to join me sometimes on these occasions. When I was taken to the wards the sisters and nurses often wanted to kiss me. My mum regarded this as very unhygienic and so she told me to bow my head. In this way it was the top of my head that was kissed rather than my mouth. This did mean however that I appeared as a very shy little boy, as I tended on these occasions to walk along with my head bowed. I did not really enjoy these 'hostipal' visits as I called them. I was impressed though at the evident respect the nursing staff had for my dad. However I did like going in the car with dad to the hospital, one of the rare occasions to talk with him. In future years I was to take my own children with me on hospital visits and more recently two of my grandsons to the Royal Free on Saturday mornings.

To the present generation of young doctors, it may be hard to believe that honoraries (consultants) such as my father at that time worked for nothing in their public hospital appointments. They were truly honorary, completely unpaid. Such consultants had to earn their living, chiefly at nights and weekends in private practice, with occasional half-days during the week. For part of the War my father was the sole senior urological surgeon at Prince Alfred. The question he had to endure at that time was why had he not joined up i.e. enlisted in the services. In fact he had a severe duodenal ulcer, which at times caused him the most distressing pain. Despite this, he did in fact apply for overseas service with the army. However both his health and age precluded overseas service. He was offered an army medical officer position in Australia, but he felt he could make better use of his surgical skills by continuing his work at Prince Alfred. He personally undertook all the major urological surgery, both urgent and routine at that time at Prince Alfred. During the war he was virtually on call, at home, all the time, apart from two weeks annual golfing holiday in Leura in the Blue Mountains. The reality was that it was not uncommon for him to be phoned in the middle of the night about an emergency, which required his immediate presence at one of the three hospitals.

Of course the fact that he had such a prestigious public hospital appointment as Prince Alfred meant that he had a successful private practice. He had privileged access to the private wings at the Mater Hospital and at Prince Alfred where this was called Gloucester House. It was named after Prince Henry Duke of Gloucester who was later to be Australia's Governor-General. (In 1945 when I was at Shore, we schoolboys were taken to line the Pacific Highway to cheer the Duke and Duchess and their little sons as they drove by, my first glimpse of royalty). I remember very clearly driving in our Vauxhall down the drive around the statue of Imhotep (the ancient Egyptian described by Sir William Osler as the first figure of a physician to emerge from the mists of antiquity), to park in front of Gloucester House past the Fairfax Pathology Department on the left. Little did I realize that years later

I was to be first a medical student and then a junior doctor working in those very buildings.

The fact is that dad worked unbelievably hard, indeed sacrificially, for most of his professional time, working quite unpaid. He was to continue to do this till he retired from the public hospitals as was then required, at the age of sixty years in 1960. I believe the present generation of doctors should pause and think of their predecessors' dedication to the profession. This honorary system, inherited from Britain, finally died in NSW at the end of 1960s and the beginning of 1970s. A report from the Sydney Morning Herald on Tuesday January 19, 1960, the month of my graduation in medicine, explained the 'Honoraries were not paid for services they gave at 257 hospitals and 13 other institutions in NSW at that time.' People unable to afford the ordinary fees could be treated free as outpatients of a hospital or if necessary in the hospital also entirely free. This report from the NSW branch of the British Medical Association went on to say 'It often happens that such a patient will be operated on by a leading surgeon, while a patient able to pay fees is content with someone less eminent and whose fee is lower'. So public patients could get better care, by implication!

I myself was to be appointed as the first staff or salaried physician at the Royal Alexandra Hospital for Children in 1971, so I was there at the beginning of the end of the honorary system. This system in Australia was of course the system of medicine inherited from Britain but which lasted much longer in NSW as in 1948 the National Health Service (the NHS) was established in the United Kingdom and the honorary system abandoned.

Sometimes on Saturday mornings dad would drive down to Manly Hospital to make a post-operative visit to patients on whom he had operated earlier in the week. When he took Judith and me as well, we used to have lunch with gran and Auntie Ethel at Allowah, which was nearby. Occasionally in summer we would go down to Manly Beach and body surf once the war was over. Of course in 1944 and in 1945 until the end of the war, no swimming at all was possible on Manly Ocean Beach. The beach was defended with barbed wire and anti-tank devices.

I would like to pause now to describe the house known as Allowah, at 1 Tower St Manly. It was astonishing that after all their years in Australia, both Gran and Auntie Ethel still spoke with Scots accents. As I stated earlier, the house interior was very Scottish in feeling. This was partly due to the large dark Victorian prints of highland cattle and bleak moors in the large entrance hall but partly due to the occupants. It was a large house with a large entrance hall leading to an imposing stairway. On the right there was a smoking room where the wireless set was sited. We used to gather sometimes to listen to the BBC news. The bells of Big Ben would chime and the announcer would say 'This is London calling, here is the news.' It sounded quite dramatic and gave me a strange feeling in my stomach! Next to this room there was a beautiful drawing room with an upright piano. Dad was a great pianist for light music and popular classics. Both rooms opened onto a spacious enclosed veranda with superb harbour views. On the left of the hall were a large dining room and a small hallway leading past the toilet, a butler's pantry and on to the kitchen, scullery and laundry. It was a house built for servants, but in my time there were none. Upstairs there was a separate flat where we had once lived, as mentioned earlier. There were another two large bedrooms and a dressing room. Again there was a large enclosed veranda at the front. It was here that Judith and I had temporary beds put up for us to sleep, on the rare occasions we stayed overnight. It was a very scary house at night. When we were alone upstairs when dad (mum virtually never came to Allowah) was still downstairs with gran and Auntie Ethel, it was spectacularly scary, especially on windy nights when there were lots of strange noises. It was a rather dark and even sinister, but yet exciting, house with the prospect of mysterious unknown 'treasures'. The sinister feeling doubtless related to the presence of a 19th century 'maori's head' with cowrie shells for eyes that had been 'collected' in the South Pacific. It was placed above the washbasin downstairs. What was its true story or what has happened to it since remains unknown to me. In the large entrance hall there were three large black pieces of antique Chinese furniture. My paternal grandfather had apparently collected these in the nineteenth century from old Imperial China. They stand today in our sitting room in Woodford Green. One is a beautiful double chair carved in Chinese red wood with the Chrysanthemum of Imperial China. However there were two black and white prints on the walls, which also made a lasting impression on me. One was a print of Lord Leighton's painting 'The Return of Persephone' from an ancient Greek myth. This showed her leaving the underworld escorted by Mercury, the messenger of the gods, being received by her mother Cere with outstretched arms. Then there was the dramatic picture of 'The Chariot Race' by Alexander von Wagner, the Munich painter of the nineteenth century. This vivid picture captures all the action and excitement of the race in ancient Rome. It is packed with detail. Perhaps these pictures fostered my later enthusiasm for ancient Greece and Rome. In the nineties, I was delighted to see the original of the latter work in the Manchester City Galleries. I have also seen Leighton's original in an exhibition at the Royal Academy. It is now in Leeds City Art Gallery. The dazzling colours of the originals were marvellous to see, but it was the black and white prints in Allowah that made such a powerful impact on me as a child.

In 1944 a notable medical event occurred for my family, a new operating theatre at the Marrickville District Hospital was named after my grandfather Dr Richard Barzillai Trindall who had been the local general practitioner. His son my Uncle Roy was an honorary surgeon on the staff in his role as a local general practitioner. I and my sister, mother and grandmother went to the opening of the new building works in November 1944 by the NSW Minister of Health, the Honourable C.A. Kelly MLA. The grandchildren of Dr R.B. Trindall were recorded in the annual report to have donated £30 in his memory. There was a kind of party afterwards with cakes and jellies. I remember being impressed by the occasion, especially the food!

At the end of 1944, I left Mowbray House with many happy memories, but with some excitement to be going on to the 'Big School'. Sadly Mowbray House School did not long survive the retirement of Mr Bavin some years later. The chapel does survive. It was moved stone by stone to become the local parish church.

Over the years I kept a connection with Artarmon as I used to have my hair cut by a barber there who I had used from my time at Mowbray House. He was Mr Perry. He had been in the second AIF in the war. He told fascinating tales, while I had my 'short back and sides' hair cut followed by the application of Brylcream to keep my hair sleek in the fashion of the time. I learnt from him that the P and O Line was the Peninsular and Oriental Line and that the Peninsular in question was the Iberian one. I also learnt that POSH meant Port Out and Starboard Home, and many other odd pieces of information.

My parents had arranged for me to start as a dayboy in the first form of the preparatory school of Sydney Church of England Grammar School, a private school popularly known as Shore School or more simply Shore. It is situated in North Sydney, on the northern shore of Sydney Harbour. The boys called the local shopping area, officially Victoria Cross, 'The Shore'. Its tower dominates North Sydney even today even though it is crowded in by high-rise buildings. St Matthew 5.14 states 'A city that is set on a hill cannot be hid'.

The school was modelled along the lines of an English Public School. In Sydney such schools are referred to as great public schools or GPS schools in contrast to the government funded, state or public schools. Although the Church of England in Australia changed its name to the Anglican Church of Australia, the school authorities with the support of the old boys have retained the traditional name of the school even today. I journeyed each day to school to and fro by train. There are two stops from Wollstonecraft to North Sydney. I travelled on my own, as I was eight years old. However there was a famous school 'bully' (at least so my mum believed), at Shore, who was some years older than me, but who lived near us. To my great embarrassment mum had taken the prophylactic manoeuvre of asking him to keep an eye on me, when I started at Shore. Actually I think this request from mum did insulate me from any bullying at all in my early years. He used to call out to me 'How are you going?' but I had no real contact with him. Bullying was I am afraid far from unknown at Shore at that time. In fact my Cousin Richard was known as Bully Buzz. I began in Form I with Mr Monckton. He was affectionately known as 'monkey'. We had our morning assembly each day in the prep school but my earliest memories however centre upon the chapel.

My first recollection of Shore chapel was during my first week at school, when I was the youngest boy in the school just turned eight years. It was my first chapel service there as a brand new pupil of Shore preparatory school. The chapel was immediately next door to the main school and an integral part of the school as a whole. Sydney Harbour Bridge provided a wonderful background to this fine building.

This first service I attended, must very unusually have been a service for the whole school. Normally boys of the preparatory school attended separately on Friday mornings. My class marched in last of all. I was very last, as my surname began with W. The only remaining seats were on benches in front of the sanctuary itself, i.e. within the chancel at the east end of the chapel. Shore chapel, modelled as it is on Eton Chapel, has its congregational seats arranged parallel to the central aisle. Furthermore each row of seats rises above those in front, in the manner of an amphitheatre. This means that the progress of anyone going up the aisle, as they advance is surveyed by 'hundreds' of eyes. I have never felt smaller or more insignificant as I made my long journey from the west door, right along the whole length of the chapel to my place in the chancel. After a brief pause, the prefects marched in with arms swinging, uniformly, in military style. They looked huge, like large men. Some even wore waistcoats. Then the Head Master of the whole school Mr L.C. Robson swept down the aisle with his black Oxford gown swinging from side to side. Shortly after the robed boys' choir processed from the vestry door directly into the chancel itself, right in front of me. The school chaplain Rev. Nigel à Beckett Backhouse was the last to enter the chapel. Throughout, the school organist Mr Allman played gentle music, but once the service began the music became triumphant and the lusty singing of the assembled boys of all ages seemed to risk lifting the very roof of the chapel. The service was short with no sermon.

At Shore, perhaps surprisingly, there was only limited teaching about Christianity per se. Such formal teaching as was given occurred in Divinity classes, which were really just 'scripture' studies given by various masters with widely varying Christian convictions. There certainly was no attempt whatever at 'brain-washing'. Chapel sermons were a rarity. We were never taught anything about the Church of England per se. The daily chapel service was the basic Morning Prayer taken from the 1662 Book of Common Prayer (i.e. The Prayer Book) and the lessons were always taken from the Authorized or King James Version of the Bible. I grew in time to love the majesty and power of the words. I became very familiar with the school lesson which was read quite often. This is The First Epistle General of Peter 2: 11-25. Verse 20 has remained with me all my life:

> For what glory is it, if, when ye be buffeted for your faults, ye shall take it patiently? But if, when ye do well, and suffer for it, ye take it patiently, this is acceptable with God.

Looking back it would seem that the dictum of Dean Inge of St Paul's Cathedral London namely that 'Religion is caught not taught' was the hallmark of the attitude of Shore School to Christianity in my day. However something occurred that first day in Shore Chapel, which I had never seen before, but with which I was to become very familiar. The prefect who was to read the lesson from the Bible, first of all, turned a page in the Book of Remembrance, which listed all the names of those old boys of Shore who had so far served or died in one of the two World Wars. The Second War was of course still continuing, when I entered school in the first term of 1945. In fact 2,270 Shore Old Boys were to serve in the Second World War. A total of 231 died in both wars. The book of remembrance was placed in the centre of the chancel, where it stands today. Once I joined the senior school in 1949 until I left in 1953 this simple and impressive daily act of page turning was to be a part of the chapel service that I was to attend from 8.40 to 9.00 a.m. each morning of my school life.

The clear message that came from this to every boy was that the school regarded the supreme virtue to be summed up in the familiar words:

> 'Greater love hath no man than this, that a man lay down his life for his friends
>
> **St John 15.13.**

Shore Chapel itself was built as a memorial to those old boys who had died in the First World War. The stained glass in the body of the chapel shows the patron saints of the allied nations, St George for England, St Hubert for Belgium, St Paul for the non-European nations, St David for Wales, St Denys for France, St Gregory with the Angle children (angels not Angles) for Italy and St Patrick for Ireland. The great eastern window executed in England in 1928 by Edward Moore presents the theme 'From suffering to Glory'. The central figure is Jesus Christ holding a sphere representing the Heavens and under His feet is the Earth. Underneath the window is a modern representation of the first stirrings of Our Lord in the Tomb on the first Easter Day by Andor Meszaros. Thus the chapel is visually Christ centred. However two large flags hang high above the chancel on each side, the Union Jack and the Australian Flag, as in Mowbray House Chapel. The sacred in the centre and the secular at the sides.

Later on when I moved to the senior school, in 1949, I joined the school choir as a boy soprano until my voice broke aged 14 years. I did not sing in the senior choir after that. The organist's wife Dora (always called Mrs Allman), who was a distinguished organist herself, assisted her husband who also acted as the choirmaster. The Allmans made a great husband and wife team and were very loyal to the school. I remember them coming to the Ingleburn Army Camp for our Cadet open day, bringing food and drinks for us. We sopranos were usually called trebles by Mr Allman, in contrast to the altoes. The first money I ever earned was when we sang at weddings on occasional Saturdays. The fee was usually half a crown (2/6) for each choirboy but some bridegrooms were more generous. It was only on such special occasions that we wore surplice and cassock, on normal weekdays we wore school uniform and only the clergy were robed.

I was not a brilliant 'voice' and the acme of the chorister, singing a solo, was not for me. I was given, to my surprise, though, in 1949, the choir prize (*Kidnapped* by Robert Louis Stevenson, one of my favourite books). I was told privately it was for 'effort'! I really did enjoy singing the anthems. One has stuck with me forever. This is Samuel Sebastian Wesley's 'Blessed be the God and Father of Our Lord Jesus Christ.' It was especially familiar as one part for sopranos namely 'Love one another with a pure heart fervently' we sang as an anthem at chapel weddings. However it was always best when we sang the whole anthem including the tenor and bass voices of the older boys, who did not attend at weddings. Most exciting of all, after the sombre words sung by the basses 'Trass witherth, and the flower thereof falleth away' was the spine tingling moment, when after a pause, the organ crashed out triumphantly as the words were sung 'But the Word of the Lord Endureth forever'. Two other particular favourites were 'Jerusalem' (And did those feet in ancient times) with William Blake's powerful words set to Hubert Parry's music and also 'Jesu Joy of Man's Desiring'.

There were many memorable moments in Shore Chapel. Amongst these was the day after the King died in February 1952, when for the very first time we sang God Save the Queen. How very strange it sounded to us all. Darcy Grigg, one of the masters I most admired, gave a remarkable oration concerning the very much mourned King George VI. Other special occasions were the annual polished pennies services, on each Remembrance Day Service on 11 November, when every boy offered a polished penny as a personal act of remembrance for all those old boys who had died for us.

I remember how powerful was the memory, in Shore Chapel of Gallipoli and the ANZACS who had died there. Fourteen old boys of Shore died, in the Gallipoli campaign. They are all buried there. In June 2001 with my wife, we went on a Medical History cruise to the Black Sea. As we sailed into the Dardanelles Colonel John Richardson, a retired British army Medical Officer and fellow historian of medicine, was able to point out to us, some of the features of the Gallipoli peninsular. In October 2011 I was very fortunate to visit the actual Gallipoli battlefields, with a small group led by Antony Bird, the brother-in-law of John. I was able to visit the graves of several of the old boys of Shore. Two I found in the cemetery at Shell Green above Anzac Cove. We walked up from Anzac Cove. There the beach is so narrow that the cliffs and slopes seem to almost rise out of the sea. We climbed up "artillery road" to the heights. Even walking up the track was quite hard going for us. We found the grave of a Shore old boy, Captain Rupert Richardson of the Australian Light Horse in the Shell Green Commonwealth War Graves Cemetery. As I stood there I recalled that a stained glass window in Shore Chapel remembers him. I reflected that he had died so very far from home on the other side of the world in an alien land but that his memory lives on in the land from whence he had come.

Especially memorable was the last service at the end of each year for those boys who were attending chapel for the last time, as they were about to leave school. I remember feeling quite choked as we sang the hymn.

Lord, dismiss us with Thy blessing,
Thanks for mercies past received.
Pardon all their faults confessing.
Time that's lost may all retrieve.
May Thy children
Ne'er again Thy spirit grieve.

My own last service was of course very special it was a rite of passage.

The occasion most personally memorable for me in the chapel was my own confirmation service by Bishop Venn Pilcher. Most of my friends and I were confirmed together on that memorable day. Amusingly we boys had had a message from the Bishop not to wear Brylcream on our hair. This was to avoid his hands becoming too greasy after laying hands on the heads of more than 50 boys.

The Bishop's words of confirmation:

> Defend O Lord this thy servant with thy heavenly grace that he may continue thine for ever and daily increase in thy Holy Spirit.

remain very special for me.

My local C of E minister at St Giles, Greenwich, Mr Blumer, kindly came to my confirmation service, but he thought I should have been confirmed at his church. Actually there was a brief hiccup before I attended the confirmation classes, which preceded confirmation, when the chaplain discovered I had been baptized by a Presbyterian minister. I had to make clear to him that it was now my own choice to be confirmed in the Church of England, which in future would be my church. This I was very pleased to do. I had grown to love its service and music.

Then there was All Saints Day on 1 November, the one occasion each year when those boys who were communicant members of the church took communion together, for me yet another memorable occasion. However I must emphasize that despite all I have written, I was not an especially religious boy, unlike some of my evangelical friends. Apart from them, some at least of my friends, but certainly not all, felt similarly to me about the chapel. I however looking back now, it is clear that these daily acts of worship, with their times of prayer and quiet reflection accompanied by beautiful words and music meant a great deal to me. For me now and always, the chapel and its order of service epitomize what it means to be an Anglican. If there is such a thing, I remain a Shore Anglican. However the term Anglican is not one which Shore boys of my day would have ever used. We were C of E. This is what we stated our religion to be, when filling in our applications for concessionary rail travel to the school of our denomination.

However the 'great thing' at Shore in my time certainly was not the chapel but 'Sport'. Sport dominated school life. High achievers in sport were those most admired by boys and masters alike. At least that was what appeared to be the case to me. Nearly every prefect was a distinguished sportsman. Sport was compulsory.

Now I was not very good at sport. I was not well co-ordinated. By contrast my father was a passionate and successful sportsman, as is my son James. I was sadly quite a disappointment to dad with my failure to excel in sport. The Shore sport year was basically divided into two, cricket in the summer and rugby football in the winter with a brief intermediate time for athletics. There was also an annual swimming carnival or gala held in the Olympic Pool at Milson's Point once a year and some opportunity for tennis but it was the big two, namely cricket and football, that counted. I in fact at some point attempted all five sports, but without much success.

The term rugby was hardly ever used. The game we played was simply called football. Soccer was regarded as a game largely played by immigrants i.e. New Australians (post-war immigrants to Australia). Shore was, and is, very fortunate to have wonderful playing fields at Northbridge, some miles north of the school, and there was also one playing field at school. There was one afternoon of sport each week and sport on Saturday mornings in the season, when playing other schools at school or away. In football there was one sporting activity that I could do well. This was tackling below the legs, so bringing down the ball-carrying player. My father had taught me well. It did not need good hand-ball-eye co-ordination for that. In fact as a result I rather enjoyed playing football. I continued to play occasionally up to second year medicine. I was often a five-eighth. However the truth of the adage 'the bigger they are the harder they fall' frightened me very much when once my tackling brought down a large well built boy running fast for a goal. I made a well-placed tackle below his knees. He fell to the hard ground with a terrible thud. For a few moments he did not move. Had I killed him? Certainly I had almost knocked him out. In the event he was all right and he recovered quite quickly. However my greatest moment was when I myself was kicked in the head with a resulting laceration of the scalp. This lead to fresh blood streaming over my face. I left the football field and walked to the changing rooms feeling like a great warrior of old, receiving admiring looks from friend and foe alike.

The changing rooms themselves could be quite threatening for a very small boy as I was when I started in 1945, especially if by mistake, one attempted to undress in a place where the 'big' boys normally changed. This happened at my first football practice and to my distress some of the older boys aggressively tried to shove me out of the place I had selected to change. However Leggett, probably the biggest boy in the Prep School, said 'Leave him alone!' This act of kindness I have never forgotten.

Sometimes we played away from school. This could be a bit intimidating especially when we were playing St Joseph's Christian Brothers' School, usually called Joey's. They were a tough lot and there was always an edge to matches between Shore and Joey's. Was it the protestant catholic divide? Dad thought so, especially as many of the staff both brothers and priests were from Southern Ireland. The other Roman Catholic GPS school in Sydney was St Ignatius College at Riverview. It had been founded by English Jesuits and in contrast to Joey's the boys had a reputation as 'gentlemen'!

Cricket I hated. I was completely hopeless. After standing for what seemed like ages as a fieldsman, with nothing to do, a ball would come my way. I would miss catching it and face boos and angry words from my fellow teammates. I did however play regular sport right through the preparatory and main schools including cricket and indeed most of the sports on offer. I did not want them to defeat me, but they did in fact most of the time!

However the highlight of the sporting year was an occasion that my family and I enjoyed very much. This was the annual GPS rowing regatta held west of Sydney on the Nepcan River at Penrith, at the foot of the Blue Mountains. It was quite a long journey by car or train. This was the one occasion of the year that dad drove the whole family to a school event in the old Vauxhall. We had a picnic on the banks of the river with our friends and I shouted for Shore in every race until I was hoarse. Shore was well known as a rowing school and so we often won, which added a celebratory note to the occasion.

1945 saw the final victory in the war with Victory over Japan or VJ day as the great celebration. I don't remember the celebrations personally apart from the fireworks display on Fort Denison in Sydney Harbour one evening. We viewed the marvellous display from Cremorne where 25 years later we were to observe a similar fireworks display in 1970, to commemorate the Captain Cook bicentenary. However on the actual Victory Day itself, my dad had to walk home all the way from Prince Alfred Hospital to Wollstonecraft, many miles. This was because masses of people walked into the city, even walking across the Harbour Bridge, so closing it to car traffic. It was the greatest party Sydney had ever seen.

Going back to my progress through the prep school, in 1946 I moved up to Remove B. Our master was an eccentric Englishman Bill Brierley. He did a very unpleasant thing to me, one occasion at football practice. He called out my name and when I came over to him he unexpectedly pinched both my cheeks and almost pulled me off the ground. 'So Walker-Smith does not think I can coach football,' he said. It then dawned on me that my Cousin Richard had told him my frank opinion of his football coaching skills. It can be imagined how doubly angry I felt.

Brierley had several canes in his collection, which he swished around the classroom from time to time. One was called ice cream! Corporal punishment was still used at Shore throughout my time, in fact during the tenure of L.C. Robson as Headmaster (he was Headmaster throughout my time at Shore) there was a great emphasis on discipline and respect for authority in general. This was shown in the emphasis on the importance of school uniform which had to be complete. It consisted of a grey suit with short trousers for the younger boys and long trousers from those aged 14 years and over. Changing over to long trousers was known as 'being pulled through'. Boys themselves policed the way the uniform was worn. It was a terrible solecism to have the upper button of one's jacket done up. For headwear during the wartime years a soft felt hat was worn with the traditional alternating dark blue and white school hatband. After the war there was a return to the wearing of a boater with the same hatband. The Shore boater remains emblematic for the school. It is interesting that wearing of school boaters has almost died out from English public schools but continues even in the 21st century in their Sydney equivalents.

Next year I moved up, although still in the B stream, to IIb with H.C.W. Prince. He was also an Englishman but temperamentally quite different from Bill Brierley. He inspired me with an interest in both Latin and English Literature. I especially remember him reading aloud *Puck of Pook's Hill* by Rudyard Kipling. When I finally visited Southern Sussex many years later it had a curious familiarity. At the end of the year Princie, as he was affectionately called, took the view that I was too young both chronologically and in my ways, to leave the prep school and to go on to the senior school. With my parents' agreement I repeated a year. So in 1948 I moved sideways to Form IIa. This meant I had moved from the B stream to the A stream where I remained for the rest of my school career. K.D. Anderson, an Australian, was the form master, as well as being Headmaster of the prep school. He was quite a disciplinarian and also used the cane. It was forbidden for boys to be in the classroom during the lunch hour except on raining days but one day a friend and I had wandered inside on a rather dull day. Shortly after Mr Anderson swept in, berated us for being in the classroom and ordered us to his study. He then asked us each to bend over in turn and he gave us 'six of the best' with his cane. It did hurt. We tried to be unflinching. That afternoon we were greeted as heroes in the changing room at Northbridge when the red wheals on our white bottoms were visible in the showers. The only other time I was caned was by 'Bish' Forster for reading a book when I should have been listening to the lesson, the following year in IIIa. I deplore corporal punishment and can see no merit in it.

In Form IIa for the first time we now studied French, taught by another master, Mr Butler, a dynamic young man whom I remember saying very often 'Vite, vite monsieur!'. In that year I also remember learning and really enjoying Australian poetry taught by K.D. Anderson. I particularly remember Dorothea Mackellar's poem, 'My Country'. The second verse I found very evocative.

> I love a sunburnt country,
> A land of sweeping plains,
> Of ragged mountain ranges,
> Of droughts and flooding rains.
> I love her far horizons,
> I love her jewel-sea,
> Her beauty and her terror -
> The wide brown land for me!

I have a tenuous connection with the poet as I have a beautiful Book of Common Prayer in my possession, which was hers. It was a souvenir edition produced for the Coronation of King George V and Queen Mary in 1911 and given to her by Ada MacCormick on June 22, 1911.

Also I read for the first time the ballads of A.B. (Banjo) Paterson, the poet so beloved by nostalgic Australians when they are far from home. He of course wrote the words of '*Waltzing Matilda*', but my favourite was '*Clancy of the Overflow*'. It was also in that year that I met my oldest continuous friend Garth Setchell. We have remained friends ever since, even though he took up architecture and I medicine.

Finally after four years I entered the senior school to form IIIa where Jimmy Burrel was the master. He was one of the most popular and well loved masters in the entire school. He was an older man, a real gentleman of the old school and a great anglophile with a real love of the old country. He dinned into us the importance of 'Good Manners'. He cited the motto of Winchester in England namely 'Manners Makyth Man'. Shore in fact had close links with another English public school, Shrewsbury, at that time. A young clergyman, Mr Forster, was seconded from there to Shore. In Form IIIa he taught us geography. He also caned me on the occasion I mentioned earlier. He had a rather grand manner, so was popularly called Bish, short for Bishop. He was quite a sportsman and was clearly an advocate of muscular Christianity.

It was in that year that for the first time I took part in a theatrical show, a Gilbert and Sullivan production of *The Mikado*. The show was performed in a commercial theatre, The Independent, North Sydney, This made the performances very realistic and exciting. Boys took all parts. Boy sopranos and boy altoes took the parts of girls and women and the older boys whose voices had broken were the men. The school orchestra provided the music. Darcy Grigg and Wilbur Sawkins were the masters responsible. In my first Gilbert and Sullivan I was in the 'female' chorus as one of the Japanese young ladies. The following year we did *Merry England* instead of G and S, as that year J.E. Williamson did not grant permission for a school production. Then in 1951 I tried to sing in the male chorus of *Iolanthe* but my voice, after breaking, was a bit unstable, so Darcy told me to take a year off from singing. Then the following year I was in the male chorus of *The Gondoliers* and finally in my last year in the sailors' chorus of *Pinafore*. I am afraid my voice was never good enough for a part as a principal. Furthermore I remained rather too shy for that. However it was all marvellous fun. Dad loved Gilbert and Sullivan too and played the piano effortlessly. So we used to have good 'sing songs' at home whilst I was learning the choruses. I think of all my activities at school, I most enjoyed performing in Gilbert and Sullivan.

From IIIa, I moved the next year in 1950 to Form SaI with Darcy Grigg as master. I really respected him. Through Latin and history classes he inspired me with a love of ancient Greece and Rome, having already inspired me to enjoy Gilbert and Sullivan. Maths was becoming my black spot at school and I was often struggling. In 1951 we had to sit the intermediate certificate and we had Peter Jenkins (Tojo was his unkind nickname) as our master to prepare us. He had been at Shrewsbury and so unlike most other masters he always wore a black gown. He was active in the army cadets where he was a Captain.

I now joined the cadets as a private. I disliked cadets. I liked nothing about army life but I was determined to succeed. So I quite soon attended a corporal's course, which I passed successfully, and finally, a year later in 1952, I went on to an Officer's Course at Singleton Army Camp. I passed this successfully and so became a cadet-under-officer. This course for trainee officers included boys from other GPS schools such as Kings School, Parramatta and so I met Sam Stevens again. I in fact came top of the course in the examination, but that week felt like a kind of hell for me. Not a single one of my own friends had been accepted for the course. Most of those attending were boarders who were high achievers in sport. I felt quite alone. Until then I had lived a rather sheltered life as a dayboy. The school boarders in those days had a much tougher time. The boarders dominated the Shore contingent at the Officer's Course. I had hardly ever encountered bad language before. That changed very quickly. During that week I became aware of another harsher much more unpleasant world 'out there'. Fortunately this was only as a spectator. Some of my innocence had been lost. I also discovered that unexpected kindness from strangers also could occur.

There was an annual cadet camp each year, my first was at Ingleburn and thereafter at Singleton in the blasting heat of summer under canvas. Singleton is some distance north of Sydney, requiring a long train journey. We trained with the .303 Lee-Enfield rifle, which had been the standard issue rifle for the army in the First World War. The rifle was rather heavy for fourteen-year-olds learning all the intricacies of presenting arms, sloping arms etc. It had quite a recoil on the shoulder when fired. I was very fortunate to have Peter Bradhurst as the officer for my platoon in my first year as a cadet in 1951. He was very understanding and helpful to us younger boys. I have never forgotten that, yet I have not met him again since I left school. In my last year at school in 1953, I was officer in charge of my own platoon for the year and at Singelton. I am not sure I was by any means an unmitigated success as an officer. I was aware that some of the boys in my platoon appreciated my leadership and a few became particularly attached to me, but others did not like me. One boy I upset unjustly and I remain guilty about it. He had had rather a dirty belt, which had not been blancoed properly. I ordered him to correct this. Next day he came back 'brisk of step' but I petulantly found fault with what he had done, perhaps to assert my own authority. He was deflated and rebellious and I may have made an enemy. I was very glad when the camp was all over and we took the final train journey home. That was the end of the army for me fortunately. I had first joined the cadets in 1951 at about the same time as we moved house to 68 Shirley Road. My mother forbade me to wear my cadet uniform for my first visit there! If I had she would have regarded that as a bad omen for the future need for me to be in the army. Looking back now I find it hard to understand quite why I put myself through the ordeal of wanting to succeed in the cadets when I disliked the army so very much.

Our new home was also situated in Wollstonecraft, not far from Milner Crescent. This was another bungalow but larger and grander with fine rooms with tall ceilings built circa 1904. It had a traditional Australian curved corrugated iron verandah roof. The wood columns of the verandah were finely carved and there was stained glass in the front door.

At the end of 1951 I passed the intermediate certificate examination and then went on to the fifth form where one had to chose which subjects were relevant for future courses of study. Clearly chemistry and physics were essential for medicine. Biology was not an option at Shore. I gave up Latin but rather unusually elected to study ancient history. Darcy Grigg had left me with a real enthusiasm for the ancient world. In fact the one career I did consider at all seriously other than medicine was archaeology. In my final year at Shore, I went with dad to visit the Nicholson Archaeology Museum at the University of Sydney. At that time architecturally it was a work of art itself with its gothic architecture and vast windows. Inside there were plaster casts of antique sculptures as well as the genuine artefacts of archaeology. For me it was an exciting, indeed marvellous place, very evocative of the ancient world. When we returned home my mother said, 'Archaeology would make a nice hobby!' That seemed to be that. Apart from briefly toying with the idea of diplomacy, thereafter it was medicine for me. However archaeology and the ancient world were and are an abiding interest. When I finally set foot on the shores of Greece years later in 1963, I do remember thinking of Darcy Grigg. I felt grateful to him.

I also liked English literature and a rather eccentric but great master at Shore was Pat Eldershaw, I remember well him telling us of the importance of the distinction between sentiment and sentimentality. The former was good and the latter bad. I was disappointed when he gave as an example of sentimentality the 'Far, far better thing that I do today' speech by Sidney Carton, from Charles Dickens *Tale of Two Cities* which I had myself found very moving. Was he or I correct? The power of sentiment per se rather than self interest as a potent motivator for human action has been a lifetime interest.

I rather enjoyed chemistry and had a chemistry set at home but I could not abide physics. Our chemistry master was Toby Pascoe, a quiet retiring man, who presided over our quite exciting laboratory experiments. Some of these I tried to repeat at home. He was also the pianist for the Gilbert and Sullivan performances. Clem Tiley was the rather laconic presence who tried to teach me the physics of motion, light and sound etc, etc. Curiously he used to use Latin tags. One of his favourites was 'Tot homines quot sententiae' meaning 'so many men so many opinions' when he despaired of getting so many answers to a simple question. Physics all seemed very remote and too mathematical for me. I would have to endure a year of physics at University later on.

I cannot ever remember agonizing about the content of medicine, i.e. what doctors actually did. I just knew that I was going to do medicine and that was that. I had some experience of personal illness. I had as child recurrent bouts of vomiting between the ages of seven and ten years. These were diagnosed as 'bilious attacks'. Incredibly my mother used to force a reluctant me to take the terrible tasting castor oil, the vilest, most nauseous medication I have ever been given. It also caused terrible diarrhoea. She endeavoured to ameliorate its awful taste with fresh orange mixed with bicarbonate of soda. I could never abide fresh oranges thereafter. On occasion I had such a bilious attack when I was staying with my Auntie Lell in Killara. She never did give me this medication but gave me plenty of fluids with a little dry toast. I certainly loved her for this! Looking back on these attacks, they were probably mild episodes of cyclical vomiting. My most significant encounter with the medical profession was when at the age of 14 years I tripped and fell through a glass windowpane at home, gravely lacerating my left wrist, severing my ulnar nerve and artery. The latter gushed blood but my father rapidly applied local pressure and a surgical dressing. That night it was surgically repaired at the Mater Misericordiae Hospital. I am left however with a partial left ulnar palsy.

One clear influence was the example of my uncle. I admired my Uncle Roy Trindall very much. He was a somewhat quixotic general practitioner with anti-establishment views and unusually for our family an agnostic. He had served as a medical officer in the First Australian Imperial Forces (AIF) during the First World War as a medical officer on HMAS *Kanowna*. Yet he would never ever discuss his wartime experience or attend any events on Anzac Day. He was quite an intellectual and had lots of interesting ideas and influenced me considerably in favour of medicine. He reinforced my own decision.

I should perhaps mention 25 April here, Anzac Day, the anniversary of the terrible events at Gallipoli in the First World War. Even now in Australia this is still a great day, a sad day. Although this anniversary recalls a defeat, commemoration of this day signalled to the world that Australia had arrived as a nation in its own right. It was the rite of passage of the young federation which had been founded on 1 January 1901. I attended an Anzac Day ceremony as recently as 2001 in Cairns and it had lost none of its old sadness, dignity and pride.

The poet laureate John Masefield wrote a very moving account of the Anzacs (The Australian and New Zealand Army Corps) at Gallipoli. He wrote of them:

> The finest body of young men ever brought together in modern times. For physical beauty and nobility of bearing they surpassed any men I have ever seen they walked and looked like the kings in old poems, and reminded me of the line in Shakespeare: 'Baited like eagles having lately bathed'.

These are fine words, especially from an Englishman.

The highlight of each Shore year was the Annual Speech Day. In the early years between 1945 and 1949 I received prizes. Two prizes for divinity, one for the choir and two form prizes. One of these was the John Scott Memorial Prize in 1948 in memory of a young old boy 'lost on active service' whilst in the second AIF. Thereafter I had no more prizes. Yet in 1953 based on my leaving certificate result I was awarded by the government of the Commonwealth of Australia a Commonwealth Scholarship, which would pay for all University costs for my medical course. My results were Chemistry A, French A, General Maths A, Ancient History A, Physics B and English B. Speech Day was a memorable day each year, when parents and family visited the school and so had a chance to meet and talk with the masters at the end of the school year.

Speech day was held under a large marquee on the school playing field. The proceedings at that time were presided over by Dr Howard Mowll, Lord Archbishop of Sydney and referred to by the Headmaster as My Lord. He was a formidable figure, a tall big boned man who was overweight, not unlike Charles Laughton. He had a commanding presence. He always wore, to these events, the knee breeches and eighteenth century kit of an English Bishop. He did however have somewhat bowed legs and a large paunch, so the spectacle of Archbishop Mowll in his very tight knee breeches walking down the steps onto the school assembly ground from the marquee had been known to raise some discreet sniggers. He was an Englishman educated in Cambridge and a committed evangelical, appropriate for Sydney, the most evangelical diocese in the Anglican Communion. He had also been Bishop of West China from 1926 up to his appointment in Sydney in 1933.

The Speech Day Guests who gave the principal speech, by contrast, I find hard to remember although it was sometimes the State Governor Sir John Northcott. However there was a great speech I heard at Shore after I had left. On 4 May 1954 I came back with dad, mum and my Auntie Lell (my mother's sister) to see the new Memorial Hall opened by the Governor-General of Australia, Field Marshall Sir William (later Viscount) Slim of Burma, a war hero. This was most appropriate as the Hall was a memorial to all Shore Old Boys who had served in World War II. My father held him in particularly high esteem. I have never forgotten some words that Slim said on the occasion of his visit. The exact words of course escape me, but it was along the lines of 'You boys are having a very privileged education. You, yourselves have done nothing to deserve it. You need to spend the rest of your life paying back the debt you have incurred.' He is the only Governor-General of Australia to be commemorated in the crypt of St Paul's Cathedral, London, because of his distinguished record in World War II, especially in Burma. His words were a challenge for my life and me.

On reflection, in preparation for this autobiography, I have come to realize just how much my life has been shaped by the influences of my education at Shore. The school gave me an excellent general education in both science (albeit no biology) and humanities and lauded the ideals of service and sacrifice. Yet in relation to my own decision to study medicine, it was quite neutral without any influence at all. There can be no doubt I had a very privileged and fine education at Shore, which has stood me in good stead throughout my life. The school motto which comes from Lucretius (99-55 BC) is 'Vitai Lampada Tradunt'. 'They hand on the torch of life'. This motto has been a theme for my life.

Shore in my day was a school which emphasized the importance of discipline both personal and institutional. There were great pressures to conform, especially in sport, but there were also some opportunities for music, as I have outlined and the arts (indeed an Art School was founded whilst I was there). Interestingly taking part in Gilbert and Sullivan was almost 'mainstream', whereas the choir and the library were certainly not. I look back on my time at Shore very positively, but it certainly was not all joy and happiness, for I felt I was always part of some minority group or other such as the choir, the stamp club etc. Clearly my school days were not the best years of my life. Nor in the main did I form most of my closest and long lasting friendships there, these came later in University and more recently. Many good school friends like Gerald Bartlett, Richard Mountstephens, Phil Stewart, Tony Styles, Peter Somerset, Colin Woodley and George Gillard, I have not seen or rarely again. Garth Setchell and Ron Scott were the two I kept in touch with over many years. I did also experience real moments of pain such as sporting failures, unhappiness at Army Cadet camps etc. There was bullying at Shore in those days but in general I experienced at school more kindness than unkindness, from both boys and masters alike. Shore opened my eyes to an exciting world of the intellect, especially in history, both ancient and modern, English literature and chemistry with the excitement of actually doing laboratory experiments. It was a positive experience.

The school in my day was both vigorously Australian in its way of life and powerfully British in its traditions. In reality these traditions were chiefly English in origin, indeed several of the masters, and indeed Archbishop Mowll himself, were English. To my mind, looking back this represented Anglo-Australia at its best.

With all this description of school life I should also mention our annual family annual holiday. From 1944 to 1955 mum, Judith and I went every year to Newport Beach for a summer holiday, shortly after Christmas. Dad drove us down and picked us up but never accompanied us. He always had a separate golfing holiday in Leura, at another time. This was sad for us. In the early years we had a joint holiday with my Auntie Lell, Uncle Haydn and the

Buswell family, with my Cousins Joan, Betty and Richard and nana too. I have kept closely in touch with Joan and Betty and after her marriage her husband John Allerton ever since. John was also an old boy of Shore who served in the Royal Australian Navy with his name listed in the Book of Remembrance. I also have kept in touch with their children Mark, Tim and Chris. Mark once stayed some months with us after we had settled in England. He introduced me to a common enthusiasm for Rennie MacIntosh and his Glasgow School of Art.

Each year we would rent a large family house and lots of friends, boys and girls of both families would stay with us from time to time. We had a great time. We still all remain a close extended family to this day with reunions, albeit infrequent, as we now are continents apart.

Throughout my schooldays, my immediate family never travelled outside the environs of Sydney. I did however have one holiday trip during my school years in the Blue Mountains with Tony Styles and his family and Graham Leonard from Mowbray House. My first trips interstate occurred when I was a university student. My first international visit was to England, for further training.

I should also mention that Christmas afternoon and evening was always celebrated with the extended family, just before our annual Newport Beach holiday. For most of my childhood this was at the home of the Buswell family at 16 Birdwood Avenue, Killara. The Christmas celebration also included the birthdays of nana and her brother Uncle Tom. Looking back it is clear that nana was the Matriarch of the extended family. She tended to dominate family affairs and her influence was everywhere. Her daughter-in-law, my Auntie Dot Trindall, called her Mater. Her son-in-law my father referred her as 'the old lady' when speaking to me, making little attempt to conceal his hostility. As I grew older I found these Christmas gatherings increasingly irksome, especially when there was so often a game of cricket on the nearby oval, after our huge traditional Christmas dinner in the blazing heat. Such an occasion only emphasized to all the family and dad, in particular, how bad I was at sport! However I was quite good at body surfing and I loved our happy summer each year at Newport Beach.

Throughout my schooldays I was lucky to have my sister Judith as a companion. We were very close and this continues to the present. She attended a Church of England school for girls called 'Abbotsleigh' which was rather similar to Shore, although she had to travel for a longer distance than I did to school, travelling each day by train to the upper North Shore to Wahwonga, but the school was also close to the station. In early childhood we played a lot together and as we got older we used to go into town to the pictures together to '5 o'clock sessions' on Saturdays, i.e. between the matinees and the evening screenings. This continued after I was at University. We liked going to the 'Embassy Theatre' which specialized in British films, particularly Ealing Comedies which we liked, especially those with Alistair Sim and Alec Guinness. I particularly remember really laughing at Alistair Sim as the bishop in *The Titfield Thunderbolt.*

When we were younger, mum used to take both Judith and me on a regular excursion into town during our school holidays. A pattern emerged of going by train to Town Hall station and then walking across Hyde Park with its striking Anzac Memorial and the statue of Captain James Cook, to the Australian Museum. There we saw a host of wide ranging exhibits from a skeleton of a huge whale to geological, botanical and historical exhibits. Then mum would take us to nearby St Mary's Roman Catholic Cathedral with its two huge statues of local Cardinals/Bishops in front. Mum would lead us into its dark cavernous interior (what my father called a dim religious light). There we saw images of Christ crucified and the Virgin Mary, partly lit by flickering candles. My mother whispered to us words such as superstitious, sinister and idolatrous. Nothing more than a whisper was ever permitted. I think the purpose of these visits was to show us children how different the Roman church was from our protestant Church of England. St Mary's certainly seemed to be very alien and foreign to our young eyes. It was not till I began to visit Roman Catholic churches in Europe years later that I began to feel that these churches were really Christian too and came to appreciate their own appeal. Then the best part of our excursion was the visit to the NSW Art Gallery. I developed a particular fascination with some of the paintings in the permanent collection, as we visited them so often. Two stand out particularly in my memory these were 'The Defence of Rorke's Drift' and 'The Deaths of the sons of Clovis II' by two French painters of the late nineteenth century Alphonse de Neuville and Evariste Luminas respectively. The first was an evocative portrayal of a great Imperial event and the latter was a very frightening painting that almost haunted me. Apparently the two sons of King Clovis of France had rebelled against their father and as a terrible punishment they had had their hamstring muscles in their legs severed. Then as the painting showed, they were set adrift lying on a raft in the river to ultimately die! After visiting the gallery we paused by the statue of the Scottish bard Robbie Burns and then finished at Mrs Macquarie's Point (called after the wife of the visionary Governor Lachlan Macquarie) overlooking the harbour and the bridge, before walking to Wynyard Railway Station and thence home.

It was always a memorable excursion.

It would be incomplete to end an account of my childhood without mentioning our dogs and cats that played such an important and happy role in our family life. Puppy Smut mentioned earlier was followed by Chips, Mac, Jip, Toby and my favourite and the one who lived to the greatest age Cobber, a black cocker spaniel of great courage and devotion. We also had two cats, Winkie and Boots. For a time we also had a parrot and we always had lots of goldfish.

So to conclude, my childhood was happy and remarkably quiet. I hardly ever left Sydney. I was sustained and supported by a loving family. I had a very good education, which placed me well, for my onward move to the Medical School at the University of Sydney.

CHAPTER THREE

University of Sydney and its Medical School

DURING THE FIRST FIVE of my years at university, uniquely in my life, I kept a regular diary from 1 January 1954. Curiously this was triggered because Admiral Walsh, dad's old friend, gave me a diary for his annual Christmas present. This he repeated until 1958 when he stopped. I then stopped keeping a diary, except for my voyage to England in 1962. So in this chapter I shall be drawing from these diaries, rather than memory alone.

I started at university (most often called Uni at the time) with high hopes and in a mood of considerable optimism and excitement, but I must also confess to being apprehensive and scared. What I had not anticipated was the size of First Year Med in 1954, nor the loneliness I would experience with the loss of all my school friends, none of whom had elected to study medicine. Although other old boys from Shore were in my year, none were my friends, but one, Gordon Stokes, was to become a good friend. Although some of my school friends, Garth Setchell, Robert Steel and Ron Scott were up at Uni with me, they were studying other courses. Very occasionally we met to have lunch in the University Union, Kerry Goulston who had been a year ahead of me at Shore from 1946 onwards and whose home was further along Shirley Road was in Med II. He gave me very practical advice for coping with Med I and gave me his lecture notes. Fortunately after a while very good friendships did emerge in First Year Med, especially with Peter Thom (my first Roman Catholic friend) and Michael Nicholls. Both were to become very close friends, especially Peter. But in the end, they were sadly both not to continue with medicine, and so I was again to feel real pangs of loneliness when I started Med II. But I am jumping ahead.

So I began my medical career as a first year undergraduate student in March 1954. The University of Sydney had been founded in 1850 and the medical school opened its doors to students in 1888. My grandfather Trindall enrolled in 1889. Most of the founding fathers of Sydney Medical School were Scottish, and from Edinburgh in particular. The most notable was Sir Thomas

Anderson Stuart, founding Professor and first Professor of Physiology. My father and both uncles (Hugh Walker-Smith and Roy Trindall) had also been medical students at this medical school.

The course began with an Orientation Week, which was quite an exciting time. It started in a formal manner with a welcome from the University Chancellor Sir Charles Bickerton Blackburn, 'resplendent in his gold-covered robes in the magnificent Great Hall'. Magnificent indeed is the Great Hall of the University of Sydney, modelled, as it is, upon Westminster Hall, the oldest part of the Palace of Westminster, where Queen Elizabeth, the Queen Mother's body lay in state in April 2002. Construction of the Great Hall of the University of Sydney began in 1854 but was not finally completed with its marble floor till 1879. Its architect was Edmund Blackett, a Londoner who resigned as Colonial Architect to take on this monumental undertaking. It was built in what he described as Tudor Perpendicular Gothic and indeed it is a masterpiece of Victorian Gothic and a remarkable monument of the age of Empire. It is both imperial and royal in its decoration. Most notable examples of this are the stained glass windows showing the Kings and Queens of England plus Mary Queen of Scots and Oliver Cromwell. There are also the Oxford and Cambridge windows as well as others showing great literary and scientific figures etc., including William Harvey. Sir Charles Nicholson, a Scottish doctor who became Chancellor of the University, secured donations for these windows and journeyed to England to supervise their manufacture. On completion of the stained glass, before its journey to Sydney, he arranged for it to be conveyed to Windsor Castle, where Queen Victoria and Prince Albert admired it. This was very appropriate as the glass is a remarkable example of Victorian Imperialism. Nicholson himself was an extremely generous benefactor to the University and gave it his own collection of antiquities to form the nucleus of the Archeological Museum which still bears his name, as mentioned in the last chapter.

Orientation Week continued with talks by the University Union and the Medical Society who arranged a symposium entitled 'The Medical Student' which I found quite helpful. When I began medicine, the curriculum was basically unchanged from the time of the foundation. It was largely based on the old University of Edinburgh curriculum. It was a six-year course, with First Year really a pre-med course. In that year we studied four disciplines, namely: Chemistry, Physics, Zoology and rather incredibly Botany. However it is only our Botany lecturer Dr McLuckey, an elderly voluble Scot, whom I can remember at all clearly. He had lectured dad in 1918. I found his lectures fascinating. I also enjoyed Botany Practicals, looking down the microscope for the first time. I had never done Biology before, and I have ever since enjoyed microscopic work. Years later, a good deal of my own gastroenterological research involved histology. This term means the microscopy of body tissues, which have been sectioned and then stained with various dyes (often haematoxylin and eosin), to colour the tissues and make the microscopic structures clear and distinct, when examined with the light microscope. Of course in Zoology too, we looked down the microscope, involving, in fact, histology, but in practical classes we also dissected the stingray. At first I also found this interesting, albeit a bit smelly and not exactly aesthetically pleasing. By April 2, I was writing 'we dissected the stingray once again, this time doing the heart and eye. I am getting a bit tired of it and when I think of the number of times I will have to go over it, it is pretty awful.' We later were to dissect the sheep's brain, the ox's eye and the rat. In one Zoology Practical my mother horrified me by suddenly appearing with my cut lunch, which I had accidentally left at home. I was so embarrassed. What would fellow students think? Her intentions were good but she had not realized that her son had left school and was a young man! Although in fact I had only just turned seventeen years old. Indeed I lived at home throughout my university education. At that time most other students also lived at home if they came from Sydney. Only a few privileged ones lived in one of the four residential colleges, all denominational in foundation. These were St Paul's for the Church of England, St Andrew's for the Presbyterians, Wesley College for the Methodists and St John's for the Roman Catholics. Staying at home did mean I studied a lot but I believe it held back my general development and achievement of an independent life. However I was able to arrange some great social occasions at home, especially dances with my growing number of friends both male and female. This was the first time that I had been educated with girls.

Academically it was a successful year for me. I passed with a distinction in Botany, and credits in Chemistry and, to my surprise, Physics. Only 135 out of a total of approximately 360 undergraduates passed, an extraordinarily high failure rate. During the vacation I had my first job working in a stamp shop in the Royal Arcade, with the firm of A.C. Campe. I was a keen philatelist, so it was really fun and I earned my first pay.

Second Year Medicine at last ushered me into medicine itself. We were based in the Old Medical School, now known as the Anderson Stuart Building, a remarkable example of Scottish Tudor Gothic architecture. With its massive stonewalls, the building was always cold even on the hottest of Sydney days. Its long corridors were lined by busts of famous figures of medical history from Hippocrates to Sydenham, and Scottish notables such as Sir James

Young Simpson of Edinburgh, the discoverer of chloroform anaesthesia. There were eponyrmously named lecture theatres: Vesalian, Hunterian and Anderson-Stuart. There were also stained glass windows with figures from medical history. One such is a picture of Aretaeus the Cappadocian. He was an historic figure who years later was to interest me, as it was he who first described what he called the Coeliac Affection in the First Century AD. More extraordinarily and not planned by the original architect, the men's urinal was looked down upon by stained glass figures from the medical history. All these architectural features were redolent of the distant past and northern climes. This gothic building with its echoes of northern Britain stood in complete and remarkable contrast to the hot southern environment where the building actually stood. Yet it did give us students a powerful message that we were engaged in an ancient and indeed noble profession.

It was particularly in Second and Third Year that lifetime friendships were made, often amongst those who dissected together on the same cadaver or body for a whole year.

Amongst those dissecting with me on my cadaver were three students who were to become life-long friends. There was John Turtle, who was to become probably my best friend at medical school and who was eventually to become the Professor of Medicine in Sydney. Then there was Phil Thompson who became a plastic surgeon, and Phil Southwell who was to become a radiologist. In addition there was George Vakkur from Estonia, Ehe Treufelt from Latvia, and there was another girl who I recorded as 'quite nice but she cut away all the superficial nerves and arteries on one side!' We even played 'interbod' rugby football. This was the last time I played the game, as I twisted my left knee during the match, injuring the medial meniscus on that occasion.

The cadaver was, I am afraid, usually called the 'bod'. This term bore no disrespect for the dead but was one way of coping with an experience, which certainly was not at all pleasant. Looking back I am surprised that I cannot remember any of the staff preparing us for this exposure to death in the shape of these dead bodies. Most of us had never seen a dead body before. For me seeing one of these bodies during Orientation Week at the beginning of First Year was the first time I had seen a dead person. Bearing in mind we were mostly still teenagers, I believe this was rather heartless, probably being justified on the basis of 'being thrown in at the deep end', a quite popular philosophy among doctors at that time.

In fact our grim dissecting room provided a rather horrifying scenario. My stomach heaved when we first entered the vast gothic room with its sickly sweet stench of formaldehyde emanating from the row upon row of bodies in various states of dissection. An unforgettable and indeed quite unpleasant memory is of the extraordinary gothic environment with little groups of white clad students gathered in tight groups around the cadavers, pouring over their Cunningham's Anatomy texts covered by protective plastic covers in a vast room. Yet in another way the dissecting room seemed sometimes like a temple of arcane mysteries. In fact we had a very tough and rigorous teaching programme in anatomy including detailed knowledge of the skull and the skeleton. Anatomy of the brain was reserved for Third Year Medicine. We were taught in the dissecting room by young trainee surgeons who wanted to brush up their anatomy. One such was a young Chinese surgeon from Singapore who worked with my dad. He was our most effective teacher.

In relation to the above account of the dissecting room, I was astonished in March 2002 to read and see on television Gunther von Hagens' extraordinary Body Worlds exhibition in Brick Lane, London. He has developed a technique he calls plastination for preserving cadavers. The exhibition appeared to be like a glamorized version of what I described above, attempting to remove the horror. However whilst he claims an educational value for the exhibition (which of course is the only justification for the dissecting room for medical students), he clearly is using bodies for entertainment. Why else would the cadavers be placed in the poses he has used for some, such as a flayed figure holding his own skin? Andrew Renton in the *Evening Standard* struck the right note for me, when he stated that as he walked past cadaver after cadaver, he felt diminished by the experience. 'Every individual is rendered anonymous by von Hagens' production of innominate carcasses, seeming to me like cattle in a slaughterhouse.' What surprises me, is that this the Government, in view of the Anatomy Act, permitted this exhibition especially after the outcry related to the uncontrolled use of body parts in Alder Hey Hospital Liverpool, which cannot be defended. Yet the intent of the latter was for medical research rather than idle entertainment.

The TV account of that exhibition reminded me of the body of an aboriginal woman which had been sliced horizontally at the time of Sydney's first Professor of Anatomy, J.T. Wilson, and was placed along one wall of the Anatomy Museum. It was used to demonstrate the relationships of one organ to another and sometimes was used in the anatomical Viva Voce examination. My father remembered well being asked to point out an anatomical point on one of the body slices. In the present age of the CT scan such knowledge would have been of value to radiology trainees, but in 1955 such precision of anatomical knowledge did not appear relevant to anyone except those few of us who were to become surgeons. Whether these sections are still there today

I do not know, nor do I know why the fact was mentioned that this was an aboriginal woman.

So anatomy was a key subject. We also studied physiology, biochemistry, histology and embryology with formal lectures and practical demonstrations. Peter Bishop was the newly appointed Professor of Physiology, so he personally gave nearly all the lectures himself, and these were good value. His own field was the physiology of vision. N.W.G. McIntosh, Professor of Anatomy, known as Black Mac, gave his lectures arrogantly with an almost Oxford accent. A surgeon from Prince Alfred Hospital, Dr Norman Wyndham, known, poor man, as Foetus Face because of his youthful appearance, gave meticulous lectures on embryology with little chalk drawings on the blackboard but these were difficult to understand. I was to write two papers with him years later when a Research Fellow at Prince Alfred. Dr Clelland gave the dreariest lectures I have ever heard on histology. The most aggressive lecturer of all was Dr Bill Hensley in Biochemistry, talking frequently of the American Cyanamide Company. He rightly, continually emphasized biochemical basis of much of modern medicine at that time. He became quite excited when talking of Selye, with his concept of stress and also the role of steroids in treating patients. The practicals were variable in interest and value. A young cardiologist Dr Gaston Bauer taught those in Physiology. These were like going back in a time warp with the tracings of rabbits' intestinal contractions on smoke blackened rotating drums, as described at the end or the nineteenth century.

In Third Year Med, in 1956, as I said earlier, we studied the anatomy of the brain in detail whilst continuing with the other subjects of Med II. In Biochemistry we had lectures from Professor J.L. Still who raised in me a new enthusiasm for biochemistry. It was a short but intense year. It was possible in those days to visit the post-post-mortem room at Prince Alfred and get a human brain to take home for private dissection. Like many of my friends I did this, and put the brain wrapped in newspaper in my suitcase. On the way home at Town Hall station a quite dreadful thing happened - my bag burst open and the brain rolled out, falling out of its newspaper. I was appalled and rapidly placed it back in my bag with great embarrassment. Looking back on it now I feel very embarrassed that I should have been myself party to the idea of taking home a human brain for dissection.

Then in the spring we began Junior Fourth and so we moved over to the 'New Med School', now known as the Blackburn Building. This was a time of intensive lecturing and practical demonstrations in Pathology, Bacteriology and Pharmacology. For the first time we visited the postmortem room for demonstration of actual autopsies of dead bodies. If the dissecting room was unpleasant, this was diabolical. The sanitized images on television bear no relation to the bloody gruesome business of the postmortem room, at least in the memory of those young eyes now grown a lot older. A veil must be drawn over the details. There were searching examinations in each of these basic subjects. 1956 was a very tough year.

Teaching in clinical medicine at last began on 11 March 1957 in Fourth Year Med. This was the introductory course in medicine, therapeutics and surgery, with mornings in the university and afternoons in the hospitals. Both the Professors of Medicine and Surgery were new appointments, so we were their guinea pigs. In medicine we had Professor Ruthven Blackburn, the son of Sir Charles Bickerton Blackburn, the then aged Chancellor of the University (a distinguished physician himself who had graduated in England in 1898). For surgery we had Professor John Loewenthal who had been Hunterian Lecturer of the Royal College of Surgeons of London. After they both had given their introductory lectures in the New Medical School (The Rockefeller Building, as it was then officially called), Dr William Morrow (later Sir William) followed with a therapeutics lecture. He was the doyen of Sydney physicians at the time and specialized in gastroenterology. He later was to become one of my principal mentors. Then we went next door to the Royal Prince Alfred Hospital to be welcomed by Sir Herbert Schlink, the Chairman of the Board of Directors, whose wife Meg Mulvey was a dynamic young obstetrician. We proudly wore our new short white coats for the first time. This dress was compulsory and demonstrated our lowly status. There was a hierarchy of dress. Junior resident medical officers wore short white coats and white trousers, the girls wearing white dresses, senior residents and registrars and the University staff wore long white coats, whilst the 'honoraries' (honorary consultants) wore blue suits.

Of key importance for our future was the formation of our clinical teaching group. Yvonne Holcombe, Josephine Glen-Doepel, Don Tindall, Bob Rundle and Peter Sinnett joined four of us who had dissected together, John Turtle, Phil Thompson, Phil Southwell and me. Peter was to become a very good friend and best man at my wedding in 1969. He was to become Professor of Geriatrics at the University of New South Wales.

The following day at Prince Alfred, this group attended our first ward clinical teaching session in surgery, given by Dr Tomlinson, our clinical tutor in surgery (in Sydney surgeons usually did not use the title Mr as they did in London and Melbourne). I rather disgraced myself by 'coming over faint', related to the combination of his demonstration of a series of patients with colostomies, and the heat. I was ashamed to have to sit down with my head between my legs. Next day I went with Bob Rundle and Don Tindall to see Dr Tomlinson perform an amputation and then an appendicectomy. I accepted the invitation of the surgeon to come onto the operating floor, and I felt I had redeemed my shame of the previous day.

Later in the week we had our first clinical teaching in medicine by Dr Richard Harris, our clinical tutor in medicine, which I enjoyed much more. Dick Harris, was indeed a formidable, albeit young, physician. He was of the old school. He in fact was portly and looked a bit like James Robertson-Justice in the film *Doctor in the House*. From the first he taught us to pronounce the word abdOmen with the emphasis on the O as a kind of signal that we were now clinicians. He abjured us never to have our hands in our pockets. With subtle humour, he remarked 'That is my prerogative alone!' He gave us classical instruction in the clinical art. This has served me well throughout my professional life. Sometimes when he was away we had a very dynamic young cardiologist, Dr Dick Richards, to teach us. He was brilliant. We were well taught in clinical medicine. Yet I did find auscultation (listening) of the heart to be rather difficult. I wrote on 13/9/1957: 'Unfortunately I listened to a heart and said it was a systolic murmur, when in reality it was diastolic. I am afraid I find listening to hearts and clinical medicine in general the most difficult thing I have ever had to do so far in the medical course.' In fact I also did find it difficult and awkward going up to patients and interrupting them, just to let me examine them and listen to their hearts etc. I found C1 Ward to be particularly intimidating. This was a very long Nightingale Ward of male medical patients, with an elderly sister in charge, who had early Parkinson's disease and thus showed no facial emotion. I had to ask her for permission to see a patient and then go up to the patient, ask their permission and then draw a screen round the bed. I was conscious of many eyes watching my every move. I soon realized it was best to go in pairs, so I often went to the wards with John Turtle. At the end of 1957 I was able to write 'I feel that medicine is indeed my life's work and that I must settle down for the next 4-5 years and endeavour to become a first class clinician.'

1957 was the year for me, when for the first time I travelled outside New South Wales. First of all between University years, in January, I went with dad, accompanied by my friend John Turtle to tour Tasmania. We flew first to Launceston and then travelled around most of that beautiful island with its historic echoes of England, especially obvious in Hobart. Then at the end of the year after the exams, in December, I drove with several Uni friends including John Turtle, Peter Sinnett and Phil Thompson. We drove across the country to Adelaide in South Australia. We then motored along the very beautiful Ocean Road with its rugged grandeur to Melbourne where we stayed a few days. Then we returned to Sydney along the coast via the Prince's Highway.

In fifth year, 1958, we began the 'specials', as well as continuing with medicine and surgery. These consisted of obstetrics, ear nose and throat (ENT), ophthalmology, psychiatry and paediatrics. In psychiatry we were privileged to have Professor Ian Trethowan, recently arrived in Sydney from England. He had come to help reform NSW's archaic psychiatry laws and to so abolish terms such as 'Master in Lunacy' and 'Lunatic Asylums' which were still current in the 1950s in Sydney. His lectures were exciting, almost thrilling. However it was paediatrics that I was to most enjoy. We went to the marvellous Royal Alexandra Hospital for Children, often known simply as 'the kids', a ten minutes walk away from Prince Alfred, in Camperdown. This was a wonderful place to go. The charismatic Professor of Child Health, Sir Lorimer Dods, taught us. He was an inspirational lecturer and clinical teacher. I can remember his clinical demonstrations/lectures as if they were only yesterday. Demonstrations on Pink Disease and tuberculous meningitis stand out. Pink Disease is a disease of children long gone, as it was due largely to mercury poisoning from mercury contained in teething powders or in medicaments for napkin rash. The baby with tuberculous meningitis was later tragically to die. Little did I know then that paediatrics was destined to be my life's work, but what I did know, was that I liked the idea of caring for sick children.

A notable event during the year was the opening of a new Elizabeth II Research Centre for Mothers and Babies in the Department of Obstetrics by the Queen Mother. I and some of my friends acted as ushers for the impressive open-air ceremony. We had a rather charismatic Professor of Obstetrics, Professor Bruce T'oomba Mayes who had written a textbook, which was the sole base of his lectures and the basis of our course, jokes and all. What was wonderful about obstetrics was the fact that we as students actually delivered babies, supervised by the midwife. We then gave them their first bath ourselves. One amusing observation I made on a newborn baby I bathed was that the baby's breath appeared to smell of garlic. When I went back to his Italian mother I found she had been eating garlic not long before the baby was born. Does garlic cross the placenta? It is a much-hackneyed observation. But there is nothing as wonderful as the first cry of the newborn baby, especially when it is somewhat delayed. The first time I heard such a cry from a newborn baby whom I had delivered myself, I must confess to feeling quite 'choked'.

It was in Fifth Year that I began my lifetime interest in the history of medicine. I was one of the student founders of the Medico-historical Club. Its evening meetings had a wide range of topics and sometimes even had an international speaker. 'I once gave a talk on John Snow of cholera fame and another on our founding professor, Anderson Stuart. I was encouraged very much by that very kind gentle and underestimated man Sir Edward Ford. He was Professor of Preventive Medicine and lectured us on the dreary yet important topics of 'Deep pit latrines and disposal of sewage' etc. He was however a medical historian too and had a wonderful library He invited the Medico-historical Club to visit his library for one of our meetings. I was quite overwhelmed when he later sent me personally two books from his library, which are still precious components of my own library of books. First and most remarkably from the personal library of Sir Thomas Anderson Stuart with his bookplate, there was a book dating from 1735 entitled *The Archbishop of Cambray's Dissertation on Pure Love*. As Sir Edward wrote 'the subject may be of little interest to you, but it will be a memory of a great doctor'. Then he gave me a copy of Anderson Stuart's own booklet '*Report on the Koch method of Treating Tuberculosis, 1981*'. Anderson Stuart had been sent by the NSW government to Germany to investigate Koch's claims for tuberculin as therapy for TB, which sadly were false. These books became the nucleus of my own collection of medical history books and were the catalyst for this bibliophile interest.

Two notable visitors of international fame came to the University that year: Michael Ramsay, Archbishop of Canterbury, and by contrast the American evangelist Billy Graham. We were allowed to cut short lectures to go and hear them. Both speakers from such widely different perspectives of Christianity, were able to hold the attention of large gatherings of young students remarkably successfully.

Final Year followed with intense teaching in medicine and surgery plus obstetrics and gynaecology. There were very few occasions for social activities. Looking back I really did work quite hard with at least four hours of solid study at home each night, yet I would not have admitted this to my friends! We had an exceptionally good teacher in the Honorary in charge of our medical firm, Dr Billy Bye. He had a great gift of stimulating his students and his continual insistence that common things commonly occur was an excellent foundation for future years in the profession.

The final examinations in the midst of a very hot summer were a gruelling ordeal. The joy of passing the exams just before Christmas could not be confined. I passed with Class II honours and was ninth in the year, immediately after my friend John Turtle, from a total of circa 160 graduates. My entire fourth year clinical group passed. Shortly afterwards I had a particularly fine summer holiday surfing at Newport Beach. The graduation ceremony occurred in the gothic splendour of the Great Hall of the University of Sydney in January 1960 on an extremely hot summer's day, after we had already begun our life as junior doctors on 2 January 1960.

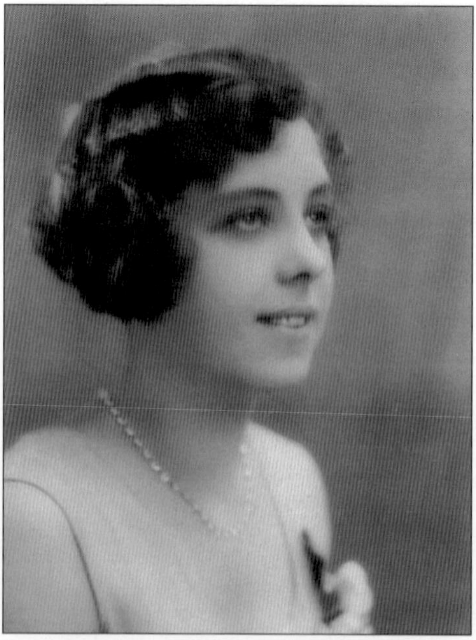

1. Alexandra (Alix) Buckingham Walker-Smith (née Trindall) BA (Sydney), (1901-1970)

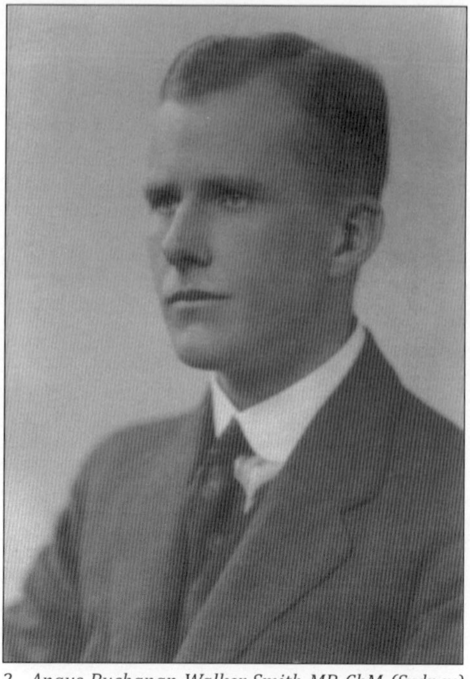

2. Angus Buchanan Walker-Smith MB ChM (Sydney) FRCS (Edinburgh), (1900-1975)

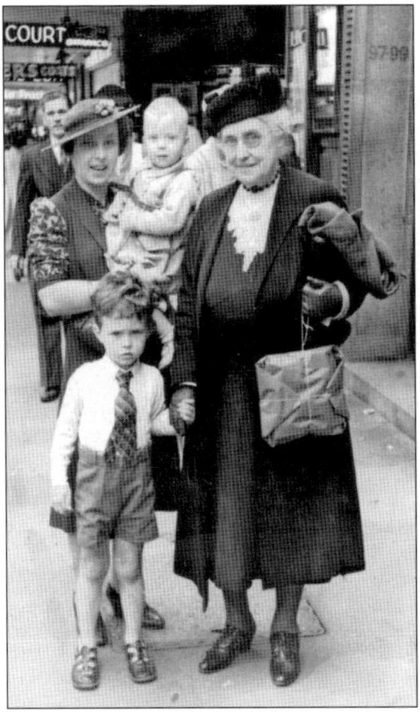

3. Author aged five years with mother, sister Judith and grandmother (nana) in George St, Sydney, 1941

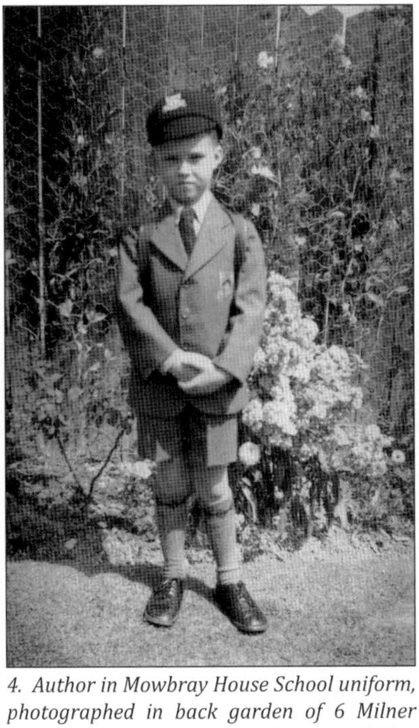

4. Author in Mowbray House School uniform, photographed in back garden of 6 Milner Crescent, aged seven years, January 1943

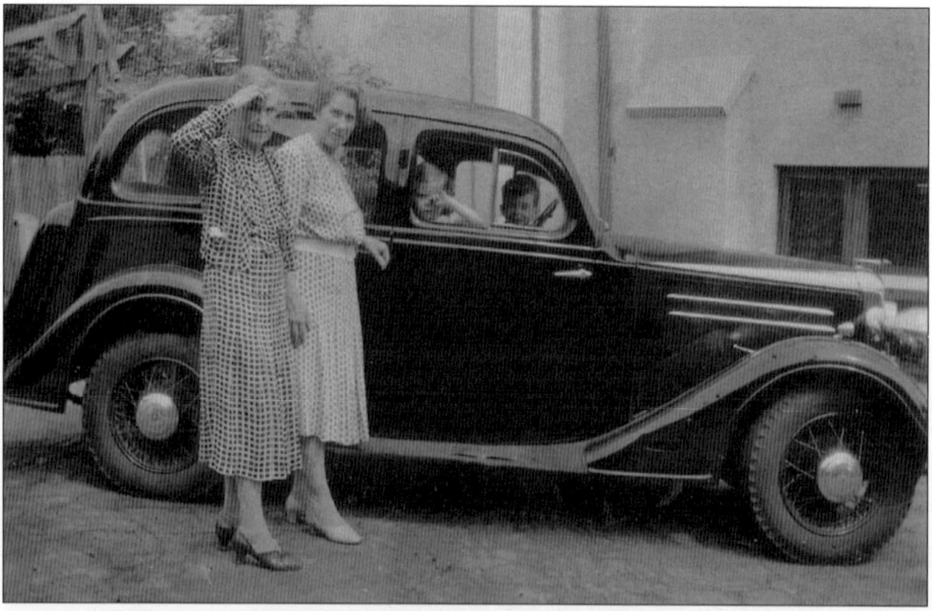

5. Gran, auntie Ethel, Judith and Author with 1935 Vauxhall at the back of Allowah

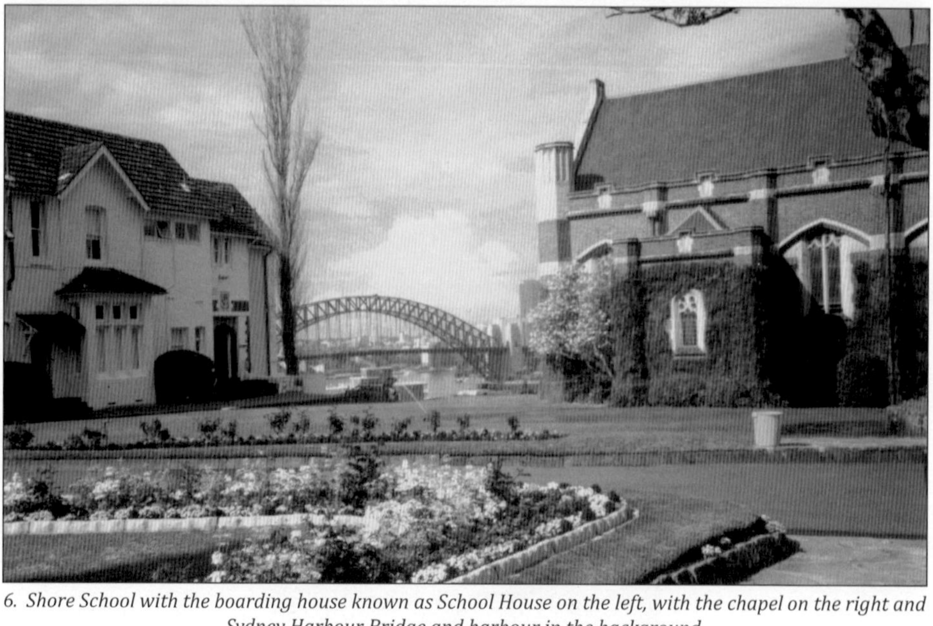

6. Shore School with the boarding house known as School House on the left, with the chapel on the right and Sydney Harbour Bridge and harbour in the background

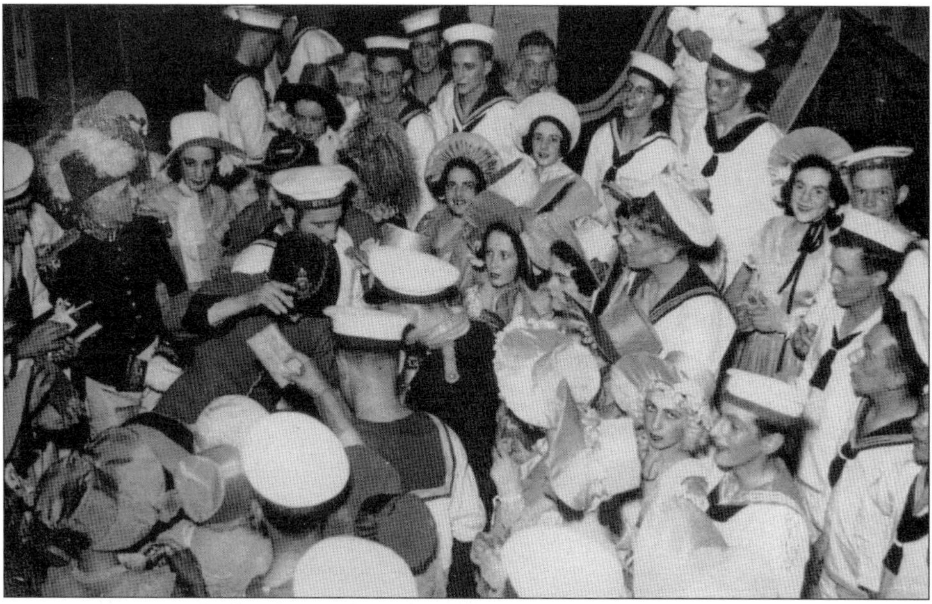

7. Shore boys as the 'Ladies and Gentlemen' *of Pinafore, 1953.*
The Author is on the far right, second from the top

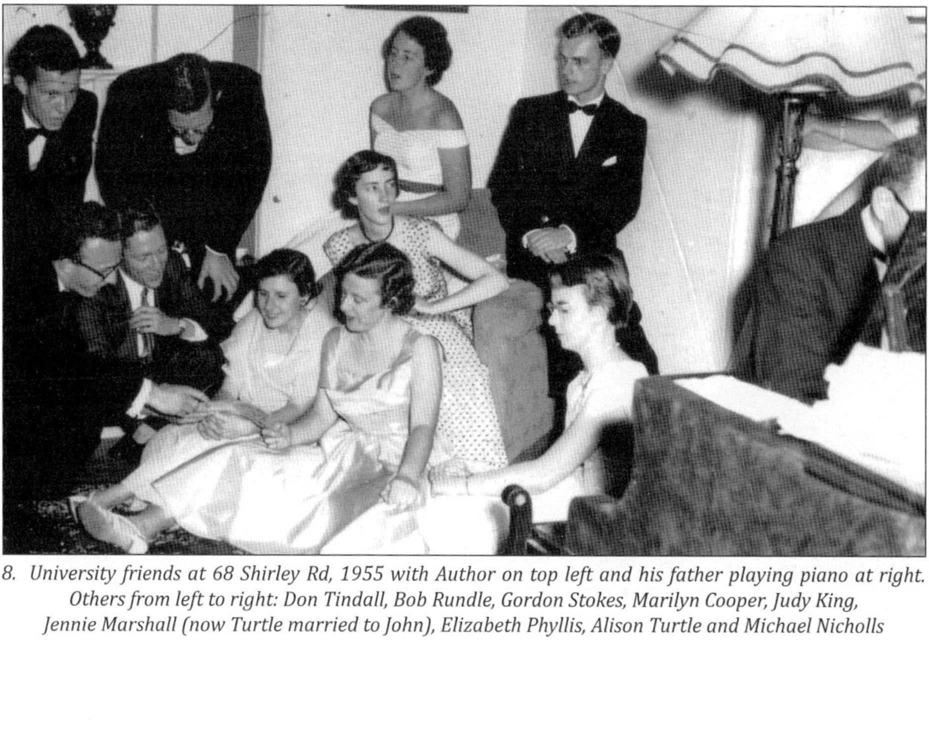

8. University friends at 68 Shirley Rd, 1955 with Author on top left and his father playing piano at right.
Others from left to right: Don Tindall, Bob Rundle, Gordon Stokes, Marilyn Cooper, Judy King,
Jennie Marshall (now Turtle married to John), Elizabeth Phyllis, Alison Turtle and Michael Nicholls

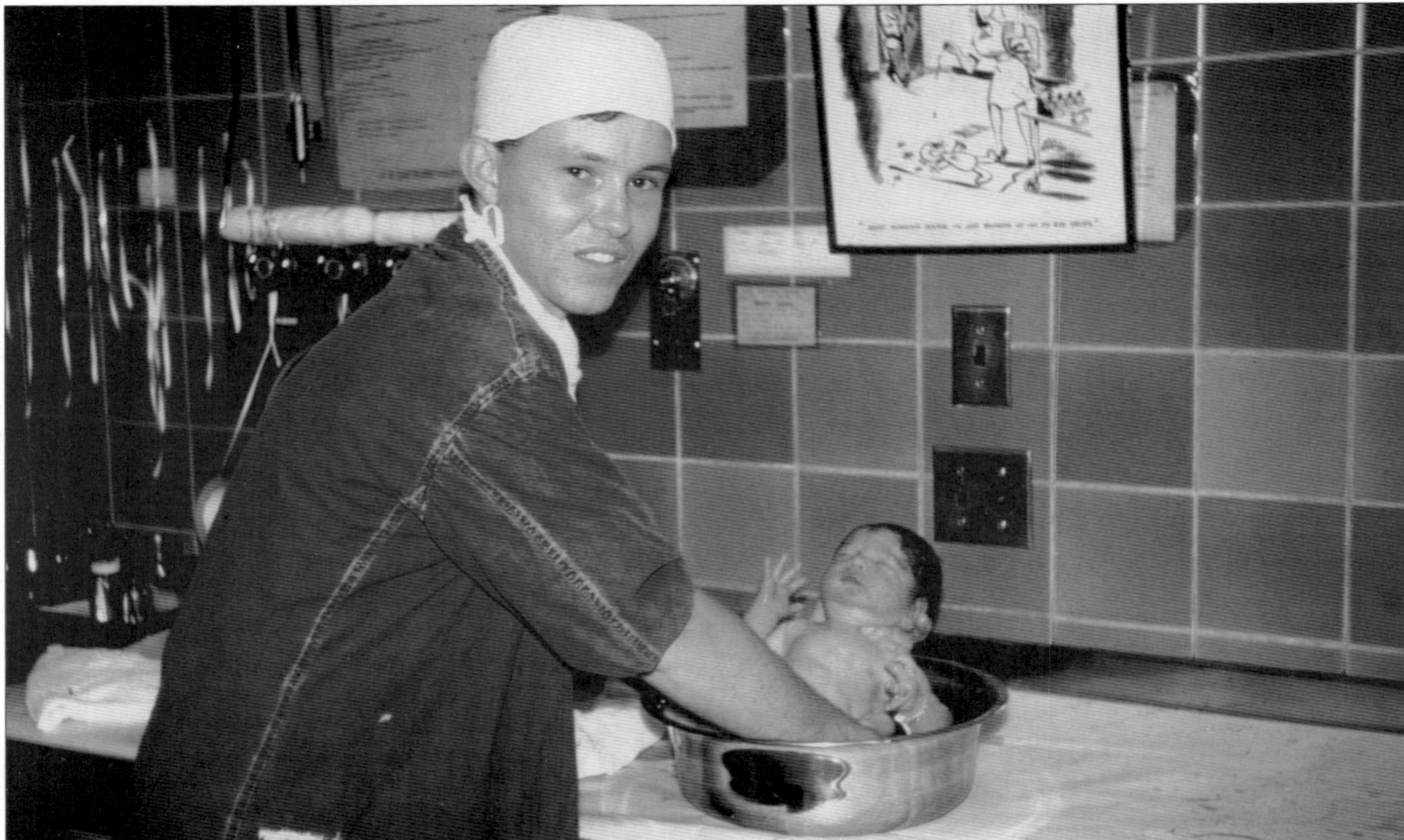

9. Author as fifth year medical student bathing a baby he had just delivered at King George V Memorial Hospital, 1958

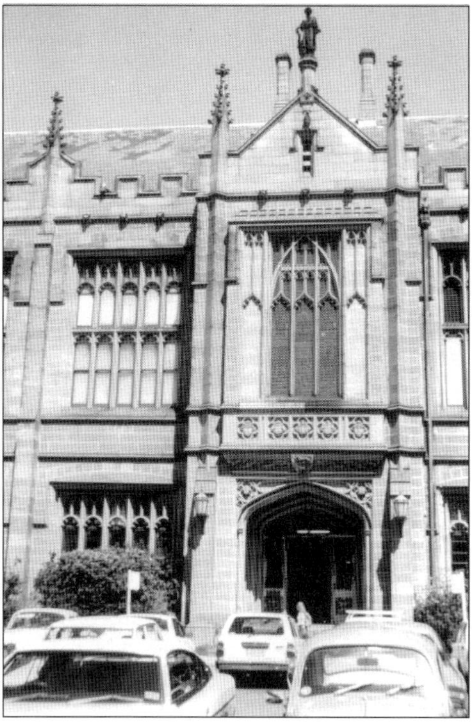

10. The front of the Old Medical School, with the dissecting room on the first floor on the left, 1955

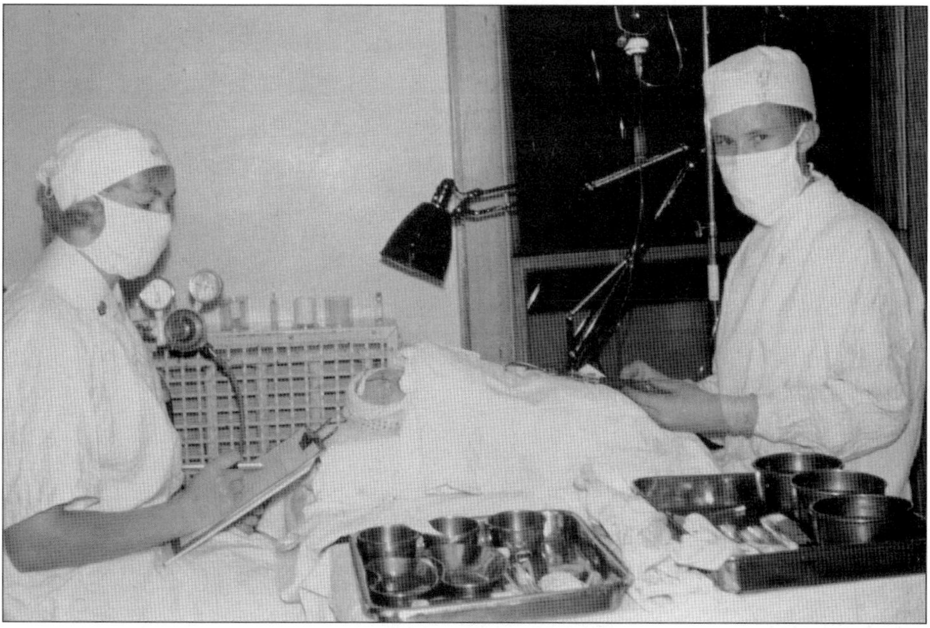

11. Author assisted by nurse performs an exchange blood transfusion on a newborn baby at King George V Memorial Hospital, 1961

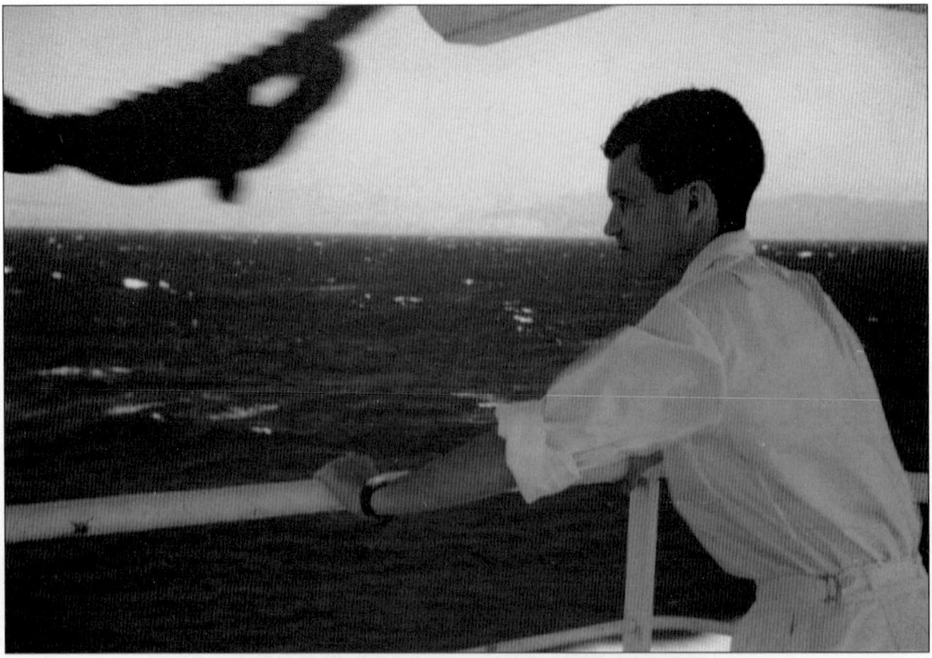

12. Author on MV Aramaic *in the Red Sea, 1962*

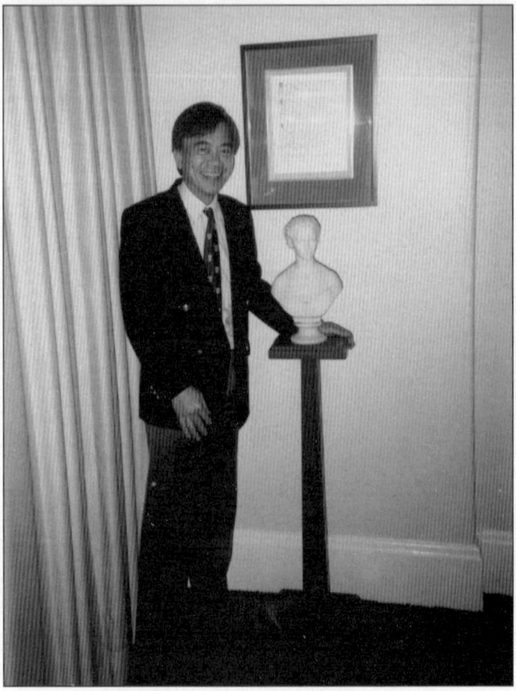

13. Dr John Samuel Yu, general medical superintendent of the Royal Alexandra Hospital for Children, with the bust of Queen Alexandra, 1990

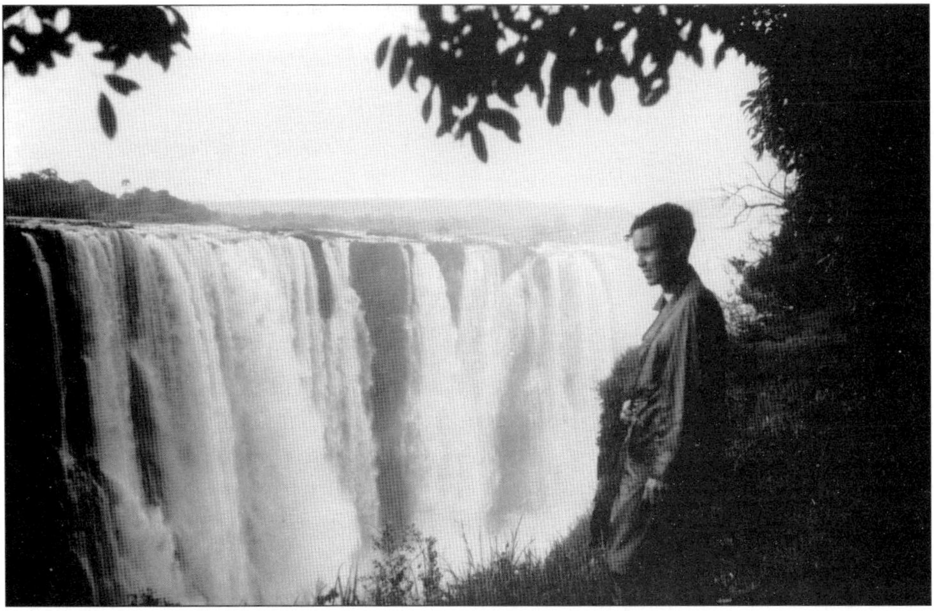

14. *Author visiting Victoria Falls, December 1966*

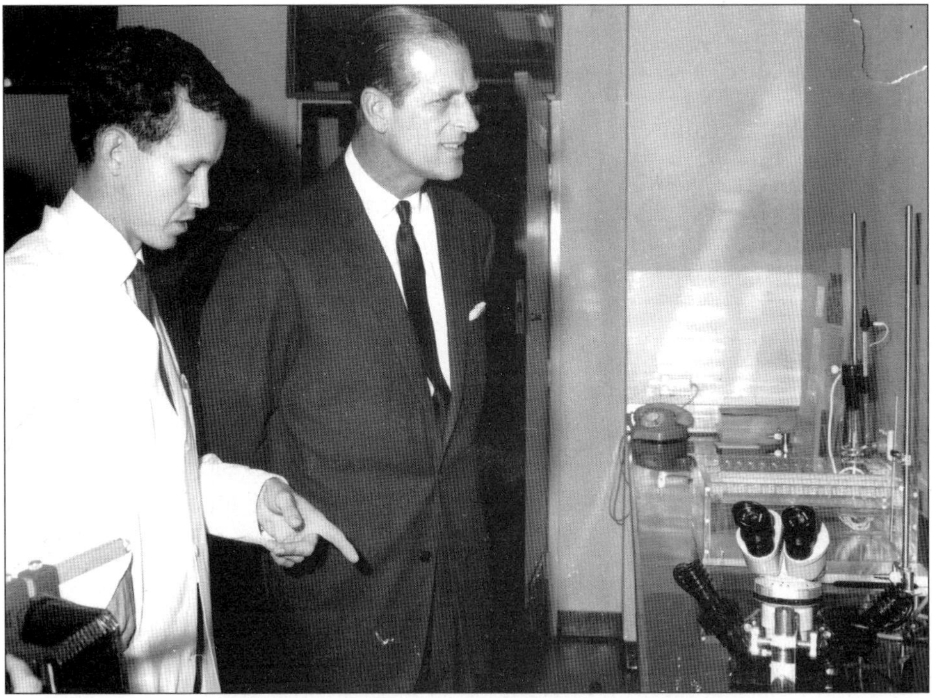

15. *Prince Philip being shown the gastroenterology laboratory in the Institute of Child Health in Sydney by the author, with the dissecting microscope on the right, 1968*

CHAPTER FOUR

Junior Doctor in Sydney

My LIFE AS A DOCTOR began in January 1960 at the Royal Prince Alfred Hospital where I had been lucky enough to be appointed as a houseman or junior resident medical officer (JRMO). Resident, we surely were. I lived in a spartan room in the Resident Medical Officers Quarters at RPAH for the next two years.

I should first just recall how the hospital founded, in 1876, came to be named after Prince Alfred, Duke of Edinburgh. He was Queen Victoria's second son. During his Royal Visit to New South Wales he was shot in the buttock by an Irish Fenian O'Farrell at Clontarf, a pleasure resort in Middle Harbour 'in an assassination attempt'. The bullet was removed and he recovered uneventfully, but the loyal people of Sydney were outraged that this attack should have occurred upon their very first Royal Visitor. Therefore they raised a large sum of money to build a hospital in his honour. In due course, the Royal Prince Alfred Hospital was built and eventually opened to patients in 1882. Six pavilion blocks were originally designed after the plans of St Thomas's Hospital, London.

On their round the world trip, the royal brothers, Prince Albert Victor, Duke of Clarence and Prince George, Duke of York (future King George V), sons of Edward Prince of Wales (future King Edward VII) visited Sydney in 1881 and laid the foundation stone of the Princes' Block still standing today. A further royal connection occurred when Prince George, then Duke of Cornwall and York returned in 1901, after inaugurating the new Federal Parliament Building in Melbourne, to lay the foundation stone for the Queen Victoria Memorial Block (the Vic Block). The new maternity hospital within RPAH was in due course to commemorate his memory, as King George V Memorial Hospital (KGV), opening in 1940. My mum and dad attended the opening ceremony. They both wore academic dress, a unique event in the wartime years. I remember their excited chat on returning home after the event. My first child Louise was destined to be born there in 1970.

In due course, the Royal Prince Alfred Hospital became a teaching hospital of the University of Sydney. Its position next door to the University campus was very convenient for students. In my time, Sydney Hospital, St Vincent's Hospital and Royal Shore Hospital were the other three teaching hospitals of the University. The students at these hospitals had to travel regularly some distance from the University unlike us at Prince Alfred.

When I was a student there, most of the original buildings were still intact. It has since then had several major re-developments. Linked to it at that time was a more modern annexe, the private wing, Gloucester House, as mentioned earlier in relation to my father. Across Missenden Road were separate parts of the hospital the King George V Memorial Hospital for Mothers and Babies and the Page Chest Pavilion (named after a doctor politician, Sir Earle Page).

The post of JRMO involved rotating through a number of 'firms' during the course of a year. The training was very broad and comprehensive, more so than provided by the NHS in the UK. In my case medicine was my first term with that doyen of Sydney physicians Sir William Morrow, then surgery with Dr Stan Lovell, followed by neurosurgery with Dr M. Morson. There I met Dr Gordon Roden, an anaesthetic registrar who was a good deal older than the rest of us. We became good friends and he became a kind of father figure for me full of sage advice. His Daughter Dillon ten years later was to stay for some time with my family in London. The next term was Obstetrics with Paediatrics, and then Casualty (Accident and Emergency). Casualty on Saturday night was mayhem, an introduction to a slice of life I had not seen before. This was followed by Blood Bank and finally Urology, my father's specialty, but he had retired by then. In fact he retired on his sixtieth birthday, 25 January 1960, at the then compulsory age of sixty years required for the honorary staff. The hospital's chief executive Dr Edgar Thomson, had startled me on that day by paging me and telling me to come immediately to Vic 2 North, my father's ward. He was a rather grim faced man with black horn rimmed glasses with an aggressive manner. So when I arrived, I was both surprised and pleased to find a tea party was being given by dad's colleagues in his honour, to mark his retirement. I was proud to hear the tributes paid to him by his peers, especially concerning the respectful courteous manner he always used to address patients. Elderly men he always addressed as 'Sir', no matter their occupation. The hospital marked his retirement by commissioning Andor Meszaros, who sculpted the resurrection scene for Shore Chapel, to sculpt his profile for a bronze plaque for the hospital library, with a copy for himself which I am honoured to now have.

At this point it may be helpful to describe the composition of the firm or team at RPAH in 1960. Leading a firm was a senior honorary medical officer (HMO) supported by several less senior honoraries. Then leading the junior doctors was the registrar supported by a senior resident medical officer (second year graduate) and finally the most junior member of the team the JRMO or houseman. As explained earlier, the honoraries did all their public hospital duties unpaid, earning their living in private practice. In 1960 this honorary system was still flourishing and doctors of the generation of my father and Sir William Morrow approved of the system, but for younger consultants wanting to make their way in the world they wanted the system changed. However there was no enthusiasm for a UK style NHS, as this did not have a very good reputation in Australia at that time or indeed ever since. There can be no doubt that in 1960 very high quality care was delivered for patients at RPAH. The equal of anything in the UK, as I was later to discover for myself. The honorary system was of course based upon the old system which had existed in Britain from the nineteenth century. Perhaps the motto for this old order might be 'Miseratione non mercede', which means, 'From consideration not gain'. This motto dated 1822 still stands on the wall of the old St Thomas's operating theatre in London, which has been so remarkably preserved. This was a charitable way of practising medicine and was clearly ripe for change, but this did not occur in NSW until the late sixties and early seventies.

JRMOs worked hard and of course were salaried, albeit modestly. We were the general 'dogs' bodies' of the firm. We took all the histories and examined the patients, writing up the notes. We wrote all the pathology, X-ray request forms etc. We performed all the venepunctures necessary for the investigations. We gave regular intravenous medications such as heparin. We were on duty for our own patients at 1 p.m. every night otherwise we generally worked a 1 in 2 rota. We could be up most of the night when our firm was 'on take' i.e. accepting medical emergencies.

Once I got on top of it, I found this hard work was quite exhilarating. It was wonderful to at last be doing something practical. Yet, at first performing all the venepunctures was a terrible burden. Fat elderly patients with fragile and difficult veins were a nightmare. I hated hurting patients. When one elderly lady started praying to God, out loud, that I would find a vein, it was terrible. I had virtually no training in venepuncture, the only training being some desultory advice from anaesthetists when we spent our weekly half day off the ward, in the theatre giving anaesthetics. Another untrained burdensome duty for the JRMO was to inform patients or their relatives concerning the diagnosis and prognosis, unless Sir William as he glided by had already responded to a patient's query. This could be an unsupervised and a frightful burden when one was required on occasion, to tell patients, and or their relatives, that they had cancer. At that time cancer patients were often not told the diagnosis, if the family did not wish it. We were often summoned to the front hall of the hospital when relatives arrived requesting information about the family member who was an in-patient. At first this task of breaking bad news was an ordeal, but with experience one became progressively more skilled and whilst never pleasant it ceased to be an ordeal.

We, as very young, inexperienced doctors, were very dependent upon our junior doctor colleagues (not much older) and the nursing staff, especially the sister. My first ward was C1, an enormously long Nightingale Ward, for male medical patients. These were mostly elderly men and were lying in symmetrical rows on either side. The sister in charge was known to be a 'dragon' who could devour young doctors, but she was also known to have a heart of gold. This she revealed when one asked for her help, without pretending to have experience which one did not possess. Sadly, she had early Parkinsonism and so showed almost no facial expression, as I mentioned earlier when I had encountered her as a student. Eventually we got on well, and I valued her help. Some months later she honoured me, by inviting me to visit her flat, with a number of lady artists including the well known artist Thea Proctor, who asked me to sit for a portrait. I still have a sketch she made on that occasion.

I was also fortunate to have Bruce Connolly as my SRMO, who really looked after me in those stressful first days. At that time, it seemed I had to do a thousand and one venepunctures all at once, telephone all the laboratories at once, and go to the X-ray department at once, to try and find all the latest X-rays for Sir William's formal ward round. This round was a very difficult occasion for the JRMO because one had to have everything ready, know everything about the patient and be responsible for everything that went wrong. Sir William himself, supported by registrar and SRMO, proceeded elegantly along the ward with his kindly manner talking gently and reassuringly but briefly to each patient. Many were so pleased 'to have a Sir' as their doctor. He was indeed the only medical knight at RPAH. Sir William's diagnostic ability was legendary.

The following year I was appointed as a Senior Resident Medical Officer (SRMO). I again did a term in general medicine with Dr Ralph Reader but this time I also did terms in thoracic medicine and cardiology in the Page Chest Pavilion. My future brother-in-law Howard Peak was my registrar in cardiology. This dominance of medical firms was because I had set my goal to be a physician. I also did more obstetrics at King George V Hospital doing countless dilatations and curettages in women following miscarriages. I even did one Caesarean section under supervision. I also performed many exchange blood transfusions for haemolytic disease of the newborn, usually at that time due to blood group Rh incompatibility. In this procedure, by 'exchanging' the baby's blood with other compatible blood, the level of bilirubin circulating in the baby's blood, which could damage the brain, was lowered and there was time for baby to recover from the anaemia. This disorder can now be prevented. I also quite often had to give anaesthetics in King George, including open ether. With this technique the sedated but un-intubated patient had the anaesthetic administered via a muslin mask on a metal frame. We first dropped on ethyl chloride as an induction and then open ether drop by drop. It was often very difficult to know how deep the anaesthesia was. I once nearly feel asleep having almost anaesthetized myself during a gynaecology list! It was not an ideal mode of anaesthesia. It has long since been abandoned.

There is one procedure I performed in the Obstetric term, whose memory embarrasses me. This was the routine circumcision of newborn baby boys by means of bone forceps without any anaesthesia! A nurse would hold the baby very firmly on her knee, and the baby's foreskin pulled forward and a bone forceps would then be applied gently, at first making sure it was well clear of the glans. Then the bone forceps was brutally snapped shut and the foreskin chopped off. The poor little boy would scream lustily for a few minutes, then quietly whimper and was taken back to his mother. At the time I did not like the procedure at all but our seniors told us 'Neonates do not feel pain like older children and adults!' This is now known to be quite untrue and neonatologists like my future colleague Kate Costeloe at Barts and Homerton Hospital, in London, have emphasized neonates do feel pain and require pain relief. In the 1960s circumcision was quite routine for Australian boys. The story put about at the time was that Australian soldiers in the desert during World War I developed bad balanitis, i.e. infection of the foreskin, related to the heat and sweating of Egypt. It was considered good for personal hygiene. Paediatricians have been fighting against such a view for years and now this routine practice in Australia has been abandoned.

I also did a surgical term, performing several appendicectomies myself and suturing many wounds for the honoraries. However despite my surgeon father, I had no vocation for surgery. I planned to be an adult physician. However during my surgical term there was a landmark event for me, I contributed as a junior colleague with a veterinarian and a bacteriologist to a medical publication, a case report, in the *Medical Journal of Australia* (1961 2 395). Looking back this was a notable event for me, my first publication, albeit not yet as first author (the next landmark). This report concerned a man of 43 years who had been admitted with an axillary (under his arm) abscess and swollen ankle with periostitis (inflamed lining surrounding the bone) following a bite from a dog on his right hand. A very unusual bacterial pathogen Pasteurella multocida was cultured from the pus in the patient's abscess and from the mouth of the dog. The patient fully recovered with surgical drainage and the appropriate antibiotic, but the case was the first time Pasteurella multocida had been identified in Australia. This occurred only because the bacteriologist Phyllis Rountree in the Fairfax Institute of Pathology (I mentioned earlier in my childhood visits) used a special culture technique, having been informed that the abscess followed a dog bite. I provided the clinical details for the report and I was proud to be associated with a publication. It whetted my appetite for the notion of clinical research but it was to be five years before I published again, but thereafter, medical writing became one of my mainstream activities.

My greatest short-term ambition was to further my training by going to England. In fact for years longer than I could remember, my burning ambition was to visit England for both non-medical and medical reasons. My father before me had trained to be an urologist, largely in London, but also in Edinburgh and in Harrogate in Yorkshire. He had regaled us with 'stories' as the family put it, of his days in Britain. We became especially familiar with some of his teachers in London at St Peter's Hospital for Stone, in Covent Garden where dad had been RMO 1932-3. He had to pay a mess bill for the privilege as in those days there was no salary! Sir John Thomson-Walker, Swift Joly, Ogier Ward, A.H. Harkness (who my sister and I were to meet in due course in London), Cuthbert Dukes (who I was to meet in London) all became household names, but above all Barrington. Dad regarded Barrington as a kind of hero, but clearly a great eccentric, mum did not like to hear about him, as he was clearly a misogynist and a man with a caustic wit.

The long and short of all this was that dad had inspired me concerning the quality of British Medicine. Clearly his years in Britain had been the greatest years of his professional life. So I applied to do the famous Hammersmith Course in Medicine in London and I was accepted for the autumn of 1962. This was known to be a course where people from the Commonwealth and Empire could come to learn the latest in scientific medicine. However before then I wished to extend my overall training by working for six months at the Royal Alexandra Hospital for Children, again as a lowly junior resident medical officer. In those days it was considered good experience for a physician in training to spend at least six months caring for children. The time I spent at

RAHC was quite marvellous. Although I did not realize it at the time, this move changed my life.

So for another six months I lived in a hospital residence, making a total of two and a half years with a hospital as my home. I worked often on alternate nights, many times without sleep, especially during the Obstetrics term. Little social life was possible. Often on those weekends when I could get to my parents' home in Wollstonecraft to be with my family, I mostly slept! Perhaps we worked too hard but it did provide wonderful continuity of care for the patients and provided a fantastic experience for me throughout my life.

At the children's hospital I had a wide range of exposure to medical and surgical specialties. Diseases such as scurvy and rickets still occurred occasionally but infectious disease, in particular gastroenteritis and respiratory infections, were the largest part of clinical practice. Urgent tracheotomy for children with acute epiglottitis (swollen inflamed epiglottis at the back of the tongue) still occurred, albeit rarely, requiring urgent tracheotomy. When a child with severe respiratory distress was admitted to the relevant ward the nursing staff would ring the 'trache' bell, which meant every medical officer available, had to rush to the ward and consider doing an urgent tracheotomy. We all used to run down the hill but some of us were hoping we would not get there first! This custom dated back to the times when diptheria was a common problem often requiring lifesaving tracheotomy to prevent children dying from asphyxiation.

I concluded my experience at RAHC with a term in the Professorial Unit, lead by the Englishman Professor Tom Stapleton. My teacher as a student, Sir Lorimer Dods, had retired and with his support, Stapleton had been appointed as his successor. Sadly by the time I worked in the Professorial Unit, relations between the two were not good. Working in lower Todman Ward as professorial JRMO was an interesting time, but the atmosphere was erratic and enigmatic. Little did I realize that in five years time I would return as professorial registrar! However a great asset was that John Yu was professorial registrar. We became lifelong friends. He had been the year ahead of me at medical school.

Two clinical vignettes occur to me as illustrative of the demands made on junior doctors at that time. These concern two patients, one adult, at RPAH and the other a child, at RAHC. I 'specialed' these two patients for two weeks each, twelve hours on and twelve hours off. They were both managed in side wards, their breathing being taken over by an artificial respirator, in an intensive care mode, but not in a modern intensive care unit. At RPAH the young man, unusually, had developed tetanus (he had not been immunized) with major breathing problems and required a period of therapy producing paralysis. So the newly developed Bird respirator took over his breathing artificially. It was responsible and demanding work. The second concerned a girl of 11 years with a poliomyelitis-like illness due to an unusual virus. She had developed generalized paralysis below the neck and so she also needed artificial respiritation with a Bird Respirator. One amusing thing happened. I had the perhaps eccentric desire to reassure her by sometimes singing to her. One night she began to pray to God aloud that the doctor would stop singing! That was the second and last time that a patient prayed out loud above me.

This training as a junior doctor in Sydney over a two and a half year period was very broad, embracing many disciplines both medical and surgical. I had obtained direct surgical, obstetric and an aesthetic experience as well as mainstream medicine and paediatrics plus some laboratory experience in the blood bank at RPAH. I also had good holidays far away from it all with my friends either in the country or by the sea, with holidays on Lord Howe Island off NSW coast and on the Barrier Reef in Queensland. These hospital years were great times for forming new friendships and sustaining old ones. I made new friends at RPAH from the year immediately senior to me, with John Burgess, he was to become an Endocrinological Consultant Physician at Prince Alfred and from the year junior to me, with Bob Dick, whom years later was also to settle in England and at RAHC with John Yu. He was later to be a colleague at the Hammersmith Hospital and was to help me years later, to make the decision to change from medicine to paediatrics. He was to become Chancellor of the University of NSW.

So as I determined to leave Sydney for London, I looked back with some satisfaction on a period of good broad training in medicine in its wider sense. However I still had so much to learn about medicine and the greater world that I could hardly wait to set forth on my journey abroad.

CHAPTER FIVE

Ship's Surgeon

FROM MY EARLIEST DAYS, my dream had been to go to England. I had read so much about England. I had heard so much about England. I had met so many wonderful English people. For many years this was my primary long-term goal. My sister had gone on ahead of me to England for a working holiday, working to begin with as a legal secretary in Bedford Square, London in 1962.

Following my father's example before me, I elected to travel to England as a ship's surgeon or doctor. Other friends such as Bob Dick were in due course to make similar journeys. Dad had been a ship's surgeon several times, in his young days, even memorably sailing around Cape Horn. I was lucky enough to be appointed by the Shaw Savill Line to be a ship's surgeon on their ship, the MV *Aramaic*. She was docked in Sydney a week or so before I was due to board her. So I first visited the ship in Sydney before I embarked, as she was travelling around the Australian coast en route to Adelaide, where I was to join her. Dad accompanied me, for moral support, on my visit to meet Captain Williams, a short red-faced Englishman. I felt incredibly gauche and inexperienced and was glad to have dad with me. I sampled tinned English biscuits for the first time. They were rather good.

So my actual departure from Sydney for Adelaide was by air from Kingsford-Smith airport on 12 July 1962, with mum, dad and Auntie Lell waving me farewell on it rather dull day. My great adventure really began when I boarded the *Aramaic* at 4 p.m. that day. The *Aramaic* was a cargo ship for general merchandise. She was a motor vessel built in 1957 with a gross tonnage of 6,533. She was built in Germany at the Bremen Vulkan Yard. She was single-screwed, with nine cylinder super-charged diesel engines. She was 475 by 54 feet long. The Shaw Savill Line had been founded in 1858 by two young Britons, Robert Ewart Shaw and Walter Savill. The Shaw Savill company flag was the original national flag of New Zealand, which consisted of the cross of St George with another red cross in its first quarter, on a blue background and with a white star in each of its quarters.

I was allocated a rather fine deck cabin. After stowing my gear, I met some of the young officers and I was immediately asked to join a game of poker for small sums of money. My puritan upbringing made me refuse and I sensed a little frisson as a result, but this was a wise decision. However for the next day or so I certainly felt like a fish out of water. The next morning I met the captain and signed the articles as ship's surgeon (Article 22). I was to be paid one shilling a month, just as my father had before me, i.e. I had a free trip but no salary. I investigated the small hospital bay and clinic room, checking what drugs etc. we had in the pharmacy, and saw several crewmen with minor problems who were waiting to be seen. One sailor had a high temperature and I recommended sick leave from his normal duties. Later that day, he was caught going on unauthorized shore leave. In fact, I had been deceived by my first malingerer. Apparently he, unbeknown to me, had slipped his thermometer into hot tea.

I went ashore to see Port Adelaide in the afternoon and recorded in my diary 'nothing much to see in the town'. I was surprised next morning at 6.30 a.m. to be summoned to examine a prisoner who was to be repatriated to the United Kingdom. I was asked to decide whether or not he was fit to travel. No one in my medical school had ever told me what needed to be done in such a situation. We were to leave port at 7.00 a.m.! Common sense dictated that I should make a quick routine physical examination after a brief enquiry as to his health etc. I adjudicated he was fit. This simple clinical decision was the first occasion in my medical life that I had acted without any back up or support from a hospital colleague. This made me appreciate clearly that, as the Americans say, 'the buck stopped with me' on the *Aramaic*.

We duly sailed out of Port Adelaide on 14 July on a perfect clear day with a sea continuing calm, even as was commenced crossing the infamous Great Australian Bight. My great sea voyage had begun. It was to last five weeks before we finally docked in Liverpool on 20 August. As a complete novice to the sea I was indeed lucky with the weather, as the good weather continued for two days. However by 17 July, after we had left the Australian coast and started our passage across the Indian Ocean, we encountered a heavy swell. I missed breakfast that day but was 'able to deal adequately with lunch and dinner'. The swell was to continue for the next three days but I became adjusted to it and was not seasick, unlike some of the crew. I was now settling into the routine of shipboard life. I had all my meals with the Captain and ship's officers in their Mess. Luncheon and dinner were quite formal affairs with very interesting and wide ranging conversations. A typed elegant menu was produced for each of these meals, which I have kept as a souvenir. Each morning I conducted a clinic but there was not much medical need. Biweekly, I joined the Captain for a full inspection of the ship. My responsibility was to advise on general public health measures etc. One of the young officers told, me that he had not been immunized against smallpox. At that time this was essential if one were to go ashore in a Middle East port etc. We had the vaccine on board. When I vaccinated him it was for me a first time. I was a bit worried some days later when the skin lesion looked red and inflamed but that was really par for the course, indicating vaccination had taken successfully. On 20 July we had a message from a ship 200 miles away seeking a medical opinion. The problem sounded acute intestinal obstruction, requiring surgery, so I radioed what little appropriate advice I could give. We were too far away to directly help. In event of more practical importance to me occurred one night. I was awakened from my sleep in the early hours one morning, by a very anxious young crewman clutching his abdomen because of severe pain. He told me he was scared he had appendicitis, at first I was too. I immediately recalled the little glass bottle on the desk in dad's study at home which contained the appendix he had removed whilst at sea, the skipper having administered the anaesthetic. On taking a history I soon discovered he had had several previous episodes of abdominal pain before, even on one occasion having been admitted to the London Hospital for observation. After careful examination, I concluded he did not have appendicitis, thankfully I was correct.

By the 22 July the weather had completely changed from cool or cold, to very much warmer weather. The ship's company changed from blues to whites. For me, I began to wear white shorts and shirt with long white socks, very similar to the officers, but with no cap. This long crossing of the Indian Ocean was a very quiet time for me and I was able to both study and read with occasional sunbathing. In fact I got a bit sunburnt. On 26 July I celebrated 'crossing the line' i.e. crossing the equator by hosting a 'beer party' in my cabin for the Captain, Mate (Jim Glyde), Chief Engineer, Second Engineer, Radio Officer and Chief Steward. I had been warned or jokingly threatened that I would suffer some more traditional ordeal, being dressed up in a strange costume and forced to do something stupid, as this was my first crossing. In the event, evidently the officers had decided to be kind to me and omit this treatment. Indeed I became aware that I was generally known on the ship as 'the young doc'. Everyone called me 'doc' except the Captain who invariably called me doctor. I was treated throughout the voyage with notable consideration by all the seamen on the *Aramaic*, both the officers and the crew, perhaps they sensed my vulnerability but chose not to take advantage of it. Some of the latter were pretty rough and ready merchant sailors. A few were really tough characters that had seen much life, but everyone was very decent to me. Some of them unburdened themselves to me concerning their many and varied problems, such as marital complications etc. I hope I provided a good ear and expressed some common sense, despite my own relative lack of experience of life at that time. This experience of counselling, again a first for me, was unique and immensely worthwhile. I also felt that as I was trying to care for them they were certainly caring for me too. There was a marvellous spirit of camaraderie on the MV *Aramaic*. My father had experienced something similar in his days as ship's surgeon.

On 27 July bad weather hit us with the hot wind of the South-West Monsoon but the next day I had the great excitement of seeing for the very first time a coastline which was not Australian. We had encountered the African coast at Cape Guardafui in Somalia. The coast initially was precipitous with cliffs of a dark reddish-brown colour and no green vegetation at all. It was wreathed in a dense heat haze. This was followed later by more gentle slopes and then relatively flat land when we saw the little town of Alula with its white buildings gleaming in the sun. Then came the mass of Cabo Elephante where we left the coast to cross the Gulf of Aden for our landfall in the crown colony of Aden.

We entered Aden Harbour at 4 a.m. In my enthusiasm for the very first time, I went up on to the Bridge uninvited, although I had been told by the officers that I should never go on to the Bridge without the Captain's invitation. The Captain ordered me to stand in the corner of the Bridge and not to move or to say a word! It was a great privilege, which I appreciated to see our skilled harbour entry directed by the local pilot who was a white clad Englishman, very much part of the Imperial system. In fact I and the radio officer Don Bray were to go ashore in what can only be described as imperial splendour. We left the ship in a company barge protected from the sun by a while tarpaulin, with the flag of the Shaw savill line flying proudly from the bow the four arab crewman clad in loose dark blue tunics and trousers with red sashes around their waists and a dark blue fez-like hat and each proudly held a staff. One stood at the prow, as we rapidly travelled across the harbour.

There were two large passenger liners anchored in the harbour. At that time Aden was a major bunkering station and tourist port on the way to and from Australia. We were the only two crew members privileged to go ashore from the *Aramaic*, the radio officer for ship's business, me as a tourist! The streets of Aden were a revelation to me. The sight of a beggar girl, one-legged men walking with crutches, blind people obviously suffering from trachoma contrasted with the rich goods from an affluent society for sale to the tourists. I purchased my first tape recorder with great anticipation and also a silk prayer rug, which I kept for many years. I had never seen before the great contrast between affluence and poverty. This was combined with the almost 'Aladdin' like atmosphere of the Arab streets and street markets. I also glimpsed the British officered police force, men and officers immaculate in khaki with black gleaming boots as if on ceremonial parade, patrolling the streets. My sojourn in Aden was all too brief. I gave my colleagues at lunch a breathless account of my experience, which they received rather laconically, as might be expected. The crew had however some experience of Aden themselves, as they had traded over the shipside with the bumboats which had come alongside the ship, as it was anchored in the harbour. The skipper even allowed some of the Arabs on board with their wares, to the delight of the crew. I wrote in my diary 'What a fantastic place, Aden.'

We left Aden at 11 a.m. and then moved out round into the Red Sea for our journey to the Suez Canal. As we sailed through the Red Sea, the atmosphere was incredibly hot and dry. The only way to get cool was to put on a swimming costume, get under a cold shower and then walk out onto the deck in the hot wind. We arrived at the southern end of the canal on 1 August at Port Tewfik to await the convoy, which we had to join to pass through the canal. As we were a British ship we had to go to the end of the convoy where all British ships were relegated at that time. This was an inconsequential gesture of hostility residual to the Suez Affair of 1956. The Egyptians spitefully demonstrated their continuing hostility to Britain by insisting her ships should occupy the humblest position at the end of the convoy. Likewise the Captain gave the order that unlike Aden, no Egyptian traders etc. were to be allowed on board and if they tried to force the issue, hoses were to be used! We had of course to fly the Egyptian flag, which at that time was the flag of the United Arab Republic as Egypt was notionally united with Syria in that republic.

We spent the next day travelling through the Suez Canal and a marvellous sight it was. For the first time I climbed the mast and achieved a superb panoramic view of the canal on either side. We paused at the Bitter Lakes and there we saw several British troopships carry men back home from East of Suez, part of the ongoing retreat from Empire. Some of the men were swimming from the ship in the lake, as we were to do later in Genoa harbour. Along the way it was pointed out that all British monuments including the statue of De Lesseps in Port Said, the original builder of the canal, had been destroyed following the Suez Crisis. The one exception, thankfully, was the massive Anzac memorial which we saw near the Canal. Although the

Egyptians had tried hard it had proved too large to destroy. For Australians the continued existence of this memorial is so important as the Anzacs spent much time in Egypt, for training, before the Gallipoli campaign.

We passed the town of Ismalia where one of the young trainee officers Ken Saville pointed out where British soldiers had been garrisoned in what had been the Canal Zone. At this point it is perhaps of interest to mention that the Suez crisis in 1956 had strongly polarized Australian society just as it did British society. My father strongly supported Anthony Eden's decision to invade Egypt to secure the Suez canal, whereas my mother was opposed largely on humanitarian grounds, fearing the loss of life. Our Prime Minister, Robert Menzies strongly supported Eden and had been an important player in the affair. Many of my fellow Sydney university students in 1956 had enthusiastically supported the British move and were even eager to go and fight the Egyptians. Although there were others passionately against. In the event the British had to withdraw. I myself wonder what would have happened if a quick dramatic military success had been achieved.

I was to visit Egypt some years later, as a guest lecturer and visitor to the children's hospital in Cairo. I had a very unpleasant and frightening experience one morning where I had left my hotel very early, to photograph the British Embassy, which during the First World War was the military centre where Lawrence of Arabia had had to report. As I was taking my photograph, two armed Egyptian soldiers suddenly seized me. They gestured vigorously that photography was banned, but spoke no English. They were very young and what really frightened me was that they had a scared look in their own eyes. Naively, I gesticulated pointing to the Union Jack flying overhead that I was British, implying it was OK for me to photograph the building. At first I did not know what to do. I realized that I had not told anyone in the hotel that I had left the building. Suddenly I came on the idea of offering a bribe, the hallmark of old Egypt. So I took a £20 note from my wallet, all that I had. I gave it to one of the young soldiers, who to my great relief grabbed the note, then roughly pushed me aside. I made way back to the hotel as fast as my legs could carry me i.e. short of running. My hosts told me I had taken a great risk, the British in parts of Cairo were as unpopular as they had been in 1956!

Our journey through the Suez Canal finally ended when we arrived in Port Said where night had already fallen. We sailed straight on and the Captain was glad to be leaving Egypt.

So the *Aramaic* made her way out into the Mediterranean Sea. Next day across its beautiful dark blue waters I was to see the island of Crete. Many years in the future, I was to have several pleasant holidays there with my future wife. Sicily was our next landfall and the journey through the narrow Straits of Messina between Scylla (monsters) and Charybis (whirlpool) of antiquity, negotiated with such difficulty by Ulysses (as I had learnt from Darcy Grigg at Shore). This time I was invited by the Captain up onto the Bridge to see the skilful navigation through these straits separating Sicily from the Italian mainland. We passed the island of Stromboli with its active smoking volcano on our port side, followed by the storied island of Monte Cristo and on to Genoa, our first port of call in Europe.

We docked at first in the outer harbour in the afternoon. The weather was warm and perfect. The sea was a marvellous green blue, so I and some of the young officers decided to swim from the ship. This was both delightful and refreshing, albeit tinged with a little risk, as it was quite difficult getting back onto the metal platform with sharp edges at the foot of the ship's ladder, as the sea was a bit choppy and I needed some help from my mates. We noted a vast American aircraft carrier, apparently nearby. The youngest officer suggested we should swim over. Clearly it was farther then he realized and we wisely did not. The pilot guided the *Aramaic* into the inner harbour that evening. I went ashore as soon as I could and was fascinated by my first glimpse of Europe, but I was irritated to find so many American sailors apparently everywhere, as so many US naval ships were then in port. The wonderful piazzas with their fountains and the street markets were all a revelation to me, filled with the vigour and vitality of Italian life.

I was delighted next morning to be invited by Captain Williams to be his guest for the day, to see something of Genoa. A chauffeur-driven car provided by Shaw Savill, picked us up to see the sights. Strange as it may seem, the first sight, he took us to see was the elaborate, and quite extraordinary cemetery of Genoa, one of its principal sights. Genoa and Zagreb are the only two cities where the locals have recommended to me that I visit a cemetery, as an important tourist visit. Both proved to be fascinating, with a range of architectural styles and beautiful gardens. We also saw what is reputed to be the house of Christopher Columbus, Genoa's most famous son. Then we were driven to the beach resorts and residential areas, thence to lunch in the city. In the afternoon we visited the eleventh century cathedral of St Lorenzo, the first cathedral of the old world I had ever seen. I was struck by how tall it was and how dark it was inside, in contrast to the brilliant light outside. This darkness was just like St Mary's Roman Catholic cathedral in Sydney. However all my prejudice fell away and I was delighted by the experience. Afterwards we visited a couple of bars, finally sitting in the Piazza Ferrari, sipping Martinis and watching the passing parade, the first such occasion for me. This was the European way of life! We returned to the ship at 10 p.m. It had been a memorable day for me, with my introduction to continental Europe and the Mediterranean way of life. I have since visited Italy many times and it is one of my favourite countries.

Next morning we set forth on our journey past Gibraltar, which we did on 10 August. I was delighted to see the great rock for the first time. A long white cloud stretched out westerly from the top of the Rock. Years later we were to have two happy family holidays in the Caleta Palace Hotel on the eastern side of the Rock and discovered how fortunate we were not to be on the western side with its frequent overhanging cloud, a common feature of Gibraltar weather. Later we passed Tarifa the most southerly point of the Iberian peninsular and then the *Aramaic* sailed out of the Gibraltar straits into the Atlantic Ocean. By next day the weather had changed completely. It was cold and overcast with a choppy sea. The crew sadly changed back into blues, apparently they had been hoping to arrive in the English summer still wearing whites. In fact the northern weather being what it is, this had hardly ever happened to anyone on board.

Our next port of call was Dunkirk in France. As we approached we could see the Dunkirk beaches and I found it hard to imagine the scenes in 1940 when the British army was being evacuated, often in small pleasure boats. We arrived on 13 August for a brief visit having to negotiate the locks between the outer and inner harbour. I went ashore in the afternoon for a couple of hours and noted that the town appeared to have been virtually re-built following war damage. Although there were reminders of the past, still present, such as the war damaged medieval church and an obviously restored Hotel de Ville. Then on we went along the coast to enter the River Scheidt in Belgium and up river to dock in the heart of the wondrous city of Antwerp. The harbour itself was interesting with a large four-masted sailing ship, used for naval training, directly opposite where we had berthed. The Hotel de Ville and the cathedral were nearby. The cathedral was so much more impressive than that of Genoa. Its much-decorated tall tower and sublimely beautiful gothic interior lifted my spirits to new heights. I also had time to briefly visit Antwerp's famous zoo. Describing Antwerp in my diary, I wrote 'magnificent'. I was beginning to have difficulty finding new epithets to describe all my new experiences. I was only ashore for a short time but what a beautiful city with so much to see and do.

Next day after sailing along the coast we entered the River Elbe on our way to Hamburg where we arrived on 16 August. I spent most of the day ashore seeing the sights with one of the young officers, Ian Skene, a young

Scot. Once again there had obviously been a huge amount of war damage and much ongoing re-building. Fortunately St Michaelskirche had survived and its baroque interior with its beautiful organ was a completely new style for me, my first Lutheran Church. We had lunch outside in the continental style with light German beer. I was indeed taken to a beer hall with my shipmates that evening and I had a great time, even meeting and dancing with a charming German girl. Next morning I was ashore again, but in the afternoon, we left bound for our final port, Liverpool.

Next day, it was with some emotion that I had my first glimpse of England herself. The first sight of the old country was a vista of the White Cliffs of Dover themselves. Thereafter the southern and west coast of England were covered with mist and sadly invisible to us. We finally arrived at our destination, Liverpool basin, near the 'Liver' building, at 3.30 p.m. on 20 August. One fascinating chapter of my life had closed and another was now to begin.

However to my sister in London's surprise I decided to stay on board for one further night, so I could go ashore with my shipmates to see something of Liverpool and say goodbye to my new friends. Although I kept in touch with some of them with Christmas cards for one year, only one of them, Ian Skene, I was to see again. I saw him only once in Aberdeen with my sister in the following September, during our Scottish tour. I wonder what has become of them all. As I walked with my friends I was impressed by the massive scale and beauty of the old buildings such as St George's Hall and the Walker Art Gallery in the heart of Liverpool but otherwise the city seemed to be in decline, a glorious past but what was the future? I hoped this would not foreshadow my own future experience of England. Had I come fifty years too late?

In fact in future years, I was to visit Liverpool a number of times as external examiner in the Diploma of Tropical Paediatrics at the Liverpool School of Tropical Medicine, itself a great echo of Imperial times. I was to develop a particular affection for the Walker Gallery but did not think much of the 'Wigwam' as the locals call the Roman Catholic cathedral. The interior of the great Edwardian Anglican cathedral designed by Sir Giles Gilbert Scott (one of my favourite architects) is for me, another marvellous sacred space.

Finally on 21 August I took the train for London to meet Judith at Euston Station. The sea journey to England had been a memorable rite of passage for me. I had grown in confidence and experience. Looking back now it was the greatest journey of my life, physically and emotionally. I believe I grew into a new maturity during the voyage. I also had seen something of historic continental European civilization and way of life for the first time.

What I had seen I had liked very much. Indeed much of what I had seen had exceeded all expectation. As I journeyed to London I looked to the future year or two in England with mounting excitement, would England also exceed my expectations? I had not planned to come to settle, but like dad to be trained in a more cosmopolitan environment than the parochialism of Australia for about eighteen months to two years. I also wanted to sample British life and to explore the nearby continent, learning more of the European way of life which I had briefly sampled on my voyage with such pleasure.

CHAPTER SIX

Physician Trainee in London

ON ARRIVAL IN LONDON, Judith met me at Euston Station. We travelled to the Overseas Visitors Club at Earl's Court, the Mecca of young Australians in London at that time, where we were to stay overnight. As we were due to go the next day to Scotland, I was very eager to see something of London that night. I wanted Piccadilly Circus, at night, to be my first port of call in London, as dad had talked about it so much. Judith took me there by tube that evening. As we came up from the underground station, my eyes were dazzled by the splendour of the lights of Piccadilly. Dad had always described this free show of a multitude of changing lights as a feast for, the eyes for any thrifty Scotsman! Unsophisticate that I was, I did indeed marvel at the dazzling display. The advertisement lights were much more extensive in the sixties than they are today. It was really great to see London, for the very first time and at night too. I won't bore the reader by further descriptions, but that night I told Judith I was glad I had come. First impressions had certainly lived up to all my anticipations. Indeed this was to be a continual theme of my first visit to Britain.

Next morning Judith and I were at the Victoria Coach station early, for our holiday trip to Scotland, the land of our paternal ancestors. We had an uneventful trip to Glasgow except that disastrously I lost my Zeiss Contina camera on the coach. Amazingly some kind benefactor returned it to my address some weeks later, blessings on him or her. I still have it. However it meant that awkwardly, Judith and I had to share her camera on our trip. We hired a car in Glasgow and stayed at Youth Hostels throughout Scotland, journeying over 2,000 miles in 3 weeks. Our guide for this pilgrimage was a very practical free book called *A tour by car through England, Scotland and Wales* by Jessie Sisson and published by the Bank of NSW, for its travel department. At that time, very many Australians were coming to Britain, partly to seek their roots and partly just to see what the old country was actually like, having heard so much about it. So a travel book like this was essential. To this day, I find it to be a most useful gazetteer with its snippets of history. An example is given by the description of Dunollie Castle near Oban, which we were to see on our second day in Scotland.

> 'About a quarter of a mile from Oban beach are the ruins of Dunollie Castle (admission 1/- weekdays 10-1, 2-6). This 12th century fort perched on an isolated rock overlooking Oban Bay was a seat of the McDougalls of Lorn. The present house, at foot of the Rock, was built in 1750 of stones from the old castle. Among its treasures is the Brooch of Lorn torn from the plaid of Robert Bruce at Tyndrum.'

When we saw this beautiful little ruin our enjoyment was greatly increased by these well-chosen pieces of information.

I shall not tire the reader with a travelogue of our memorable trip through the Highlands and Edinburgh. Suffice it to say that a particular highlight was the brooding Isle of Mull dominated by Ben More, where my gran, (Elizabeth Walker-Smith née Buchanan) was born at Kinloch. Her forebears, via her mother, had been McLeans settled on Mull for centuries. We took the ferry across from Oban sailing past Dunollie Castle and when we arrived in Tobermory, we had to hire another car, as in those days there was no modern car ferry to Craignure as there is today. The mausoleum of governor Lachlan Macquarie at Grulins is a place of pilgrimage on Mull for Australians. He was the finest governor of New South Wales with a vision of a flourishing colony of free settlers, rather than a penal settlement. He built great buildings accordingly, such as St James's church in Sydney. He was to return to his native Mull, where he died in 1824. On his mausoleum he is described as Father of Australia.

I and my family have returned to the Isle of Mull many times since, including painting holidays to Inniemore at Carsaig with my wife, Liz. Edinburgh, too, I have visited countless times since, as Liz was born there and her mother still lived there, but that first vision of the 'Athens of the North', as gran had told us, will never be forgotten. Albeit at that time, with its dark blackened public buildings such as the National Gallery of Scotland and the Scott Monument, covered with many years of dirt and grime it was quite a leap of imagination to recall ancient Greece.

On return to London from Scotland, I was all set to start the Hammersmith Postgraduate Medicine Course. Indeed I did begin the course with great enthusiasm and excitement! It lived up to every expectation and more. It was effectively to change my life by enabling me to decide upon gastroenterology as my special interest within medicine.

Whilst attending the post-graduate course I was fortunate to stay in London House in Mecklenburg Square, London WC1. Judith was still working in London as a legal secretary and was living with two friends in Brondesbury. London House had been recommended to me both by Garth Serchell, my old school friend and Howard Peak, my colleague at Prince Alfred, who had stayed there in the past. Whilst there, I was to make a number of friends, some lifelong, notably George Soutter, a Rhodesian paediatrician and David Wollman, an American Historian and Fulbright Scholar. At that time London House for men and Goodenough House for women and married couples were halls of residence for postgraduate students from the British Commonwealth and Empire and the runner Empire e.g. the United States. I liked its motto 'Imperium et Libertas', i.e. Empire and Liberty. It functioned like a university college with library, dining hall etc. I continue to be associated with London House I dined in the hall in 2002 as a guest of Lisa Lipson, a former trainee of mine from Vancouver in Canada, back briefly in Goodenough House. Nowadays post-graduates from the European Union also may stay there, mutatis mutandis.

I had to travel each day, by tube train, to White City. I really enjoyed travelling on the underground in those days. I marvelled at its efficiency, having had nothing like it in Sydney at that time. Obviously with all the problems with signals etc, and over-crowding in recent years, my views have mellowed. At that time, bowler hatted gentlemen with rolled umbrellas were still seen on the tube trains. They invariably used to give up their seats for ladies. There were even a few young men staying in London House and working in the city, who still wore a bowler!

I liked to think of myself as a Londoner, travelling every day to White City and then walking the fifteen minutes to Du Cane Road where the Hammersmith Hospital was situated. This was Shepherd's Bush, not Hammersmith, how eccentrically British. We postgraduates in 1962 were lucky as we were able to use the new Wolfson Building for the Course. This consisted of modern lecture theatres and seminar rooms with good eating facilities. I relished getting back to formal study after thirty months of often frantic activity as a junior doctor with little time to read or reflect. Perhaps idealistically, but not so realistically, I felt my immediate goal was to expand my own knowledge and especially the scientific basis of clinical medicine for which Hammersmith was famous rather than studying specifically for, the Membership of the Royal College of Physicians of London (MRCP) known as 'the membership'. Yet this higher degree was necessary for my ultimate goal of becoming a physician and I did want to sit for it in due course, but first I just wanted to learn what the course per se had to offer.

The teachers on the Hammersmith course in medicine were great figures and good teachers especially in cardiology. Sir John McMichael was the impressive professor of medicine at the time and a cardiologist himself. The course consisted of formal lectures, seminars and bedside teaching with some clinical, demonstrations. The most memorable of these was a demonstration of the technique of small intestinal biopsy (i.e. taking a piece of tissue for examination during life rather than at death, (autopsy) from the mucosa or lining of the small intestine). The gastroenterological registrar Jimmy Stewart did this. He showed how a little metal capsule known as the Crosby Capsule, attached to a long piece of plastic tubing, was swallowed by the patient. This then passed on via the stomach into the small intestine. An X-ray of the abdomen, called a plain X-ray, checked its position there. If the position of the capsule were correct, this precision instrument was activated or 'fired' by sucking with a syringe on the end of the plastic tube. This action sucked a small piece of mucosa into the capsule and triggered the rotation of a metal block across the hole in the side of the capsule into which the mucosa had been sucked. In this way the small piece of mucosa was avulsed and the capsule was withdrawn by pulling out the plastic tube painlessly. The mucosa of the small intestine has no pain nerve fibres.

Small intestinal biopsy is essential for the accurate diagnosis of coeliac disease. This is a disorder where chronic diarrhoea with poor weight gain or even weight loss are the main symptoms in early childhood, but it can present at any age. In adults whilst chronic diarrhoea may occur the symptoms, may be quite vague. Normally in adult life and in older childhood the small intestine is lined by long finger-like villi whereas in classical coeliac disease there are no villi and the mucosa is quite flat. So biopsy is the key test for diagnosis. Small intestinal tissue obtained by biopsy is examined immediately under the dissecting microscope or stereomicroscope which enables the surface of the mucosa to be observed in a three dimensional way. If the mucosa is flat when examined this way the diagnosis of coeliac disease can be made provisionally and a gluten-free diet commenced. Final diagnosis requires in addition that as a response to a gluten-free diet, the patient must make a complete recovery. Coeliac disease is a lifelong disorder of permanent gluten intolerance and this diet is required for life. After the preliminary examination, the biopsy tissue obtained is then sectioned and stained with the haematoxylin and eosin dyes I mentioned earlier, as part of basic histological technique. It is then examined under a conventional light microscope. It is remarkable how the previously inaccessible lining of the small intestine became accessible through this sophisticated instrument invented by Crosby and Kugler of the United States, a triumph for technology.

Gastroenterology led by Dr Chris Booth (later Professor and then Sir Christopher) was one of the star firms on the course. Also of a high order were haematology (John Dacie and David Mollin), neurology (Chris Pallis), respiratory medicine (Charles Fletcher and Moran Campbell), endocrinology (Russell Fraser) and paediatrics (Peter Tizard, later professor in Oxford, John Davis, later professor in Cambridge and Leonard Strang, later professor at University College Hospital). Not only were the consultants outstanding teachers but their registrars were too. On the course, I made good friends all from the Commonwealth. Both London House and the Hammersmith course were great places for Commonwealth friendship. Particular friends were Wendy Pocock (South Africa), Tim Ashworth (Nyasaland), and François Couture (Canada). François was a great advocate for Quebec and gave me a book on the subject, *J'ai Vu Quebec.*

François and I had the great privilege to go as the guest of Dr Geraint James to the Fiftieth Anniversary Meeting of the Section of the History of Medicine of the Royal Society of Medicine meeting on 21 November, 1962. Speakers included Lord Cohen of Birkenhead, Dr Douglas Guthrie (author of *The History of Medicine,* 1945, which I knew, well) and the distinguished surgeon and historian Sir Zachary Cope. Quite amazingly as we went up in the lift, we were introduced to Sir Henry Dale, the distinguished physiologist, and Dr Cuthbert Dukes, the pathologist, both great medical celebrities, indeed living history. The latter's name was familiar to me via my father's recollections of St Peter's Hospital for the Stone in the 1930s. The meeting boosted my lifelong interest in the history of medicine which forty years later was to become my principal interest in my retirement.

At the end of the course there was the opportunity, to apply for house jobs (i.e. junior doctor posts) at Hammersmith Hospital, usually some people from the course were appointed. It had been my great dream to get a Hammersmith post as an entrée to British medicine. It was a major reason for attending the course. Fortunately I was short-listed for interview. I had never been to a job interview before as the posts I had held at RPAH and RAHC had not required interview. The interviewing panel was formidable and large, in fact including all the consultant staff. Whilst waiting to be interviewed with other applicants, I overheard that, in order to create a good impression, one had to know for which job one wished to apply. Hitherto I had not given much thought as to which branch of medicine most interested me. The teaching I had most enjoyed during the course was from Chris Booth on gastroenterology. Also, as mentioned above, I had been fascinated by the technique of small intestinal biopsy and I also had had a little experience of gastroenterology with Sir William Morrow at Prince Alfred. So when during the interview the question came 'Which firm interests you most?' I was able to reply without hesitation 'Dr Booth's firm'. I was so lucky to get the job. It changed my life and led to my abiding interest, diseases of the small intestine. I was also pleased to discover that Wendy Pocock had also been appointed from the course. One post-script to this interview, a future friend David Harvey was due to be interviewed for a paediatric post at the same time as mine. He was ordered to wait in the wrong place and so missed his interview. He was then discovered just after an appointment had been made, but was still interviewed. As he was obviously such a good candidate he was appointed but for the next post. It is good that there can be flexibility in the system but for me I am glad this happened, as our jobs were to overlap. We were to become good friends until today and my paediatric connections continued. He is now Professor of Paediatrics at Imperial College, London.

So I had to leave my comfortable room in London House and return to the austerity of a hospital room in the Residents' Quarters at the Hammersmith Hospital, into which I duly moved. For the next six months I was to work longer hours than I ever had, or ever would in my life. Basically one was on duty for one's own patients all the time. Evenings and occasional weekends off duty, were a grace and favour arrangement with my consultant Chris Booth. What this did mean was that there resulted a remarkable continuity of patient care. I got to know my patients very well indeed. Indeed the notion of 'my patients' became very real and all the house staff strove to do the best for our own patients, even in a slightly competitive spirit.

On the first day I became Chris Booth's houseman at the Hammersmith Hospital, he told me not to call him 'sir', the mode of address I had always used to consultants previously in my career in Australia. He also said in conversation that I was not a typical Australian, with that I happily agreed. I knew well that I did not fit the Australian stereotype, for one thing my accent although definitely Australian, was not very obvious. In fact his own world view and my own were, and still are, a great contrast. We had opposite views on the monarchy, Christianity and politics but we became good friends with I believe mutual respect. I have learnt so much from him. Most importantly I learnt from him a commitment to clinical science, which has under-pinned my medical philosophy, ever since. Also my vocation for gastroenterology came from him. He also introduced me to the then new concept of diseases of the small intestine. This concept I was able to adapt and extend for children, years later. He also introduced me to the idea of the practical application of newly discovered concepts of pathophysiology directly to the patient.

Chris Booth and David Mollin had earlier discovered that vitamin B12 was absorbed specifically from the lower end of the small intestine known as the ileum. Years later I was to encounter David Mollin again when he became professor of haematology at Barts medical school. We undertook some joint research, which carried the B12 story a little further. We studied the uptake of B12 in three siblings from Syria the two who had a rare congenital malabsorption of vitamin B12 with failure of uptake of B12 probably due to defect of specific receptors for the vitamin in the ileum, compared to the third sibling who proved to have normal absorption. The whole Hammersmith experience fostered such direct application of science to the investigation and treatment of patients. Many years later, at the Royal Free this approach was to be my inspiration when I encountered the problem of children with regressive autism and bowel problems (see Chapter 15).

This approach was a world away from the old rote learning which was often a feature of normal undergraduate clinical teaching of medicine at that time. The concept that progress in medicine was driven by technology was central to the Hammersmith view, of the future, at that time. The highest of standards were aspired to. This involved the need for a houseman, such as me, to have all the patients' clinical details at his fingertips on ward rounds and all investigations arranged etc. Most stressful was the occasional need to present a patient's history at the Grand Rounds in front of staff members of the Course, chaired by Sir John McMichael. If one performed badly, one's whole reputation within the hospital was at risk. Yet the great thrill of the Hammersmith experience was the exhilaration of working with manifestly high achievers in medicine.

Chris Booth was of course a general physician as well as gastroenterologist. His general ability meant that several colleagues and their families became his patients, a demanding role for his houseman following on. At first I had the difficulty of keeping up with the reputation of my distinguished predecessor, Graham Neale. He had clearly been an outstanding house physician. He and I were to become friends and he was so helpful in briefing me concerning what the job required. I was very lucky with the registrars on the firm. As well as Jimmy Stewart, there was Michael Brain (the son of the great neurologist Lord Brain) and Gilbert Thompson. They closely supervised my work. Jimmy Stewart taught me the technique of small intestinal biopsy using the Crosby Capsule. Priming the capsule before use to ensure it worked properly was quite a skilled business. I did a number of these biopsies and I became quite fascinated by the beautiful three-dimensional appearance of the normal villi with their central core of blood vessels, which could be seen so clearly with the dissecting microscope. The dramatically different appearance in coeliac disease with its flat mucosa was a fascinating contrast. This three dimensional appearance was a special interest of Chris Booth's and he had published in this area. This was to become for me a lifetime interest.

I made a number of new and lasting friends while on the house, these included Ten Feizi, Ilfra Pink, Colin Barnes, David Galton (we were to be professorial colleagues at Barts many years in the future) and David Read. David was a fellow Australian, an old Shore boy but he had been a year ahead of me, who became my closest friend in London. He was to become a distinguished academic in respiratory medicine in Sydney but was to die an early death from lung cancer, although not a smoker. In addition John Yu had come from Sydney to be a research fellow in the paediatric department. He was not resident but lived with his sister Betty Busby (a pharmacist) and her husband Colin (London Symphony Orchestra). I kept the paediatric contact by seeing John from time to time and visiting the Busbies. The registrars in paediatrics were Jon Scopes and Roger Robinson, both destined to be Professors of Paediatrics. John Yu himself was destined to be Chief Executive Officer of the Royal Alexandra Hospital for Children in Sydney. Clearly the paediatric department at the Hammersmith Hospital at that time was truly remarkable.

During this six months house job, it became clear that I needed then to study and sit for the Membership examination of the Royal College of Physicians of London. Michael Brain agreed to give us some membership teaching. I sat the exam I bit prematurely and I failed my first attempt, at Guy's Hospital. It was a traumatic episode for me. This was the one and only time in my life that I ever failed all examination. One of the examiners was Dr Boland and folk legend had it that if he took his glass eye out during the examination, the candidate had failed. He did so during my examination.

Wendy Pocock suggested I go up to Edinburgh and sit the membership there, which she had recently passed. I decided to do so. Traditional family links with Edinburgh also made this appealing but I did realize that probably I would have to pass the London exam before I went home. Going to Edinburgh would be good practice. The Royal College of Physicians of Edinburgh also offered a special subject in the exam, which included alimentary diseases, i.e. gastroenterological diseases.

In the mean time I also realized that I would have to go the special teaching sessions for the membership examination undertaken by Dr Maurice Pappworth. He ran a very popular and successful MRCP London course. He used to give his tutorials in a room adjacent to the boiler room of the baths in Seymour Street in the west end. He was opposed to the medical establishment and he was only awarded the Fellowship of the Royal College of Physicians of London, i.e. FRCP, very late in life. He wrote a popular book entitled *A Primer of Medicine,* first published in 1960, based on his course. It ran to a number of editions. I found it to be invaluable when studying for the membership exam. I still have my copy and my multiple underlining is a testimony as to how closely I read it. As he stated, his book was crammed with facts and it was facts he emphasized to us. He believed it was impossible to be a good clinician without possession of a large number of facts. His teaching style was very similar to the kind of teaching I had had at Prince Alfred as a student from Billy Bye. This was quite a different style from the Hammersmith. My chief Chris Booth referring to attempts to quantify the size of a patient's liver by palpation and percussion commented that modern imaging techniques provided much more reliable and exact information than these inexact clinical methods. He was clearly correct, but Pappworth was a very good teacher and he did give a comprehensive grounding in most of clinical medicine. However his emphasis on learning facts was out of kilter with the new teaching methods based upon reasoning. He gave us lists to memorize. I can remember one such list, the causes of radiological rarefactiom (loss of bone mineral and matrix) of the bones. I can hear him say when shown such an X-ray in the exam, the candidate should play the rarefaction record', in his harsh rasping voice. He was a physically small man with an aggressive manner. The Hammersmith Hospital and clinical researchers were his particular bête noir and he looked askance at people like me from the Hammersmith. Little did we know that he would publish a book, *Human Guinea Pigs*, five years later in 1967, which would become a landmark in medical ethics. The book has been described as a bombshell, but it certainly made clear the vital necessity of the principle of informed consent for human research. This was my approach throughout my career. I was very upset during the GMC Hearing (see Chapter 16) when the lady prosecutor suggested I was "treating autistic children as guinea pigs."

I duly travelled by train up to Edinburgh with a Canadian friend from London House, Don Wood from Toronto. We stayed at a delightfully old fashioned Edinburgh hotel, the Dean Hotel, quite close to the Royal College of Physicians of Edinburgh in Queen Street. It is a wonderful Victorian building, which not surprisingly reminded me of the architectural style of the Old Medical School in Sydney. Its statues of Aesculepius etc. hark back to the great traditions of ancient Greek medicine, rather appropriate to the Athens of the North. First we had to sit for the written examination in the examination hall in Chalmer's St. Foolishly I had drunk quite a lot of tea before the exam and I was forced to visit the toilet and I was appalled to see some candidates from overseas cribbing from textbooks. I have never seen the like before or since. For the clinical examination we had two separate exams. The first was in general medicine at the Royal Infirmary where I had a medical long case and then short cases, X-rays etc. I was fortunate to have as examiner that doyen of Edinburgh physicians Sir Derreck Dunlop with his long white hair and elegant manners. He put me at ease immediately by saying how he liked Sydney. He then said encouragingly as he showed me an X-ray of a patient's abdomen 'My dear boy, you will have no problem with this.' In fact it was so, the X-ray showed obvious gas under the diaphragm, the radiological sign of a perforated hollow viscus or organ in the abdomen. I sailed through the exam. The second examination was in alimentary diseases and unexpectedly, was held in Glasgow at the Southern General Hospital. To my surprise the college provided rail tickets for three of us travelling together from Edinburgh to Glasgow, with 'sustenance' money for refreshments. Most astonishing of all we were met at Glasgow station by a chauffeur-driven Rolls Royce. So I drove in gentlemanly state, for the first and only time in my life, in a Rolls Royce to the Southern General. Our examiner was the distinguished gastroenterologist Dr Bill Sircus. I was given a patient with a rare syndrome called Peutz-Jegher (names of those doctors who first described it) syndrome where there is characteristic pigmentation around the mouth. I fortunately noticed this pigmentation and was able to make the diagnosis. The exam went amazingly smoothly, what a contrast to the exam at Guy's. Then the final viva voce examinations were held in the columned splendour of the hall of the college. This was proceeded by an elegant afternoon tea with cakes etc. in fine china served by young ladies clothed in black with white aprons and caps. Then the major-domo announced our name as we entered the hall. We were treated as fine gentlemen and ladies in Edinburgh. The combination of elegance and courtesy inspired me. I don't think I have ever performed better in an examination. I telephoned mum and dad with joy from Edinburgh to tell of my success, the first time I had ever telephoned Australia from Britain. Dad, being a fellow of the Royal College of Surgeons of Edinburgh was delighted, but mum whilst pleased, correctly reminded me (to my irritation at the time) that I still needed to pass the London membership. I celebrated by buying a hunting MacLean kilt on the Royal Mile, which I still have today.

After my successful visit to Edinburgh I was later to pass the London membership in 1964 at St Bartholomew's Hospital. Little did I know then that Barts was to play such a major role in my future life. My first visit to

Barts Hospital had been in 1962, shortly after my arrival when I visited Jean Borthwick, daughter of Uncle Brian and Auntie Ethel. The Borthwick family gave so much hospitality to me, my sister and my friends at their home in Seaford in 1962-64 and for many years later. On weekend while I was staying in Sussex Jean suggested I might like to Barts. She was medical secretary to Mr John Beattie, obstetrician a gynaecologist at Barts. Her office on the first floor of the west wing of the hospital gave a superb view over the beautiful square and fountain at the heart of the hospital. In December 1963 I also had another Barts contact when I went with friends to see the annual Christmas show by the St Bartholomew's Hospital Students Union Drama society. This was called 'Pot Pourri' consisting of excerpts from the Christmas ward 'shows' for patients. It was held at the Cripplegate Theatre. I was very impressed by the professionalism of the students. I had never seen anything like it in Sydney. It was a very funny and very enjoyable show.

However my happiest early contact with Barts was when I passed the membership examination there. My examiners were Sir Ronald Bodley Scott (a distinguished physician, with special interest in oncology), Dr Cullinan (gastroenterologist) and Dr W.W. Brooks (chest physician). The patients I saw are etched clearly in my memory. Little did I realize that I was destined to become a consultant there eight years later. One of my friends Ten Feizi also failed her first attempt at the membership and she attributed it to Sir Ronald Bodley Scott falling asleep after lunch. She complained to the college but without outcome. Passing or failing the membership overshadowed all our lives. Yet once passed it did not really mean that much, as one had to slog on with training before one had enough experience to be a consultant. Of course like everyone else, I had to plan all my own training to be a physician and a gastroenterology specialist. There was no equivalent to the present day Calman training programme. One could consult and take advice but the decisions taken in relation to one's training were one's own, quite alone. I decided to get some more general medical training before doing gastroenterology. At that time, the Brompton Hospital was considered, like the Hammersmith, to provide great training opportunities and so I applied. Again I had to negotiate the trauma of interview and I was lucky enough to be appointed as a house physician, but best of all to Professor J.G. Scadding. I had already admired him as he did a little teaching at the Hammersmith Course.

The Brompton Hospital was a great contrast to the Hammersmith in many ways but what they did have in common was the pursuit of excellence. The hospital itself was again another architectural triumph for the gothic style of the Victorian era. To be honest the wards were antedeluvial! The hospital building has now been restored and divided into elegant flats. At that time we young doctors lived in genteel poverty. I lived in a small room high up almost in the roof, with a gas fire which gave very weak emissions of heat. The paint was peeling off the walls and the floorboards squeaked. A Canadian friend from London House, E. Barclay Simpson could not believe I could live in such squalor when he visited me, compared to the rooms of London House. Yet every morning a domestic provided us with morning tea at an early morning call. We had a small well-provided doctor's mess, which was kept clean and tidy again by domestics. We met there every evening at about 7 p.m. and then precisely at 7.10 p.m. we were lead by the RMO or the most senior registrar present to walk to the boardroom for dinner. We had a different roast every evening and the RMO would carve the joint. I remember Kevin Connolly particularly relished this task. Most weeks we had a guest evening when we could invite a visitor to join us. My sister Judith and friends from Hammersmith were my guests. Sometimes on such occasions we had a guest lecturer. One such occasion I can remember vividly was when Dr Charles Fletcher from the Hammersmith came to talk about his new television series on medicine he was producing. This was in its way pioneer TV. This evening social activity meant that the junior doctors, i.e. 'the house', bonded together very well and became good friends. As we nearly all were resident and not married we ate in most evenings and this was our home it all seemed to me to be very, very, English in a way which I liked, very much.

The twice-weekly professorial ward rounds with J.G. Scadding were the longest I have ever attended. We started at 2 p.m. and would be lucky to be done by 6 p.m. We however did have a break for afternoon tea when we went to his office in the Institute Building where his secretary poured tea for us from an elegant teapot. The round itself would begin in the ward gathering in a room outside the patient area, where the patient's history, physical findings, and investigations would be presented by the house physician. Then we would go to the patient where the Prof. would chat and usually he would listen to their chest himself. He was doing a special study on sarcoidosis, a chest disease akin to tuberculosis but different, and if the patient had that disorder, not only would he listen to the chest, but in his own meticulous handwriting record his own findings in the patient's notes. It was almost unheard of for consultants to write themselves in the notes at that time. Then perhaps, almost incredibly, considering the time it was taking, we would go back to the side room and carefully examine the patient's chest X-rays. After further discussion we then went back to the patient and the Prof. would give his opinion to the patient and discuss treatment etc. We did not have a huge number of patients but it is clear that this process took a long time, but it was a remarkably thorough process. Other consultants would look at the chest X-ray first and then discuss history etc. and would see the patient once only.

There were some very distinguished research fellows at the Brompton in 1963-64. These included Dr Margaret Turner-Warwick who would later be first woman president of the Royal College of Physicians of London and Dr Jack Pepys (later, Professor) who was a pioneer of the role of allergy in general and respiratory medicine in particular. He introduced me to the whole concept of allergy which years later was to be a major interest. Sadly he was often called 'Mad Jack Pepys' by some of the junior doctors at the Brompton, because of his enthusiasm for allergy. At that time allergy was often felt to be fringe medicine and also Jack was quite un-English in his passionately expressed enthusiasm for his subject. Years later when I had settled in London, I met him again at a British Society of Allergy and Immunology (BSACI) meeting at Barts. Jack was very hospitable and invited Liz and me to his home. This was the first of many occasions. We also became friends with his artist wife Rhoda and artist Daughter Sandra. We have several of Sandra's beautiful oil paintings at home including a view of Jerusalem from the Mount of Olives, at dawn.

Although I was not to be a chest physician, the time at the Brompton widened my horizons. I saw a good deal of tuberculosis and learnt about the modern applied physiology techniques for investigating respiratory function. By the end of my time there I was tired of being a house physician with all the associated menial tasks of history taking, ordering tests etc. Having been inspired by the Hammersmith I began to explore research opportunities for gastroenterology in Sydney.

Whilst I was at the Brompton a terrible international event occurred, the assassination of President John Kennedy in Dallas, Texas. We heard the sad news just as we were about to go to dinner. After dinner as I did my routine evening ward round I found many patients very upset by his death, some even in tears. There was even talk of 'our president'. Clearly John Kennedy had inspired a whole generation with his charisma and hope. I attended the memorial service in St Paul's Cathedral. It was a very emotional occasion with superb music in the presence of the great and the good of the nation, plus hundreds of ordinary people.

The social highlight of my time at the Brompton was the Christmas show of 1963. The junior doctors staged a show for patients, the consultants and their families, nursing staff etc. on Christmas afternoon. All the house doctors had been earlier in their own ward, carving the turkey for their patients, Christmas dinner, an age-old Brompton tradition. The show itself was great fun. My present family can hardly believe it, but I was cast in the role of one of the Beatles (pop heroes of the hour), actually Paul McCartney, wearing an appropriate wig. We belted out 'She loves you, yea, yea, yea' while pretending to play a guitar. Other acts had a big satirical aspect with sometimes snide comments concerning various doctors, senior and junior. There was lots of laughter and great fun was had by all.

On the medical side my closest friends were Ilfra Pink, who like me came from the Hammersmith and David Wright, and on the surgical side John Herman Taylor, later to be Professor of Surgery at St George's Hospital. Many years in the future we would share a major interest in research in Crohn's disease and have quite a lot of interaction. We physicians quite often had to cover surgery at nights. Mr Brock, later Lord Brock, was a distinguished surgeon on the staff who had Randolph Churchill as his patient. His father Winston, the former great Prime Minister, came to visit but sadly I failed to glimpse him. However the night before Randolph's operation he refused to take his pre-medication and insisted Mr Brock be rung. Mr Brock duly was. To our amazement, the usually formidable surgeon agreed it was not necessary to take the pre-medication! At the Brompton, Brock was famous in the operating theatre for two things, playing classical music whilst operating and rapping the knuckles of junior doctors with the back of his scalpel, when their operating technique displeased him. Another thoracic surgeon at that time was Mr Barrett who has become a famous name because of the premalignant 'Barrett's ulcer' in the oesophagus, which he was the first to describe. He was a tall, rather quiet, unassuming man and would have been surprised by his fame. They were great days at the Brompton and I was very sorry to leave when the day came. I have been delighted by the occasional reunions of 'the year of 63' which Kevin Connolly has arranged in subsequent years.

Whilst I was at the Brompton, for the first time I thought seriously of staying in Britain, although I felt it probably better to go home first. I discussed this with my parents and dad's letter to me of 29/4/64 makes interesting reading:

> I am certain you are doing the right thing by returning home in July. Some form of Health Service will certainly come in Australia, it is just a question as to when it will arrive. I trust it will not be as bad as the English system which is strongly opposed by the profession, but come it will in some form. You must realize that many doctors are leaving GB annually and well qualified men find it difficult to find appointments. I can understand your reluctance to leave GB only too well from personal experience, but in this day and age your professional future lies in this country.

I did decide to return to Sydney and after my time at the Brompton I had planned to do some locum general practice posts in England and Scotland to enlarge my wider experience of life. However I had unexpectedly quickly secured a research fellowship post in gastroenterology, back at Prince Alfred Hospital. The director, Alan Skyring wanted me back as soon as possible so I had to return earlier than planned. Still I was to be away from Australia for just on two years.

Apart from the professional training I had received, my two years in London was a memorable time for travel both in the British Isles and abroad. With David Wollman I had an easy but much enjoyed climb up Mount Snowdon, and we saw something of the beauties of the north of Wales. I travelled to the Republic of Ireland with my sister on a car trip around, its beautiful and very quiet countryside. I also returned to Scotland to visit an old friend from Sydney, Les Rae and his family. Whilst in London I had three continental trips, first I went on a car trip with two American friends Ed Daly and Bob Hunter via Paris to Rome during my first winter in the Northern Hemisphere. Then I had a wonderful two week trip to Greece, to Athens and the Pelopponese (first of many, many visits) after passing the Edinburgh membership, and a two-week skiing trip to Kitzbuehel in Austria with David Read during my second winter in the northern hemisphere.

The most notable trip of all was to the Holy Land with Orientours at the end of my time in England, as part of the Diocesan Pilgrimage of the Diocese of Gloucester. This was led by that remarkable man Bishop Basil Guy of Gloucester. We spent one week in Israel followed by one week in Jordan from 7-22 May 1964, crossing from Israel to Jordan in Jerusalem via the Mandelbaum Gate in that divided city. My old friend from Sydney, John Burgess from Prince Alfred, joined me on his way to further training in America. We were the only Australians but our fellow pilgrims from Gloucester gave us a very warm welcome. We made a number of life-long friendships including the Bishop and Mrs Guy and Judith Meath-Baker. He was the first anglo-catholic that I had met.

Little did I realize then that I was to visit the Holy Land again in the future on two further occasions, but this first was by far the most memorable and exciting. The second was to be in March 1987 to attend a medical conference on immunology and the gastrointestinal tract as the guest of Dr Serem Freier and the last was in May 1995 for the annual meeting of the European Society of Paediatric Gastroenterology and Nutrition (ESPGAN).

In 1964 we spent our first week in Israel with the highlights being visits to the Sea of Galilee, Nazareth and the surrounding countryside. We ended up in west Jerusalem and after staying overnight at the impressive YMCA building, were taken to the Mandelbaum Gate which was like a great hanger shed with a corrugated iron roof. At that time this was the only link between Israeli western Jerusalem and Jordanian eastern Jerusalem. All trace of the building has now been obliterated by the Israelis. In 1964 very few people could make this direct crossing. Christian pilgrims were one such group who could do so and our Gloucester party was in that category.

We then passed through to a no man's land where we waited somewhat forlornly in the blazing sun with our luggage. Armed Israeli and Jordanian soldiers from each side were very much in evidence at either end of no man's land. It was quite an unnerving experience. After some time of waiting in the sun several Jordanians appeared. Their chief concern was to ensure the removal of any Israeli or Hebrew labels or badges on our luggage. Then we were most cordially welcomed to Jordan. Once in our coach we rapidly sped away to our modern hotel on the Mount of Olives with superb views over the old city. Next morning we awoke to look out upon the glorious prospect of the old walled city of Jerusalem seen from the east over the Vale of Kedron. The wonder of this view lives up to all expectations with the golden Dome of the Rock standing on the old temple site and rising above the city wall. This is one of the great sights of the world. Sandra Pepys some years later wonderfully captured this view in oils and it graces our sitting room mantelpiece at home.

We made our first entry to the Holy City by walking down from the Mount of Olives and entering through the Lion's Gate. Just as the pilgrims of old, our first goal was the Church of the Holy Sepulchre, which enshrines both the site of the resurrection of Jesus Christ as well as the crucifixion of Our Lord. For many visitors, especially those brought up in the protestant tradition, the church and its occupants may be, at least at first, a great disappointment. This was true at first for me and my party in 1964. At that time the general dilapidated appearance of the church and the history of conflict between the churches to prevent restoration was responsible for this. The church was still propped up and shored up with supports of steel and wood both inside and out. This had been erected by the British Mandate Government in the 1930s to prevent the church collapsing. In fact the three principal churches which share the church, the Latin (Roman Catholic), Orthodox and Armenian agreed in 1962 on a major reconstruction and restoration programme combined with archeological excavation. So when I returned in 1987 the church had been substantially restored and the scaffolding largely gone. By 1995 all was complete, except for the resurrection shrine itself still encased in steel girders. A new harmony between the churches in this ecumenical age had at last emerged.

However even in 1964 after I had been in the church for a time I became aware of its very strange mysterious atmosphere. This feeling of mystery is very much a feature of the eastern churches. It can look tawdry and superstitious but with another eye it can tell us something of the mysteries of God. When I first saw the edicule, the shrine covering the reputed site of the tomb of Christ in 1964, the dark and gloomy scene with enormous unlit candlesticks was illuminated by a shaft of sunlight from the centre of the Dome above. This revealed a strange jumble of lamps in front of the small door opening into the Chapel of Angels, the antechamber to the tomb itself. Both this chapel and the tomb itself are very small and can at most only comfortably hold two or three people. To my surprise my heart began to beat quite fast as I went into the shrine of the Holy Sepulchre and saw the plain marble slab marking the sarcophagus itself. The prayers of the countless faithful who had been to this spot over the centuries, and others who had died in a vain effort to reach this spot over these centuries, coupled with the quiet peace, after the noise and tumult of the church itself, all had their effect on me. However the words 'He is not here He is risen' St Luke 24.6, came very much to my mind as I left the shrine. There is no space to record so much else of the remarkable two weeks I spent in the Holy Land but I have enduring memories, which will last me for all my life.

This unforgettable journey was quickly followed by a car trip with John Burgess as a prelude to my departure from England. We began by driving to the west country and a highlight was our visit to Gloucester and its ancient cathedral. John and I were privileged to stay with the Bishop and his family. We both have remained 'Friends of Gloucester Cathedral' ever since. We then drove on to Scotland, first to the lowlands and Glasgow once more. There I was able to visit the streets and houses where my Grandfather John Walker-Smith had lived and practised in the nineteenth century. I visited the addresses where he practised, 10 and 26 Pollak Street, the latter was still the sire of a doctor's practice in 1964. The street was still very typical of nineteenth century Glasgow with fine solidly built stone tenements lining a broad street. There were two stone churches at either end of the street. I was in the future to return in February 1984 and to find the scene quite transformed. I published my emotional response to this in a short piece published in the Journal of the Royal College of Physicians of Edinburgh, called '*Glasgow Revisited*'.

Quoting in part from this account;

> I crossed the Clyde via the King George V bridge and I looked down the river towards the vicinity of Pollak Street. With some apprehension I saw that there

> was now a massive motorway bridge crossing the river in that general direction. With quickening steps I walked down Kingston Street and on into Paisley Road. My heart sank as I hurried along. It was soon clear that nothing whatsoever of the old community remained. All had been destroyed partly for urban redevelopment and partly for the motorway. Pollak Street no longer existed. A modern low profile factory occupied the site. All that could be seen of the past was on the other side of Paisley Road. Here stood gauntly and alone the imposing edifice of the lending library built by Victorian worthies at the end of the nineteenth century, but it had become a refuge for male dropouts of the city. The words of the old hymn 'Change and decay in all around I see' came to mind as I walked sadly down Paisley Road, back to Glasgow Central Station. There I took a taxi which sped me via the M8 motorway over the site of Pollak Street reaching Glasgow Airport, where I took the Glasgow shuttle back to London in just over an hour! No doubt it is very convenient for the citizens of Glasgow to be able to reach their airport so quickly and to travel from one side of their city to the other in a matter of minutes. No doubt it is good that the city fathers have seen fit to give the old lending library to Talbot House so that the casualties of the late twentieth century may find some refuge there. No doubt my grandfather as an elder of the Kirk would have approved this Good Samaritan deed. Yet what of the two churches, the many houses, the pubs, the shops, a whole community that has now gone. No doubt those living in Pollak Street before re-development have been moved to one of the great tower blocks disfiguring the Glasgow cityscape. Are they happier there? Is baby battering or drunkenness any the less? I have the churches been replaced or perhaps they are not needed now because of the drift away from faith? My grandfather left Pollak Street just 100 years ago to seek for a better lift 'down-under' for himself as a widower and for his young family. He did find success, happiness and a better life. I wonder if the destruction of the community around Pollak Street has brought happiness to those who have been redeveloped.

To return to my 1964 trip, John and I drove on into the Highlands, with a return visit for me to the Isle of Mull, finally finishing our Scottish trip in Edinburgh. Then we drove down through eastern England with notable stops in York for its Minster and Lincoln for its cathedral.

After this trip the time had sadly come for me to leave England for home, this time by air, but first I was fortunate enough to have a further continental trip by car with my friend John Burgess once more, joined by my friends from London House, George Soutter and Don Wood. We drove again to Paris and on through the south of France to Turin, Milan, Verona and the wondrous Byzantine beauties of Venice and Ravenna. I left my friends after a few memorable days in Rome, highlights being visits to the Capitoline Hill and the ancient Forum. This was a second time for that wonderful city I have visited so many times since. From Rome I flew back with Qantas to Sydney.

What an extraordinary two years I had had in Britain, without doubt the most exciting and challenging two years of my life to date. Little did I realize then, that a seed had been planted, which led ultimately to my decision to return to settle permanently in the land of my ancestors. However I returned home to Sydney with great hopes to use effectively, the knowledge and experience I had acquired in London.

CHAPTER SEVEN

Gastroenterology Trainee in Sydney

RETURNING TO SYDNEY was a shock in many ways. At the airport I was astonished how much older mum and dad looked. On return to Prince Alfred, I was dismayed to find that the orientation of many staff members was now towards the United States and away from the UK. The USA was perceived to be far more dynamic than the United Kingdom, in the realm of medicine and indeed in every way. The United States was seen as the country of the future with which Australia should develop closer and closer links. The British Government had signalled its desire to be rid of the Empire and Commonwealth by seeking entry into the European Common Market.

I was now a research fellow in gastroenterology, in the A.W. Morrow Department of Gastroenterology named after Sir William Morrow. He had founded the unit in 1948, the first gastroenterology department in Australia. As mentioned earlier, I had been his house physician in 1960, my first resident post. Sir William had been very kind to me then and I had heard later that he had put in a good word for me with my chief at the Hammersmith Hospital, Chris Booth. He was a bespectacled balding man with white hair and pink cheeks, giving him an almost cherubic face. He had a gentle and courteous manner but carried an aura of authority. Although he had retired from the public hospital he was still in active private practice when I arrived in 1964. Sir William only came regularly to the department to do his early morning private endoscopy list, apart from occasional attendance at the weekly clinical meeting. My offer to assist him with the endoscopy list was generously accepted. I felt honoured to be able to assist the great man.

Dr Alan Skyring was the then director of the department (a salaried staff appointment) and was responsible for my research programme overall. Dr Steve Mistilis was the senior research fellow with whom in practice I chiefly worked.

Dr Stan Goulston was the senior honorary associated with the department assisted by Dr Bob Packard. This was a time of transition, honoraries were gradually changing to sessional salaried visiting staff positions and full time salaried staff positions were being created. In addition to the medical staff there was a nurse specialist and also several laboratory staff, including Dorothy Harrison a biochemist and Mrs Perrett a cytologist (who was English, thankfully!).

For me it was a quite depressing time. I missed London a great deal. My time there had been the happiest time in my professional life. Alan and Steve were among the most enthusiastic advocates of the American line. I found this really depressing. Alan was always going on about this issue over morning coffee, lunch etc. I had some comfort by chatting to Mrs Perrett who had an office adjacent to mine. Steve was an Australian of Greek origin who had little time for Prince Alfred's royal history and our links with Britain. He had been trained in America and was an aggressive advocate of the American way of doing things. Nevertheless, I did find it to be really exciting to be engaged in fulltime research with him, for the first time. The penalty I paid for this was a rather low salary. There was no parity at that time between hospital and research salaries. I was able to cope, as I had decided to return home to live with my parents. This was not a brilliant idea. In fact the whole return to Sydney felt a bit like turning the clock back. My mother hoped I 'had got England out of my system and would now settle down'. This was not to be.

I was infuriated to find when I was back at RPAH that I would need to pass the membership of the Royal Australasian College of Physicians (MRACP) examination. The term Australasian equates to Australia plus New Zealand. The London and Edinburgh exams were not enough! This information was told to me in private discreet conversations. Whilst possessing the membership of the London and Edinburgh colleges would be adequate for future consultant positions, I would not be able to attend medical meetings of the Royal Australasian College, so I was told. I was told of an Australian consultant at North Shore Hospital who although invited to give a lecture at a RACP meeting had to wait outside the lecture theatre beforehand and could not stay afterwards, because he 'only' had the London membership! I was told that I would be 'outside the club'. At first I resisted this pressure. I did not want to be distracted from my new exciting life in research. I had admired my father's example in relation to the surgical college. He was a Fellow of the Royal College of Surgeons (FRCS) of Edinburgh, having successfully passed the examination. He was enormously proud of his Edinburgh fellowship. In the 1930s he was offered a foundation fellowship of the newly created Royal Australasian College of Surgeons. He refused. In the 1950s he was advised he should sit the exam, as it might become mandatory for surgical practice to have the local college qualification. He was outraged and refused. Finally he was offered the FRACS as an honour. Consistently he refused. He regarded his possession of the fellowship of the Royal College of Surgeons of Edinburgh as the greatest surgical qualification he could ever possess. I admired this stand against the Australian surgical establishment. In the 1960s both the surgical and medical establishments in the respective Australasian Royal Colleges were becoming increasingly chauvinistic. To me this was a very ugly and unwelcome aspect of Australian nationalism, which was beginning to assert itself. However I was increasingly advised on all sides, including Sir William himself, that I should sit the local exam. With ill grace, I went to Melbourne, and passed the examination. Incidentally during the exam, I was shown the first case of leprosy I had ever seen, which I eventually diagnosed with some difficulty. The only positive note of my Melbourne trip was that I met Peter Phelan, another paediatric specialist in the making, who also passed the exam. He was to be a very distinguished pioneer of paediatric respiratory medicine. In fact he was to report in the future, indeed twenty years later, that the survival of patients with cystic fibrosis was significantly better in Victoria, Australia than in England and Wales. The major reason for this was because the care of the cystic fibrosis patients in Australia occurred in specialist centres unlike the UK in the 1970s.

So in 1964, I ended up with three memberships of Royal Colleges, when I had only planned one!

My research in the A.W Morrow Unit had two aspects. First I was to develop a radioisotope technique using intravenous chromic chloride to assess protein loss into the bowel in patients with a clinical syndrome known as protein losing enteropathy, supervised by Alan. This went quite well and resulted in a paper published in the international gastroenterology journal *Gut*. This was fine and the paper is still occasionally cited. Less happy was the second aspect, namely assisting Steve Mistilis in his laboratory research. This I need to explain. He was particularly interested in the liver and its pathology. Intra-hepatic pericholangitis (inflammation inside the liver around the bile ducts) was his special interest. This could complicate ulcerative colitis, one of the two main forms of chronic inflammatory bowel disease, the other being Crohn's disease. It was suggested that this pericholangitis could result from bacterial infection from the gut via the portal vein which drains to the liver. If this were true then it could be treated with an antibiotic such as tetracycline. To test this idea a rat model was developed, whereby I would inject bacteria into the portal vein displayed operatively, after opening the abdomen of an anaesthetized rat. However we tried this and it did not work until a toxic chemical, carbon tetrachloride, had first been injected several times into the rat's abdominal cavity to damage its liver. This meant that the rat's liver had to be damaged before pericholangitis could develop after the injection of bacteria. The rats had to be killed at the end of the experiment. Steve demonstrated the standard way of killing, which was basically breaking their neck swiftly, presumably with minimal pain. I found myself quite unable to do this and so the rats had to be killed by excess anaesthetic agent. This complicated the interpretation of the pathology results in the rat's liver, as the anaesthetic per se could damage the liver theoretically. I was made to feel a bit of a chicken because of my refusal to kill the rats in the standard way. This work was never published but I decided I would never again do laboratory animal work, once I left Prince Alfred. I did not have the stomach for it. I have never done animal work since. Whether others felt the same as me at the time is hard to know. It was a rather delicate matter to discuss. Steve I found an awkward colleague. He had been trained in research in America and his whole approach grated with me. He was forever criticizing clinicians for lack of knowledge and harassed our hard working Thai registrar who was trying his best to do both clinical and research work.

Later Bob Middleton joined the department as registrar. He was an outstanding and very cheerful colleague with an outgoing manner. He taught me the technique of liver biopsy and I became quite skilled in this. In an ad hoc and personally initiated way I was able to get some training in upper endoscopy with the rigid instruments in use at that time from colleagues in the department. There was no colonoscopy available (examining entire colon) but we had a sigmoidoscopy table and I was able to learn the technique of sigmoidoscopy (looking into lower part of the colon, rectum and sigmoid) with biopsy (to provide tissue for diagnostic histological analysis), largely unsupervised. There was no proper training programme either in the research itself or in the clinical field. It was a kind of apprenticeship for me.

At that time I was interested in the recent description of Crohn's colitis especially after the visit of the famous pathologist Dr Basil Morson from St Mark's Hospital in London. Little did I realize that 21 years in the future, I was to call upon his help in the unravelling the pathology of a group of children at Queen Elizabeth Hospital for Children, who had severe entero-colitis of an unusual type. A publication with him followed in 1986. As Crohn's disease is a disorder which will feature much in this autobiography, I should mention here that this is a type of chronic inflammation of the wall of the gastrointestinal tract from the mouth to the anus, first describe in Mt Sinai Hospital, New York by Dr Burrill Crohn and his colleagues. Abdominal pain and chronic diarrhoea are major symptoms, the latter being bloody when there is colitis present. Ulcerative colitis is the other major disorder included in the term chronic inflammatory bowel disease. In that disorder the inflammation is confined to the mucosa of the large bowel or colon. At the time of his visit to Prince Alfred, Morson had recently drawn attention to the fact that colitis could occur in patients with Crohn's disease as well as in those with ulcerative colitis, in an important and influential paper. After his visit I discovered a number of patients with classical X-ray features of Crohn's colitis on barium study, which had been incorrectly labelled as ulcerative colitis. I presented these to a clinical meeting after a lot of hard detective work. I was disappointed after I left the department that a clinic-pathological study of Crohn's colitis was published from the department without mention of me although I had begun the work and initiated the collection of cases. 'C'est la vie!'

I was also very involved with a clinical case of an unfortunate woman who had had most of her small intestine removed by Dr Norman Wyndham (honorary surgeon and embryology lecturer in Med II, mentioned earlier) following infarction of the gut (death of tissue due to loss of blood supply). The great clinical issue for her was, did she have enough small intestine left to survive? The related research issue concerned what was the minimal amount of small intestine necessary for survival in adult humans. The small intestine is the vital organ of the body required for absorption of nutrients from food. Total removal of the small bowel is not compatible with survival, although nowadays small intestinal transplantation from a donor is possible. It should be mentioned that the terms bowel and intestine are inter-changeable but bowel tends to be a more lay term and intestine the term used by pathologists. In the 1960s the technique of giving all nutritional requirements by veins was still being developed and was not available to us. This became known as intravenous parental nutrition but the definitive paper on this approach had yet to be published. This happened four years later in a report from the USA by Wilmore and Dudrick concerning an infant. For children especially, who were still growing, but also for adults, parenteral nutrition was to be a successful means of artificial nutrition, keeping the patient who had had massive small intestinal resection both alive and also well nourished, until adaption of the remaining small gut did occur. This process of adaption took time, usually many months. In fact parenteral nutrition was an immense advance which saved the lives of many patients, especially children. However we were able to keep our patient alive without this specific technique and two publications with Dr Wyndham in the *Medical Journal of Australia* resulted from our clinical studies in 1966. These were the first papers where I had been first author, another landmark in my career.

I also did some work with Dorothy Harrison concerning the small bowel morphology (structure) of rat small gut (gut is another alternative term to intestine) when viewed with the dissecting or stereo-microscope from specimens obtained from the animals studied with Steve Mistilis. The surface of the gut was denuded of its surface epithelium by a special technique and the three dimensional arrangements of the remaining cores of the villi could be seen. It was apparent that mature rats had broad ridge-like villi. This was well known, but what was interesting was that newborn rats before they were fed had finger-like villi, i.e. normal feeding had changed the structure of the villi from fingers to ridges. Gordon Nicholson from New Zealand who was visiting the department drew my attention to a technique of examining human gut at post-mortem to observe this three dimensional appearance of the villous cores, once the epilthelium had sloughed off at death. These cores minus surface epithelium could be visualized by staining them with Indian ink and examining with a dissecting microscope. Brian Cremer at St Thomas's Hospital in London had described a similar technique. Three years later, I applied this technique to children as the basis of my MD Thesis at the RAHC. One important question I asked in my thesis which followed on this earlier work was did something occur after birth in the human small intestine, when normal feeding occurs, which is similar to the changes that occurred in the rat?

I also made some collaborative observations with my old friend Bob Dick who was then a registrar in radiology, using the gastrocamera. This was a precursor of the modern flexible endoscope. In the future, the development of fibreoptic endoscopy, with all its facility for photography, and video but above all its ability to examine the entire colon and even the terminal ileum (ileo-colonoscopy), would by the early seventies transform gastroenterological practice in children and adults. Bob subsequently also went to England for further training. At my suggestion, Uncle Brian and Auntie Ethel Borthwick in Seaford invited him to visit them. Bob in due course married Diana, daughter of their next-door neighbour, and settled permanently in London. He became a consultant radiologist at the Royal Free Hospital. We became colleagues there once more, when I transferred in 1995. I made a number of new friends from colleagues in the hospital, especially Dick Fox and Don Cameron, whilst renewing old ones like John Burgess and John Turtle. Within the department, I made a new friendship with Owen Harris a visiting research fellow from Brisbane, who became a long-term friend, and also I became very good friends with Fung Wye Poh from Singapore. In 1969 my wife, Liz and

I were to stay with him and his family in Singapore at the end of our long honeymoon. This proved to be the first of many trips to Singapore over the next thirty years. I also renewed old friendship with Kerry Goulston who also became a fellow. He was nephew of Stan and his father was a surgeon at Royal North Shore. Kerry was destined to be Professor of Gastroenterology there and was honoured in 2002, by having the teaching facilities at Royal North Shore named after him. The Goulstons are one of a number of Sydney medical families like the MacDonalds, Blackburns and my own.

I was well on the way to planning my future career as a gastroenterologist for adults, but I did feel uncertain whether this was my true vocation. Prince Alfred itself, on my return made me uneasy. There was an unpleasant spirit of destructive competition, known locally as 'acemanship'. I was not really happy. Things had changed. The perpetual looking to America as well as a spirit of parochialism irritated me after the wonderful internationalism of medical London. Then suddenly a remarkable thing happened. My old friend John Yu asked me to give a lecture at the Children's Hospital. This was the beginning of a dialogue. As I have made clear earlier, from my student days and my six months at the Royal Alexandra-Hospital for Children, I had enjoyed working with children. Within paediatrics there was an important group of children with gastroenterological disorders. Many of these children could be treated effectively with diets. It was in general an optimistic field and furthermore it seemed particularly important to properly diagnose and treat children with gastroenterological diseases as they had so many years of life ahead of them. Failure to make accurate diagnosis and institute effective therapy could condemn them to chronic ill health over many years. Following my lecture at RAHC, John had encouraged me to consider doing gastroenterology in children and developing this specialty in Sydney. Charlotte Anderson had begun to develop paediatric gastroenterology in Melbourne, but there had been no comparable development in Sydney. John was then a medical officer in the Institute of Child Health having returned from Hammersmith Hospital. I had kept in touch with him and other paediatric colleagues, since I had left the 'kids' hospital in 1962, as I mentioned earlier.

As I looked into the subject in more detail I soon saw the huge potential for gastroenterology in children. I also remembered how happy I had been in the past working with children at RAHC. I much preferred working with children and usually young parents than with middle-aged and elderly patients.I discussed the idea with Professor Tom Stapleton. He was enthusiastic and encouraging. In October 1965 he very quickly offered me the post of Professorial Registrar beginning in January 1966. It did not take much further reflection on my part to accept enthusiastically.

In November I attended in Melbourne an International Meeting on Gastroenterology in Children organized by Charlotte Anderson. The meeting I found inspirational, especially Professor Andrea Prader from Zurich, who was visiting a lecturer speaking on disaccharide intolerance. I was to write to him the following year concerning a possible fellowship in Zurich for training in paediatric gastroenterology. My experience at the Melbourne meeting consolodated my decision to change my career goals so dramatically.

This change from adult medicine was a vast change in direction for me, because I really had to start a fresh. It was a completely new beginning, as I required training in general paediatrics as well as learning about paediatric gastroenterology. I had only six months of previous paediatric experience in 1962, as a JRMO.

Colleagues at Prince Alfred said they were sad I was leaving adult medicine. Sir William Morrow really meant it. They invited me to keep in touch and possibly plan future research collaboration together. I did in fact collaborate with Dorothy Harrison for a year or so, but there was no real enthusiasm from my adult medical colleagues. In the end, to my surprise, I was quite glad to finally leave my former alma mater, the Royal Prince Alfred Hospital. Yet I was also very grateful for all that I had learnt in that great institution. I remain proud to this day to have been a Prince Alfred man.

CHAPTER EIGHT

Paediatric Trainee in Sydney and Zurich

I AM SOMEWHAT EMBARRASSED to admit that the only formal training I ever had in paediatrics at a registrar/fellow grade was in 1966 in Sydney as a registrar, and in 1967 in Zurich as a fellow.

I was pleased to be back in January 1966 at the Royal Alexandra Hospital for children. It was almost four years since I was last there, but must of the honoraries and Institute staff were the same. I also knew many of the registrars. So it was to some extent like a homecoming. I had a warm welcome.

I was based in the Professorial Unit, whose ward was Lower Todman adjacent to the then fearfully inadequate office and seminar room facilities of the Institute of Child Health. Rather strangely the Institute was funded by the Commonwealth Government, i.e. it was a Commonwealth Health Department, whereas the hospital itself was funded by the NSW or State Health Department, reflecting Australia's federal system of government. Furthermore although a Professor of the University of Sydney headed the Institute of Child Health, the University did not fund his post or the Institute.

Professor Tom Stapleton had been appointed in 1960 to the chair. At the time of his appointment he was Assistant Director of the Paediatric Unit at St Mary's Hospital, London. In Sydney he was appointed as the head of a University teaching unit, funded directly from the Commonwealth Department of Health located in poor facilities I have already mentioned at the Royal Alexandra Hospital for Children. From the first he did his best to rectify this. Indeed to his great credit, he succeeded in achieving a completely new building for the Institute of Child Health. This was being built in 1966 when I returned to RAHC, and was completed in 1967. This was a great boost for the Institute and offered prospects of an exciting future. Professor Stapleton was an honorary physician to the hospital, but in no way was head of paediatric medicine. He thus had a complicated situation to deal with. From his perspective, it was further complicated as his predecessor Sir

Lorimer Dods continued as a chairman of the Children's Medical Research Foundation (CMRF) for many years. I myself continued to have a very friendly relationship with Lorimer whom I had known from student days. Dad and he had been junior doctors together at the Royal Newcastle Hospital (NSW) in the 1930s. Lorimer had an office in the CMRF building, which contained a small bust of Sir James Spence, a great pioneer of paediatrics in England. He had been a great inspiration and role model for Lorimer. Spence had created the first Institute of Child Health in the United Kingdom at Newcastle-upon-Tyne. Lorimer Dods had founded the CMRF in 1958 together with the then general superintendent of the hospital, John Fulton.

Tom Stapleton was a strong advocate of child psychiatry and Associate Professor Julian Katz had been appointed by him within the Institute. I was to find Julian an immensely helpful colleague and he was able to open my mind to the importance of child psychiatry in day-to-day childcare. He pointed out that few areas involving mother and baby are more loaded with emotional content than the function of the gastrointestinal tract as suggested by the words emotion and motion (faeces). Tom had also appointed Dr Graham Mortimer from New Zealand as student supervisor with honorary physician status in the hospital. He was a very good clinician. There was also Dr Bryan Dowd who was a medical officer in the Institute and also an honorary physician. It was Stapleton, Mortimer and Dowd who provided routine day time consultant cover-for the professorial ward and conducted ward rounds. During my time, Tom Stapleton did not cover at nights or during the weekend, this responsibility was divided between Graham and Bryan. Tom was in fact often away overseas, and then Bryan Dowd usually covered the ward and also acted as Head of the Institute. Tom was exceptionally fortunate to have such a loyal and reliable colleague as Bryan. Tom was a man with many international interests. He was particularly interested in developing communities and communist China. He also at that time was Secretary General of the International-Paediatric Association (1965-74). So he was away a great deal. He particularly relished travelling to places such, as communist China which were anathema to conservatively minded Australians. Curiously he had been appointed at least in part to nostalgically maintain the traditional links with British medicine. The fact that he was militantly opposed to the whole conception of the British Empire, had sympathy with communist countries and was a political radical, therefore caused some lifted eyebrows amongst those who had originally backed his appointment. There was much sadness that he and Lorimer Dods appeared to have fallen out. However his great achievement was to stimulate interest amongst medical students and young doctors in south-east Asia, long before most Australians saw the need. He developed close paediatric links with Indonesia and arranged for two research fellows from that country to work with me, which led some years later to my visiting Indonesia. From my perspective, his recognition of the future importance of specialization within paediatrics was very helpful and supportive.

Graham Mortimer was a very active young paediatrician who was later to have a distinguished professorial career ahead of him in New Zealand. John Yu was also a medical officer in 1966 and was tasked to design and fit out the laboratories in the new Institute Building. He later was to become staff physician and then general superintendent of the hospital (chief executive officer). He had a special interest in the rare metabolic disorder phenylketonuria, which could be effectively treated, to prevent severe mental handicap, by a very demanding low protein diet, if diagnosed early enough by screening in infancy. In the United Kingdom newborn babies are now universally screened for this disorder. John also contributed to the clinical service. There were also two part-time medical officers, who had been in the Institute from the time of Lorimer Dods. First there was Dr John MacDonald, with a special interest in urinary tract infection. He came from a distinguished Sydney medical clan, his brother Geoff had been a student supervisor at Prince Alfred when I started as a student and their father, the physician Dr C.G. MacDonald, was to become Chancellor of the University of Sydney in due course. Then there was Dr Helen Walsh, who had a special interest in rheumatic fever with Bryan Dowd. Her husband, Bob Walsh, was a distinguished-academic, and at the rival University of NSW. He had initially made his reputation in the NSW Blood Transfusion Service. Helen and Bob were remarkably hospitable people and I had many happy social occasions at their home. Helen was also a very valuable confidante for me. So we had a father heterogeneous group of people. Ward rounds and institute meetings could be lively, very interesting sometimes highly contentious and even entertaining on occasion.

It is strange to recall, at that time, how many child in-patients there were with rheumatic fever this very unpleasant illness which could cause permanent damage to the heart valves has now almost disappeared in developed communities. At that time there were a number of children who had severe attacks with evidence of heart damage. They were admitted to lower Todman ward rather than to the cardiology department, because of the special interest of Bryan Dowd and Helen Walsh in rheumatic fever. In fact cardiology was the first organ based paediatric specialty to be developed at the hospital, but the work largely centred upon congenital heart disease. We also had a number of children with acute leukaemia admitted as inpatients to Lower Todman, although again there was also a growing interest in the speciality of paediatric oncology by another physician, Dr Arnold Tink.

For me, my first task during the year was to enlarge my experience as a registrar in general paediatrics, and especially of neonates, about which I knew very little. John Yu was a great help, as he had had special training in neonatology at the Hammersmith Hospital. The problem was that RAHC, not being a maternity hospital, had no deliveries on site and so no normal newborn babies. As a result I had no training in normal neonates, only sick ones. My first experience of the routine examination of normal neonates was to be years later as a consultant at Barts.

My second task was to begin to develop a gastroenterology service and research programme. This was quite a difficult undertaking as I was only a registrar and most children with gastroenterological problems were admitted to other firms, i.e. under the care of honoraries. As I did not have honorary status I had to use all my powers of diplomacy with both senior and junior colleagues.

In fact my core activity in the development of paediatric gastroenterology in 1966 was to develop a paediatric small bowel biopsy service. As I mentioned earlier I had been trained in the technique of Crosby capsule biopsy of the small intestinal mucosa in adults at Hammersmith Hospital and I had continued with this technique at Prince Alfred. It had become clear that the capsule needed to be modified for children for safety reasons, using a smaller hole in the side of the capsule (2.5 to 3mm). In fact most unfortunately at the children's hospital, before I was appointed as professorial registrar, three children had had their small intestine perforated (i.e hole punched right through the bowel wall) when non-trained staff used the adult capsule with the larger port hole to biopsy children. So hardly surprisingly there was some resistance especially amongst the senior staff, against this technique. I had to sell both its value and safety for children using a paediatric capsule (it is in fact remarkably safe). The principal reason to biopsy children was to make the diagnosis of coeliac disease, a life-long state of gluten intolerance, as discussed earlier. I took the innovative view that there were other causes of small intestinal mucosal damage, especially gastroenteritis, where diagnostic information might be obtained. I was already familiar with the fact that some children had prolonged diarrhoea after gastroenteritis. I was also aware of the research studies on sugar malabsorption, especially in Melbourne and Zurich. Small intestinal biopsies had had the enzymes which split the sugars, the disaccharidases, measured in a special way known as 'assayed'. This had first been done by Dr Weijers group in Utrecht in the Netherlands in 1961. A sugar with one molecule is called a monosaccharide. The classical example is glucose. The best known examples of disaccharides (two sugars) are lactose, the carbohydrate of breast and cow's milk and sucrose, conventional 'sugar'. The enzyme splitter of lactose is called lactase and of sucrose, sucrase. Both are present in the surface epithelial cells of the normal small intestinal mucosa if lactase is deficient or even absent lactose malabsorption and lactose intolerance causing severe diarrhoea, requiring elimination of lactose from the diet, may result. Most often lactose intolerance in infants is temporary, but in adult life, a very common genetically determined fall in lactase levels is permanent. Dorothy Harrison had established the technique of lactase, sucrase and maltase assay on small intestinal mucosal samples obtain on biopsy, at Prince Alfred. So I decided my first clinical research programme would be to do an analysis of the role of small intestinal biopsy at RAHC (in modern terms, an audit) and to not only assess the structure of the mucosa three dimensionally with the dissecting microscope and light microscope but to perform disaccharidase assay in each specimen, with Dorothy's help. We worked hard and I presented a paper (for both of us), entitled 'Small bowel biopsy in children' at the Australian Society for Medical Research meeting in 1966. This was my first research presentation ever. The abstract was published in the same year, my first research publication. This was really exciting for me, a landmark event.

In this study I had noticed immediately the normal mucosa of the small intestine in children had much broader leaf and tongue-like villi than the finger-like villi of the normal mucosa in adults. This observation I extended and it was published in the *Archives of Disease in Childhood* (the premier British paediatric journal) the following year, i.e. 1967 as 'Dissecting Microscope Appearances of Small Bowel Mucosa in Children' which described the appearances of biopsies taken from 32 Australian children. This observation was to become the basis of my MD thesis in the future. The one problem with the practicalities of this study was to have easy access to the histology of the mucosa. The biopsies were processed and sectioned in the hospital's Pathology Department headed by the very distinguished histologist Dr Douglas Reye who was to become internationally known by the eponymously titled disorder of the liver, Reye's syndrome. Incidentally his name should be pronounced as if there is an R in front of eye. Now the two problems were that he was reluctant both to physically leave his department (he remained in his office, laboratory and autopsy room and did not attend meetings) and to allow histology sections to leave the department, and second he did not like Tom Stapleton. This was difficult for me as Tom's registrar. However I developed a compromise. He was prepared to have me sit in his office and both of us to look at all the sections together and also I could do my own independent review, albeit in his office. This was invaluable experience for the future, but once again I had to struggle to get, the appropriate training. From this experience I learnt for the future that it is essential to have routine clinical pathological meetings, each week, both as part of the patient service and to develop research itself. I did indeed establish this at Queens, Barts and the Royal Free, but at the latter only with some difficulty in 1995. I eventually established a good rapport with Dougie and some time later in 1971 we wrote an important paper on small intestinal biopsies on aboriginal children with gastroenterological problems which was the first of its kind. This is the first time I have mentioned aboriginal Australians, which may surprise the reader, but this was my first encounter. I simply do not recall having either seen or met an aboriginal throughout my childhood and early university life. At that time most aboriginals in Sydney lived at La Perouse and certainly not in Redfern as today. It was as a young doctor that I became interested and concerned by the very severe health problems of aboriginal children, chronic diarrhoea was especially common. Whenever an aboriginal child was brought to the hospital there was almost always a major health problem.

Quite early in 1966 it was clear to me that I had to consider what I needed to do to secure training in paediatric gastroenterology. I had had training in adult gastroenterology at both Hammersmith and Prince Alfred but this was inadequate for paediatric gastroenterology. Children were not little adults. It was already quite obvious to me, from first hand experience at RAHC both in 1966 and back in 1962, that the gastroenterology diseases of infancy in particular, and children in general, were quite different to those of adults. Tom Stapleton had generously given a promise to support me in the future to develop gastroenterology as an academic discipline in children but he had no concrete, funded post for me as yet.

At that time paediatric gastroenterology was beginning to emerge in Australia, continental Europe and the United States. There were however yet no national or international paediatric gastroenterology societies. It seemed to me that there were four centres developing across the world where I might train, if they would have me. These were Melbourne with Charlotte Anderson, Zurich with Andrea Prader and David Shmerling, Helsinki with Jarmo Visakorpi, Utrecht with Weijers and van de Kamer and Boston with Harry Schwachmann. Perhaps it might seem clear that Melbourne was the obvious choice. However there was the traditional edge to relations between Sydney and Melbourne and the Royal Alexandra Hospital for Children and the Royal Children's Hospital were competitive rivals, as perhaps in some ways they still are today. Also I had got 'the travel bug' and felt I needed more international experience. Now I had met Andrea Prader both in Melbourne at the international meeting in 1965 and on a visit to Tom Stapleton. They were old friends. I knew Zurich was a major centre for small bowel work and that there was a distinguished biochemist Semenza working with Prader and I had seen the papers of Salvatore Auricchio and Guiseppe Zoppi in the field of disaccharidases. So it seemed to me that Zurich was the obvious choice. I already had told Prof. Prader I would like to work with him. Sadly there was no one in Britain at all at that time that appeared to be developing paediatric gastroenterology as a specialty. I still reasoned London was close to Zurich and I would also be able to visit my friends and old haunts easily enough. So in February I wrote to Prof. Prader, asking him if I could work in his laboratory in the field of disaccharidases. On March 8, I was simply delighted to get his letter from the Kinderspital, stating 'I would be pleased to accept you as a fellow'. I then applied successfully for the Ewing scholarship and a Nestlé Paediatric Travelling Fellowship to cover my airfares to and from Europe and also to include a visit to North America with a visit to Harry Schwachmann at the Boston Childrens Hospital.

1966 was a good year and by the end of the year I knew I had found my life time work, paediatric gastroenterology with a special interest in diseases of the small intestine in children. I decided to travel to Zurich via southern Africa as I had two very good friends I wanted to meet there whom I had met in London. First there was Wendy Pocock in Johannesburg, South Africa and then there was George Soutter in Salisbury, Rhodesia (now Zimbabwe). I then planned to go on for a brief trip to London to visit colleagues and friends and then on to Zurich.

So in December, in fact on Boxing Day, I was once again farewelled from Kingsford-Smith airport, Sydney on another great adventure by mum, dad, Auntie Lell and this time John Yu, as well. I flew with South African Airways to Johannesburg. Our first stop was Perth and then there was the 24 hours flight across the Indian Ocean. On the way we stopped first at Cocos Island where the temperature was over 90 degrees and there was a howling gale, at midnight. We then landed, after over two thousand miles, the longest commercial flight over open sea at that time, on the beautiful island of Mauritius, still a crown colony. From the air, the island looked quite idyllic, a green and pleasant land, but at the airport was very hot and humid. Johannesburg glimpsed from the skies looked remarkable, surrounded with the yellow waste from the famed gold mines of the rand and then by remarkably green countryside further out.

Wendy met me at Johannesburg airport. It was great to see her. She already warned me in advance about the horrors of apartheid, which were obvious, all too obvious, as soon as I arrived. An army of what Wendy called Bantu porters descended on the passengers' baggage and their attitude of servility and the parallel attitude of arrogance adopted by their 'white overlords' was extremely distasteful. The racial-policy of the Nationalist South African government was well known to me and of course I was prejudiced against it, before I arrived. I must admit I also already had some degree of prejudice against the Boer, or Afrikaner people, with considerable sympathy for the English speaking South Africans whom I believed to be in a difficult situation. This was probably because I had grown up with an interest in South Africa, as an outpost of Empire with stories of the Boer war. Also I had enjoyed Rider Haggard's glamorous books of adventure in southern Africa.

Wendy showed me around Johannesburg and the University. She was then an established cardiologist in the city. The most remarkable thing that I noticed at that time, which I had never seen before in Australia or Europe, was the frequency of burglar alarms and elaborate security fences around so many suburban homes. Little did I realize that in the future, even here in London, burglar alarms etc. were to become a normal feature of suburbia. In fact at that time Johannesburg suburbia was largely white and the African workers came in and out of the city each day in fleets of buses, usually driven at reckless speeds, from the outlying African townships, as I observed.

Most interestingly, we visited Baragwaneth Hospital in Soweto, one of the African townships. The hospital was huge and housed in old army barracks. I was amazed to see row upon row of babies (totalling 55) with plaster of Paris slabs on the side of their head being given intravenous fluids via scalp vein needles, to treat their dehydration due to gastroenteritis. The plaster slabs were there to keep the needles in the veins. This technique was quite new to me, but seemed an excellent strategy and better than our technique of intravenous cutdown on leg veins, we were using for severe dehydration in infants at RAHC at that time. This was my first glimpse of the problems of the developing world. This was to be a lifetime interest, although sadly my career never permitted me ever to work in the developing world. I have however made many visits and trained a number of doctors from such communities. Interestingly the intravenous therapy of dehydration in such babies was to be replaced in the future, in all except the most severe cases, by the much simpler and safer oral rehydration therapy. This will be discussed later. We also drove to the administrative capital of South Africa, Pretoria, quite near Johannesburg. South Africa had become a republic in 1961 and had then immediately left the Commonwealth. For Afrikaners this was a kind of victory symbolizing a reversal of the outcome of the Boer War. I could never have predicted that remarkably South Africa would in the future return to the Commonwealth under the charismatic leadership of Nelson Mandela.

I found Pretoria to be a very Afrikaner city at that time I discovered that speech in English was often greeted with a surly reply. In the heart of the city stood the statue of Oom Paul Kruger, the great Afrikaner hero of the Boer war, and standing on a hill near the city was the great Voortreker, monument revered with much pride by the Afrikaner people. However for me the finest monument in Pretoria was the great Union Building, surely one of the finest buildings of the British Imperial era, only surpassed in my experience by the Lutyens buildings in New Delhi, which I was to visit some years later. I then flew on to Salisbury (today known as Harare). Now the Rhodesian government at that time had made a Unilateral Declaration of Independence from Britain (UDI) on 11 November 1965, under the leadership of Ian Smith. However the union jack flew everywhere and the Rhodesian government's position at that time was one of loyalty to the Queen, despite great hostility to the government of Harold Wilson. At the time of arrival, whilst having sympathy with the European settlers in Rhodesia, with their stated policy of racial partnership rather than apartheid, I was in sympathy too with Harold Wilson after the failure of the meeting on the naval ship the HMS *Tiger*, to agree a solution with Ian Smith.

George Soutter worked at the remarkable Harare Hospital. At that time it was the teaching hospital of the newly established faculty of medicine of the University College of Rhodesia. The medical faculty was affiliated with the University of Birmingham. The staffs of the hospital were multiracial and the relationship of the African and European staff was one of complete equality. There was an attitude of friendly bantering in strong contrast to the restrained sometimes resentful atmosphere, which was all too apparent at Baragwaneth Hospital. From the first, it was obvious to me that Salisbury was a far more racially tolerant and obviously multiracial society than was Johannesburg. I wrote a detailed report of my journey to southern Africa, which I presented as a lecture on my return to Sydney a year later. I quote the following:

> Walking the streets of Salisbury affords again a great contrast to walking those of Johannesburg. I, personally saw no signs 'Europeans only', all too apparent in Johannesburg. Africans and Europeans, together in shops, post-offices etc. even in the petrol rationing office (incidentally the only evidence of the effect of sanctions I encountered) can be seen. Nonetheless it would be foolish to say after such a brief visit that there was no discrimination against black Africans

in Rhodesia today. All I can say is, that I did not see any evidence of it whereas In South Africa one would have to be quite blind, not to observe frank racial discrimination.

George Soutter's demonstration to me of the range of children's disorders at Harare Hospital was quite eye-opening and very educational. It was obvious he was a very dedicated doctor of great humanity. In the children's wards there were many patients gravely ill with kwashiorkor and marasmus (both forms of severe malnutrition), tuberculous meningitis or measles. Measles was a severe and sometimes fatal illness. The eye complications were particularly unpleasant.

At the hospital most of the nursing sisters were Africans of the Mashona people or as they are usually called the Shona. These were regarded by white Rhodesians as a very peaceful people compared to the warlike Matabele. Some of the sisters were European, mostly British. The medical staff was mostly European, chiefly British with a few white Rhodesians and several African housemen. There were only two paediatric consultants, one was Professor Reggie Lightwood and one part time paediatrician. There was only one paediatric registrar, my host and friend George Soutter. It was obvious he did most of the paediatric work. When I met Prof. Lightwood I was surprised that such an eccentric figure who appeared to me to be quite out of touch with local needs, could be in charge. I discovered he had come from St Mary's Hospital, London. I was to meet him again in London some years later.

I found conversing with the African staff to be very interesting. One sister who lived in Highfield African Township said that Christmas 1966 had been the quietest and most orderly for years. Everyone I spoke to of all races, without exception, was against external sanctions. We also visited Domboshawa near Salisbury, famous for its ancient Bushman paintings, a great interest of George's, which gave me a different-slant on the local scene.

Later he drove me to Victoria Falls. There we flew in a small plane over those majestic and beautiful falls. The view from the air was quite an unforgettable sight, with a great cloud of spray rising up from a gorge, as vast amounts of water cascaded downwards. On the same day, we went for a short boat trip on the Zambezi River and here we encountered the Africa of story and legend. We saw elephants coming down to the water to drink, wild monkeys and the dense steaming jungle itself.

Then George and I began a great journey in his Volvo, from Victoria Falls to Cape Town. We were to travel across Rhodesia, then the Transvaal and down to Durban and finally along the coast road to Cape Town. What a journey it was. In Eastern Rhodesia we were often the only whites in the communities we visited. At Urntali we saw the new amenities built for Africans including a swimming pool and a stadium both recently constructed by the new government. We felt totally secure as the two of us travelled amongst the Shona people, where Europeans were only rarely encountered.

Next was South Africa again and the Transvaal, which was extremely beautiful with mountains reminiscent of Europe. At times it was quite cold although the season was mid-summer. We paused at Durban and swam in the sea from a beach which segregated the swimmers into three races black, white and Indian. We passed through Transkei, the first so called Bantustan, and then on to the Cape Province. We followed the garden route to our final destination Cape Town with its great table top mountain and beautiful Dutch colonial architecture. I gave an invited lecture, arranged by Professor John Hansen, at the Canadian Red Cross Memorial Hospital, on my work with small bowel biopsy. I was apprehensive but it went down quite well, with lots of questions. There I met a young Englishman, Bob Wood-Walker, who was to become in the future a district paediatrician in Colchester, referring patients to QEHC in the future. Over and over again in my career I have met colleagues in distant places, never expecting to see them again but ending up working in some way with them.

At this point I should just like to record my summation of my impressions after my journey to Rhodesia and South Africa at the time. I wrote:

> Rhodesia is a troubled land, but a traveller who passes through this beautiful country would think it was one of the most pleasant, fortunate and peaceful nations on earth, populated by black and white, working together amazingly well. Nonetheless the future of this land is shrouded in the mists of uncertainty, and unmitigated disaster could sweep across it.

Tragically unmitigated disaster did and continues. I have never visited the new Zimbabwe and could not do so under the terrible regime of Robert Mugabe. I have kept an interest in what has since happened. I have kept in touch with the Rhodesia Christian Group and through them, I heard Ian Smith speak and I met him in London at the Royal Air Force Club in London in 1997. He was then a sad figure but a man of obvious great personal courage and conviction. Then in May 2000 as an observer for the Commonwealth Association for Paediatric Gastroenterology and Nutrition to the Commonwealth Health Ministers meeting in Geneva, I joined a small group of ministers for lunch which included Dr Terence Stamp, Health minister of Zimbabwe. His vehement hostility to the British government and condemnation of the British media's coverage of Mugabe's Zimbabwe was remarkable. Then through CAPGAN we hosted a meeting at Marlborough House on AIDS and a delegate from Zimbabwe told us of the dire situation posed by AIDS. In fact the whole of southern Africa is facing a terrible crisis from all the deaths from AIDS affecting all sections of society. This includes South Africa. However in general South Africa has done much better than I anticipated after my visit in 1966/67. I wrote:

> It is difficult to take an optimistic view for the long term future of South Africa, bright though her short term future, at least economically, may be, that is unless her Government significantly modifies its policy, which of course may not be impossible. Her recent efforts to cultivate the friendship of Lesotho, Botswana, Malawi and even further north, together with her relaxation of the colour bar for visiting sportsmen, are both moves in the right direction, but at the same time her own racial laws over the past 3 years have become more rigid. For the first time Chinese people are now being forced to live in the areas of their own.

So fortunately subsequent history of South Africa was far more positive than I feared but my optimism for Rhodesia has not been borne out by subsequent events, so I was wrong on both counts! I was very sad when I finally left Cape Town for Zurich. My African journey had been a quite fantastic and unique experience for me.

I made a brief return to London, only three years after I had left. I visited Hammersmith again and saw my mentor Chris Booth, who had become Professor and Director of the Royal Postgraduate Medical School of London. The facilities had enormously improved with the addition of the new Commonwealth Building. Chris gave me some encouraging professional career advice and told me to keep in touch. I also visited the neonatal unit. It was extremely impressive. Peter Tizard and John Davis conducted the round.

I also for the first time visited the weekly ward round of Professor Sheila Sherlock, in the famed liver unit on the roof of the old Royal Free Hospital in Gray's Inn Road. There was an interesting discussion on liver transplantation and the possible place of exchange transfusion and the transfused pig's liver in the management of hepatic coma seen in hepatitis. Her blunt dogmatic and combative style was clearly a most effective teaching strategy but I observed it could be pretty stressful for those who earned her displeasure. Several years in the future I was to exam for the finals with her and observe her formidable style in action. Also in her retirement, after my transfer in 1995 to the Royal Free, we were to have some contact there. She made a great contribution to British Medicine.

Finally I visited Brian Creamer's gastroenterology unit at St Thomas's Hospital and I was particularly interested to see his technique of examination of post-mortem small bowel which was valuable for my future MD in Sydney. I was very impressed to see the new main block of the hospital and I wrote at the time 'It reflects great credit on the British National Health Service'. Then after brief visits to some of my old favourite places I was off to Switzerland.

Zurich was in the depths of winter when I arrived. I had never been there before. No one met me at the airport. I found my own way to the Kinderspital (children's hospital) with some difficulty. The hospital is situated in a pleasant suburban area of Zurich with a view of the lake, the Zurcher See. I met Prof. Prader and he welcomed me and told me with only a few words, as he was such a busy man, to join Prof. David Shmerling at 7.30 a.m. next day. This was the usual starting time for hospital work. His secretary had booked me into a guesthouse close to the Kinderspital for one week, which I duly found. However at first I had some difficulty getting in. When I pressed the bell there was a buzzing noise after a minute or so but the door did not open. So I kept pressing the bell, eventually, a rather irritated middle-aged woman opened the door and drew my attention for the first time to the usual security entry system on the continent. We did not have such systems in Australia at the time. She also told me that I only had a room for a week and that this could not be extended as the guesthouse was fully booked the following week. So I had to spend a good deal of my first week in Zurich trying to find accommodation. Prof. Prader's secretary was not that helpful but gave me a list of accommodation services. Now I did not speak very good German, the language of Zurich. I had not studied the language at school but I had attended German classes in Sydney before I left. Prof. Prader had told me that most people spoke English at the Kinderspital. At first I was quite unsuccessful in my search for accommodation. Then I did find a nice room in a family house but after I visited and it was clear my German was so poor, I had a telephone message cancelling. I was then becoming quite desperate. No one at the Kinderspital offered any help. Then I came upon the Catholisch Zimmer Dienst or Roman Catholic Room Service who were so helpful. Immediately they found me a room at Gladbachstrasse nummer 9. Ever after I have had considerable sympathy with colleagues from overseas that have come to work with us but have had difficulty in finding accommodation in London.

At 9 Gladbachstrasse, Frau Welti, who spoke no English, was very understanding of my weak German and she offered me the room that Salvatore Auricchio was vacating as he was returning to Naples after his fellowship in Zurich. He and I in future years, via ESPGAN, were to become great friends but we did not meet at that time. So at last I had a place to rest my head!

I then could concentrate on my activities with David Shmerling who would direct my work. He began at 7.30 a.m. by going around the wards to see his patients informally just with me following him. At that time he also saw any consultations within the hospital including those from the surgeons. This was an invaluable experience for me, as I would have to offer a similar service on return to Sydney. We saw complicated liver cases and children with cystic fibrosis but at that time there were no cases of Crohn's disease. This is interesting as such cases would in the future be major problems for paediatric gastroenterologists in Zurich as much as in London and Sydney. Then I was in the laboratory This was my first and only period of laboratory training. I did not know the basics apart from chemistry at school and biochemistry at University. I had to learn again to titrate, use a pipette, clean glassware etc. Fortunately there was a young English biochemist in the lab with whom I largely worked. She was married to a Swiss.

On the first day, David Shmerling came to fetch me at lunchtime. Now the city of Zurich as a whole at that time had a 'siesta' of two hours for lunch, long since abandoned. In the hospital this meant nothing happened for two hours and married doctors went home to have lunch with their wives. Shmerling took me to a restaurant near the lake and said it was a good place to eat and then to my astonishment left me on my own! In all the time I was at the Kinderspital no staff ever invited me home. I spent the long two-hour lunch break, wandering around the lake taking photographs and getting to know the beauties of the city. My first few weeks in Zurich were undoubtedly the loneliest of my life. So lonely was I, that when I heard one of my old friends from Hammersmith, Colin Barnes and his wife Marian were visiting Basel for a medical meeting, I took the train there just for the company of old friends for a few hours. However after several weeks two things happened that enormously improved the social scene for me. A young German banker Heino Meynkohn came to lodge in the room next to mine at Gladbachstrasse. We quickly became very good friends. He had a car and we started to make interesting trips together to the mountains, especially the Rigi, which is quite close to Zurich. We even drove into Germany as far as Munich where we stayed one weekend. I really liked the city, especially its antique museums, but the streets were all 'up' as a new underground railway was being built. Heino later was to come as a migrant to Australia, but ultimately returned to Germany. The second thing that happened was I discovered St Andrew's Anglican Church in Zurich, where many expatriate English people and their Swiss families worshipped. There I met Donnie Bourquin who was a medical student at Zurich University at that time. He introduced me to his wife Annette and invited me to his mother and father's home for Sunday lunch.

His father was French Swiss and his mother Scottish, of Robertson ancestry. I had such a warm welcome that I felt completely at home. I had many Sunday lunches there roast lamb, roast potatoes and gravy, wonderful. Donnie and Annette became lifetime friends visiting us as recently as June 2002. Through me, Donnie obtained a junior resident medical officer, post at RAHC some years later and after returning briefly to Switzerland, he and his family settled permanently in NSW where he has been a most successful general practitioner with four children. They, now live in Nelson's Bay, NSW. I have very warm feelings for St Andrew's church, it was a safe haven for me. After these two 'discoveries' I became very happy in Zurich both socially and at the hospital where I enjoyed the work.

The working hours for medical staff at the Kinderspital was long, 7.30 a.m. to 7 p.m., but with the two hours for lunch I mentioned. I of course had the luxury of not working nights or weekends. To avoid the loneliness I often came to have lunch and breakfast in the doctors' mess and I sometimes had the evening meal there too. Startlingly there were sometimes meatless days! Birchersmuesli and kuchen were the mainstream foods.

In the laboratory my first task was to learn how to perform the complex chemical technique of disaccharidase assay from small intestinal biopsy tissue. In the hospital, I accompanied Shmerling whenever he did a small bowel biopsy. He did all biopsies in the hospital personally, using the paediatric Crosby capsule. He used a rigid tube, which could be seen on X-ray, attached to the capsule rather than the plastic one I had been used to. He passed the capsule in the Radiology Department and did the X-ray screening himself. I extended my experience of dissecting microscope appearances of the biopsy tissue he obtained and learnt practical technical tips from him. I also learnt from him the conception of gluten challenge to diagnose coeliac disease scientifically. This process involved a second small bowel biopsy after the child had got better on a gluten-free diet to show the mucosa had improved, and then years later doing a third biopsy after the child had gone back onto gluten to show it was abnormal again. This approach both demonstrated ab initio gluten intolerance and then showed that it persisted. I was to apply this approach as soon as I returned to RAHC. Shmerling's approach was later to be endorsed at the Interlaken meeting of the European Society of Gastroenterology in 1989, which I shall mention later.

I also twice a week joined Professor Prader on his main ward round, the Chef Visite. This was a grand occasion. If there were English-speaking visitors the ward round was conducted in English. Otherwise it was conducted in a mixture of Hoch Deutsch (high German) or Switzer Deutsch (the local dialect), which I struggled to understand. At that time all house staff typed up all the clinical features in the patients' notes. Whenever a blood test was taken a mark was placed on the patient's chart and also when the result came back for the Professor's information. He swept in and out of the wards. Doors were held open, often with a bow in the old Teutonic manner, to the great Herr Professor Doctor Prader as he passed by. He was a figure of great power and influence, who not only headed the university department, but also, unlike in Sydney and London, headed the hospital's department of medicine. His only peer was Professor Grob who headed the department of surgery.

One very sad aspect of paediatric care at that time, was the limitation upon parental visiting to three times per week for an hour and a half. In the time of the 'old' Fanconi, Prader's predecessor who was still around the hospital in my day, there had been no visiting for the first week of a child's admission in order I was told, 'to break the child in'. I saw several tearful mothers walking down the Steinweisstrasse from the Kinderspital. I noticed that no one seemed to worry much if the child cried as it was generally assumed that it would do them good. Every Swiss child had to behave as a little soldier and as a result the Kinder spital had 'the best behaved children in the world'! I found it touching that despite my poor German, these children responded to a little warmth and interest.

I was astonished to find that nobody lived in the hospital apart from the two assistants on duty each night. In my own experience in both Sydney and London, 'living in' was the norm. The Oberartze, the equivalent in the UK to senior registrars at that time, were on call for medical patients but were not resident. The junior doctors were called assistenten (assistants). I made friends with two of them and I was delighted one evening when one of them Udo Dohman from Ulm in Germany came to visit me at Gladbachstrasse 9.

After a few weeks Professor Prader honoured me by the invitation to accompany him in his car as he drove for a consultation to a country hospital. He told me he wanted to find out how I was getting on and find out more about me, which I appreciated very much. It was an interesting journey and valuable for my future. He was to be key referee for me when I applied in 1972 for the post at Barts five years later.

Later on my main research project proved to be a method of testing the permeability of the small intestine of the body could disaccharide sugar lactulose, which the small intestine of the body could not split. We gave this sugar by mouth and tested the amount in the urine. If small intestinal permeability was increased this was abnormal. The difficulty of this approach was the technique of measuring the sugar in the urine. This needed a highly sophisticated technique namely gas-liquid chromatography. I worked with a young chemist M. Muller who had limited English and I had limited German, so it was quite a test for us both. Still a good paper was published from this work, which eventually appeared in 1969. In fact I had a trip to London, which I enjoyed and saw a biochemist at GOS, Menzies, to discuss this work. I stayed with David Harvey and David Wright who were sharing a flat with another friend in Connaught St at that time.

In April I had the honour to travel with David Shmerling to Sidney Sussex College Cambridge for a Colloquium on Calorie Deficiencies and Protein Deficiencies. I had the invitation via John Yu who had contacted Elsie Widdowson whom he had known from Hammersmith days. Having been in Africa recently this was of great interest, as kwashiorkor and marasmus were discussed in great detail. I was extremely impressed by a young investigator Dr Brian Wharton, who at that time came from Kampala in Uganda. He discussed treatment of these disorders. I would meet him again in 1972 at Queen Elizabeth Hospital for Children. I found it quite wonderful to be staying in a Cambridge College in the heart of that beautiful city. King's College chapel is for me one of the most beautiful places in the world.

After I had given a talk at the Kinderspital, I was very honoured to receive an invitation from Professor Ettore Rossi to give a lecture on my small bowel biopsy findings at RAHC in Berne. He, like Prader, was keen to catalyse the development of the new discipline of paediatric gastroenterology. There I met Harold Gaze and Daniel Nussle, Swiss colleagues I would meet again many times in the future.

Whilst I was in Zurich I was very grateful to receive an invitation from Professor Stapleton (on one of his many overseas trips) to accompany him to the annual European Paediatric Research Society meeting in Copenhagen in 1967. I submitted an abstract on my work on small bowel biopsy in Sydney. It was accepted and duly presented, my first at an international meeting, a landmark event in my career. It was well received. Most importantly I experienced the quality of a European paediatric scientific meeting as well as the social life. At one of the dinners I met Peter Krasilnikoff a Dane, another paediatric gastroenterology trainee like me, and we have been friends ever since. He was to become Professor and head of department in Copenhagen and I was honoured to participate in his retirement meeting in 1999.

It was not all work at the Kinderspital and the main social event of the year was the annual Ski Tag (day) at Claverdal in Davos. The skiing conditions were superb and we had a great time. However the day came when I had to leave and a small drinks reception was given for me which I much appreciated.

I had grown to like the Swiss despite their great reserve. I was fortunate that as my time in Zurich ended my mum and dad joined me on a European trip they were making. This was mum's first and only trip to Europe and Britain. It was strange to meet them at the Hauptbahnof (main railway station) on the express from Vienna. We had a memorable trip together to Zermatt and saw perhaps the most beautiful mountain in the world, the Matterhorn with its remarkable peak. We were to join up again in London in August.

My parents and I stayed with the Borthwicks in Seaford. That family were so very kind to all my family and me over so very many years, that they have a very special place in my affectionate memories. They have now all died some years ago. An example of their practical Christianity was the way they entertained in their home local German prisoners of war from the nearby camp towards the end and after the war. Each Christmas they continued to receive cards from these former prisoners over many years. Remarkably two of them with their wives and families returned to visit them in Seaford.

The three of us then drove on to the West Country which mum was delighted to see. Like me, mum found that England lived up to her every expectation. On the way we also visited Gloucester to see the Cathedral and visit Judith Meath-Baker as well as Bishop and Mrs Guy, who had been good friends since I had visited the Holy Land in 1964. The weather that summer in Devon and Cornwall was superb and the countryside with its lush greenness and ancient churches could not have been more beautiful. I enjoyed sharing this time of relaxation very much with my parents, especially mum. She and I had always been very close and I know she regretted the times I was away from home but rejoiced in my happiness and welfare. That summer dear England lived up to all the expectations of us descendants of those ancestors who had left her shores so long ago.

My parents and I were then to part company again, till we met up at San Francisco on our way home. I first went briefly to New York, my first trip to America. I was staggered at the vista of Manhattan, as seen from the top of the Empire State, which I visited with a friend of John Yu. Then I was on to Toronto where I was welcomed by Don Wood and E. Barclay Simpson who were old friends from London House. Don took me to the Hospital for Sick Children. At that time it had over 900 paediatric beds and it as the largest hospital in North America. There I met Dr Dick Hamilton. He was then a young research fellow working on an animal model for sugar intolerance and was testing the effect of lactic acid on the mucosa. Little did we know that we were destined to be co-editors of a major text of paediatric gastroenterology in the future and to become lifelong friends. Don took me to see the Niagara

Falls, which were indeed remarkable, the sheer volume of water was awesome but for sheer beauty the Victoria Falls won hands down. How privileged I was to have seen both the Victoria Falls and the Niagara Falls on one trip.

I visited Boston next as planned, to meet Harry Swachmann. I had a very useful visit with him at the Boston children's hospital my first of many visits over the years to that remarkable institution. However I was struck by the harsh competitiveness of American medicine. The chief resident was a very tough character who spoke to Harry with little respect. Some years later I was delighted when Harry enrolled in one of my postgraduate courses at Queen Elizabeth Hospital for Children. It was a great honour for me, we had kept in touch ever since my visit. My old friend David Wollman welcomed me to Boston and arranged my accommodation at the YMCA. He took me on a memorable trip to Cape Cod. Then I was on to Cincinnati to visit the Cincinnati Children's Hospital, staying with Dr Fred Silverman, a radiologist who had visited Sydney. He was clearly a workaholic and gave me an insight into the intensity of the American medical scene. I was astounded to find that he worked all day Saturday. He was a pioneer in the recognition of Crohn's disease in children by X-ray barium studies. I was also pleased to meet Dr John Partin who had written an important paper concerning the risks of biopsying the small intestine of children when a capsule with an adult sized porthole was used, as I mentioned earlier. Yet nothing I had seen in my brief trip to North America had attracted me to ever want to work there. I admired their achievements but the style and way of life were not for me. However I was to make several good friends of American colleagues in future years and I came to admire their remarkable contribution to scientific medicine.

Finally I arrived in San Francisco to have some time with mum and dad, in that beautiful coastal city so reminiscent of Sydney. Little did I realize that I would visit the city again many years in the future at a huge meeting of the American Gastroenterology Association. The Golden Gate bridge was indeed a, sight of a lifetime, but an unexpected pleasure was a visit to Grace Episcopal Cathedral, a memorable building where the Anglican traditions of music and beautiful liturgy flourish. 1967 was the time of the 'flower people' and we visited 'Haight-Ashbury' but clearly decline was already setting in towards a much sadder drug scene. After a few happy days in San Francisco together, sampling the delights of travelling on the cable cars etc. it was back to Sydney for us all with our long flight home over the Pacific. I had flown around the world. On arrival back in Sydney I felt exhilarated and keen to fulfil my mission to develop paediatric gastroenterology at the Royal Alexandra Hospital for Children and beyond.

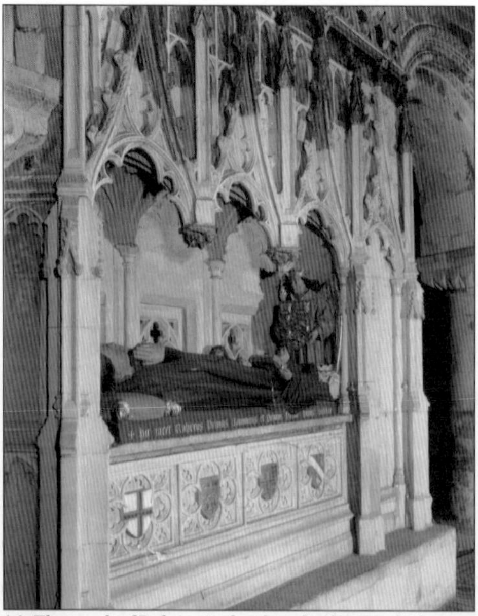

16. The tomb of Rahere in the church of St Bartholomew the Great, published with permission of Department of Medical Illustration, Barts

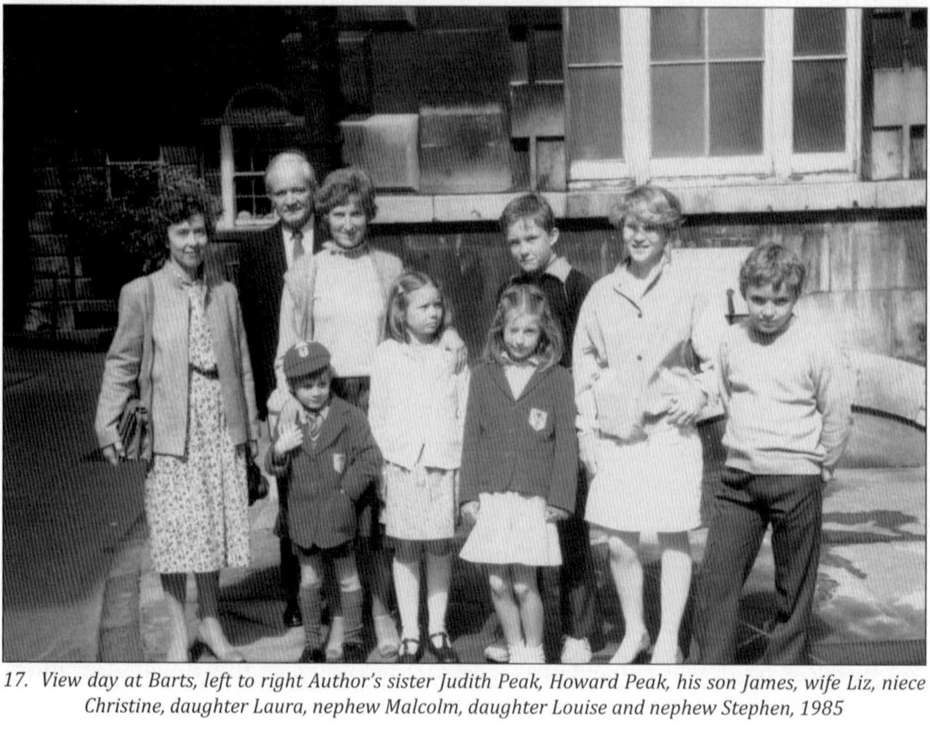

17. View day at Barts, left to right Author's sister Judith Peak, Howard Peak, his son James, wife Liz, niece Christine, daughter Laura, nephew Malcolm, daughter Louise and nephew Stephen, 1985

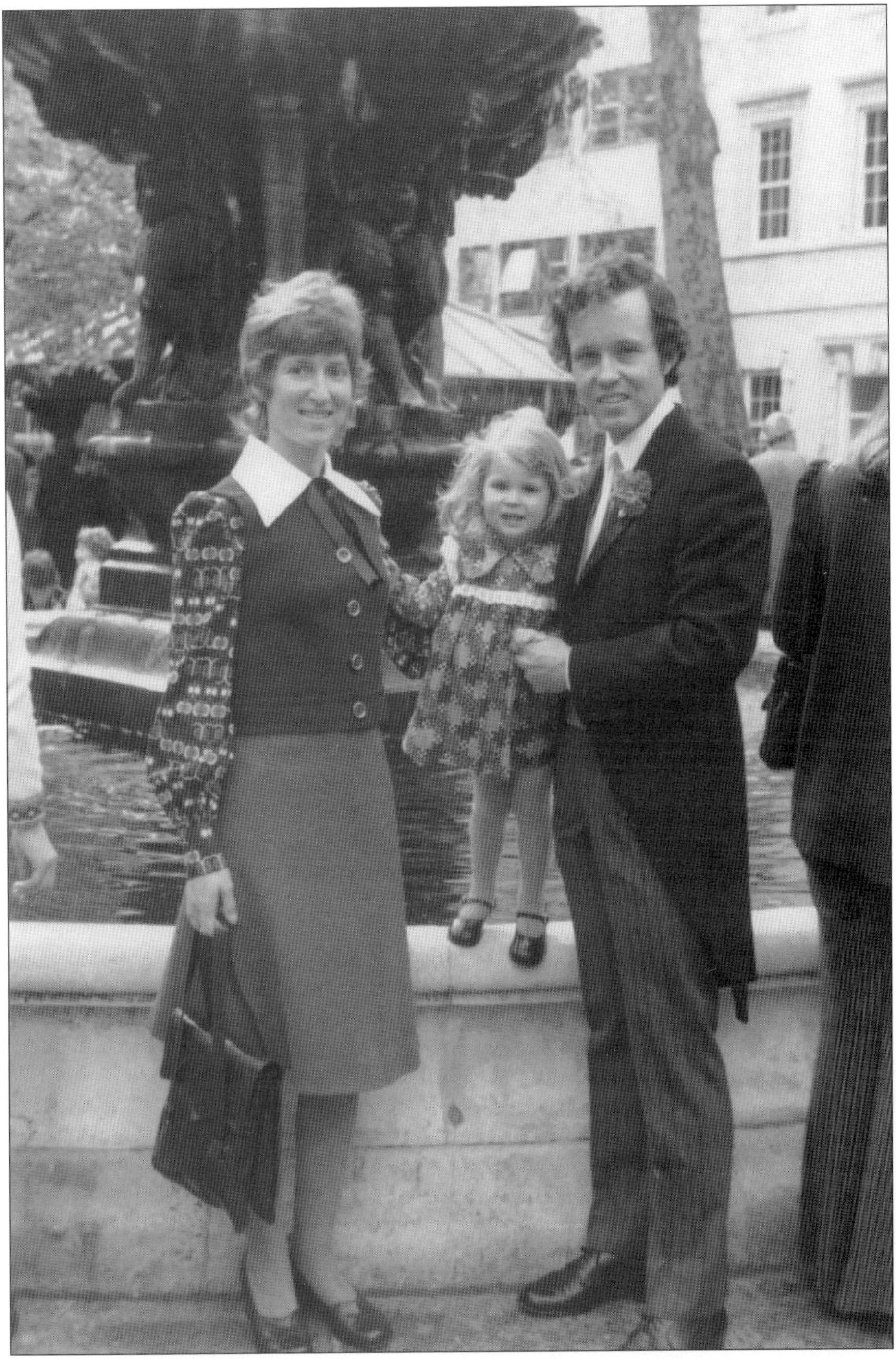

18. View day at Barts, on left, Author with wife Liz and daughter Louise, 1973

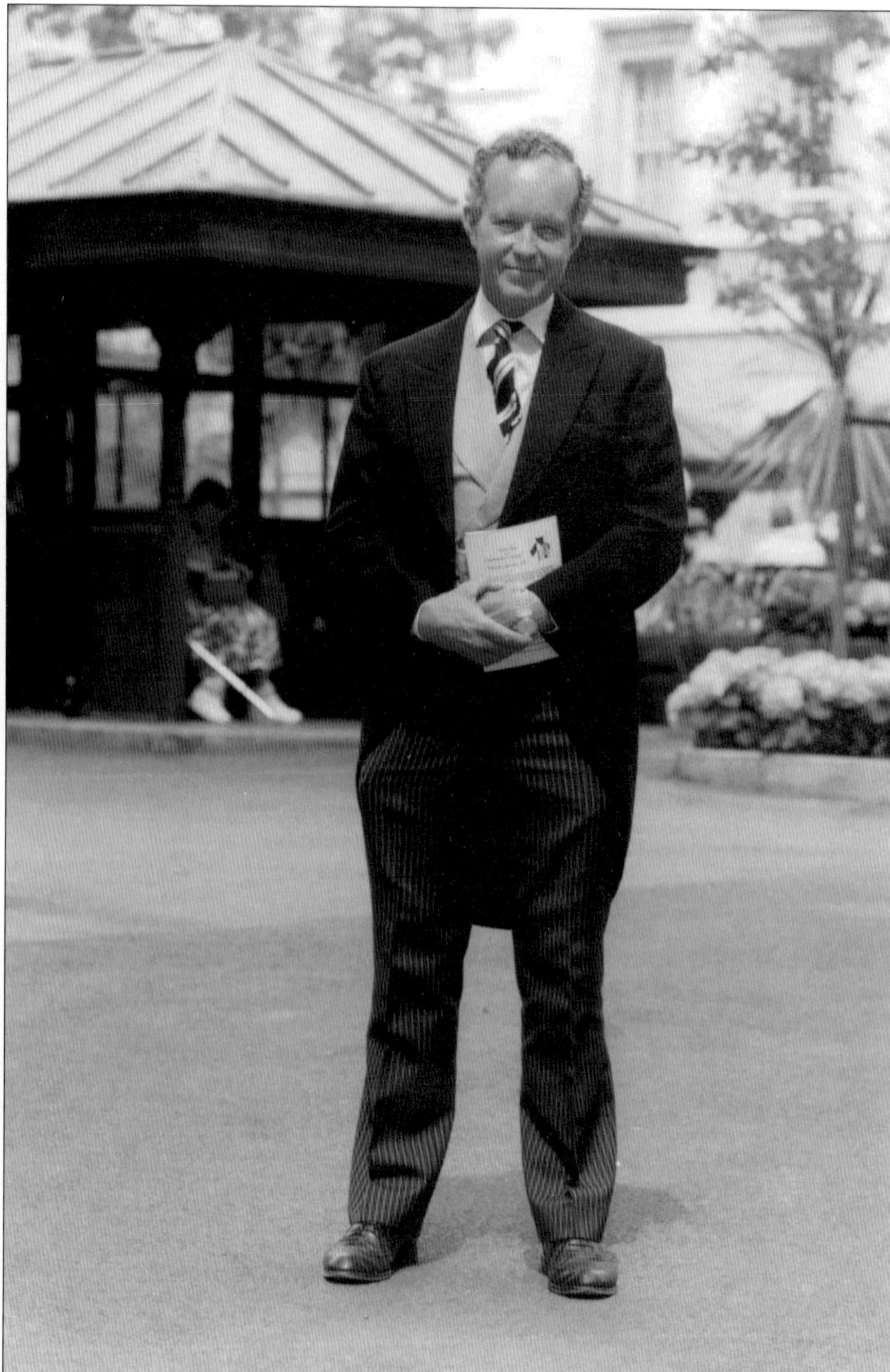

19. View day at Barts, Author, 1995

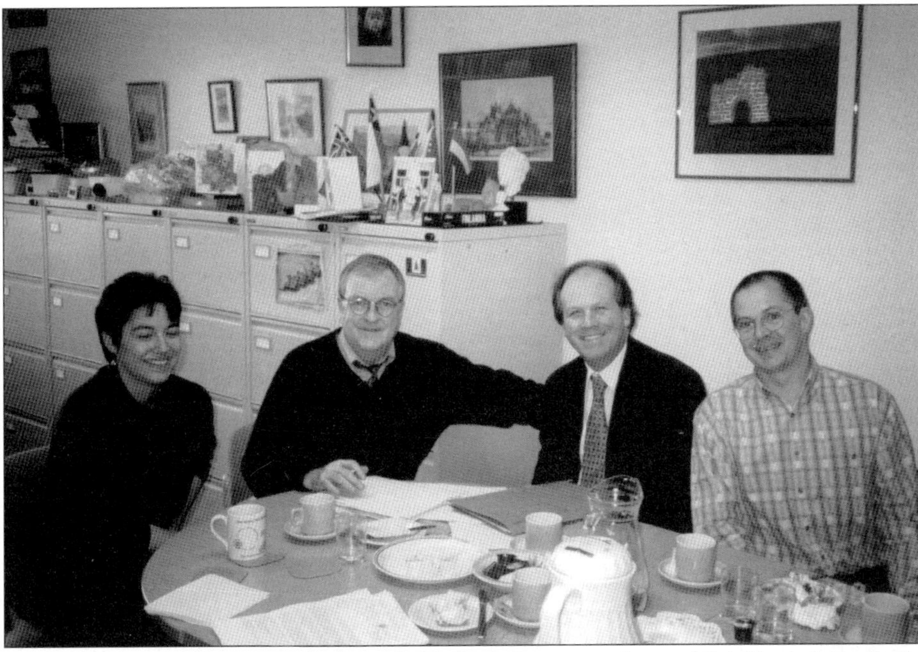

20. Ad hoc editorial office meeting for Journal of Pediatric Gastroenterology and Nutrition in Author's office at the Royal Free School of Medicine. From left to right Terry Lichay, administrative assistant, Allan Walker, Ian Sanderson and Alan Phillips, 1998

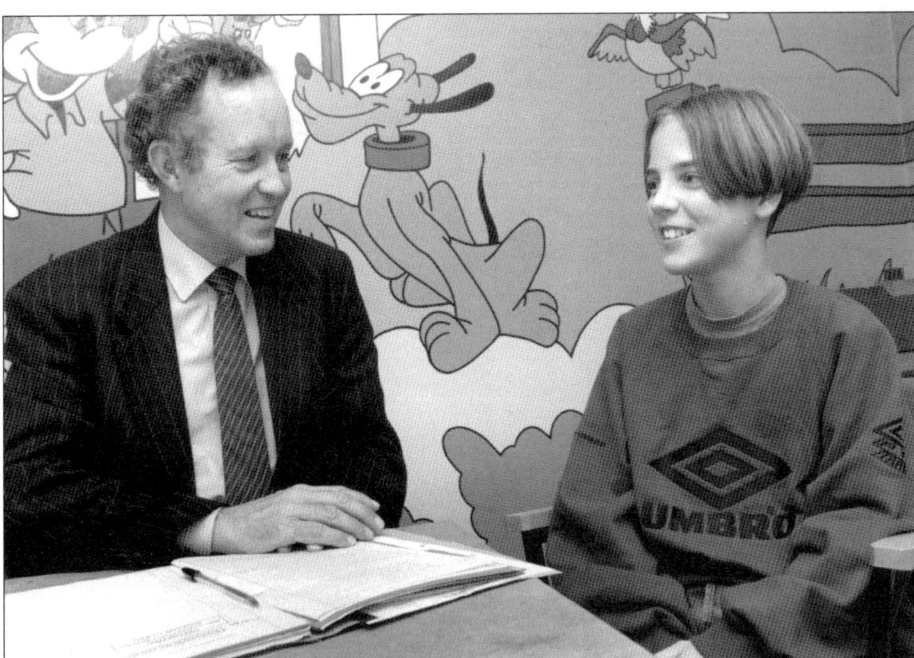

21. Author with child patient in outpatient clinic at the Royal Free Hospital, September 1995

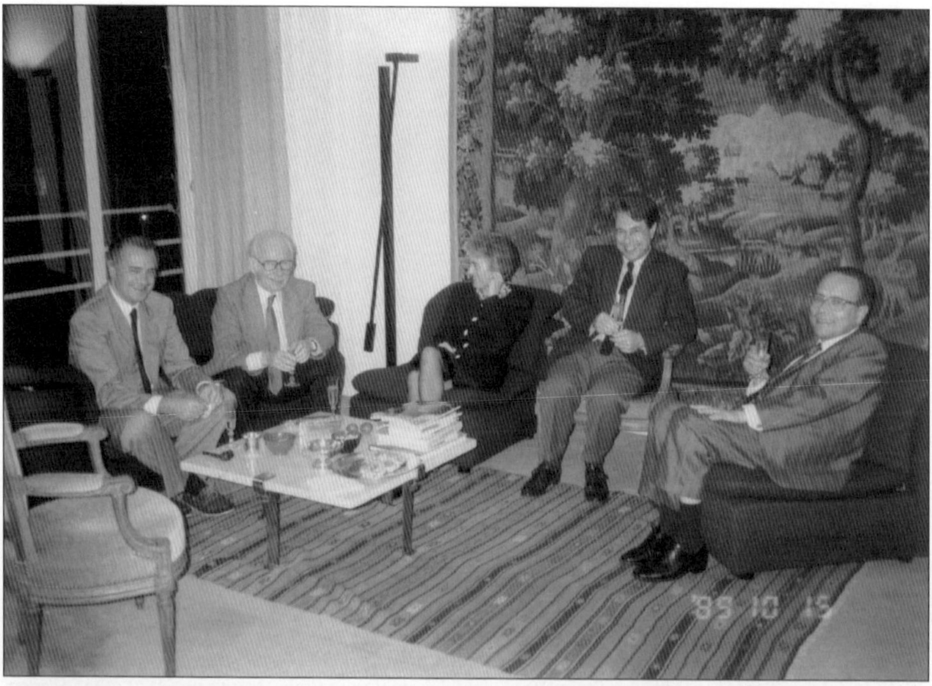

22. ESPGAN working group for coeliac disease, in home of Jacques and Françoise Schmitz. Left to right Stefano Guandalini, David Shmerling, Françoise Schmitz, Jacques Schmitz and Jarmo Visakorpi, Paris 1989,

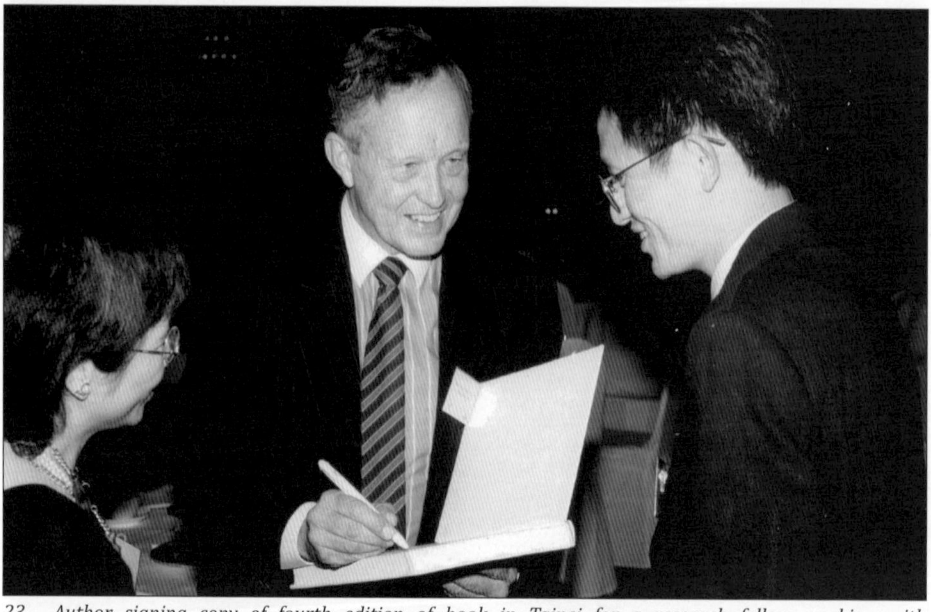

23. Author signing copy of fourth edition of book in Taipei for a research fellow working with Dr Me-Hwei Chang on left, March 2000

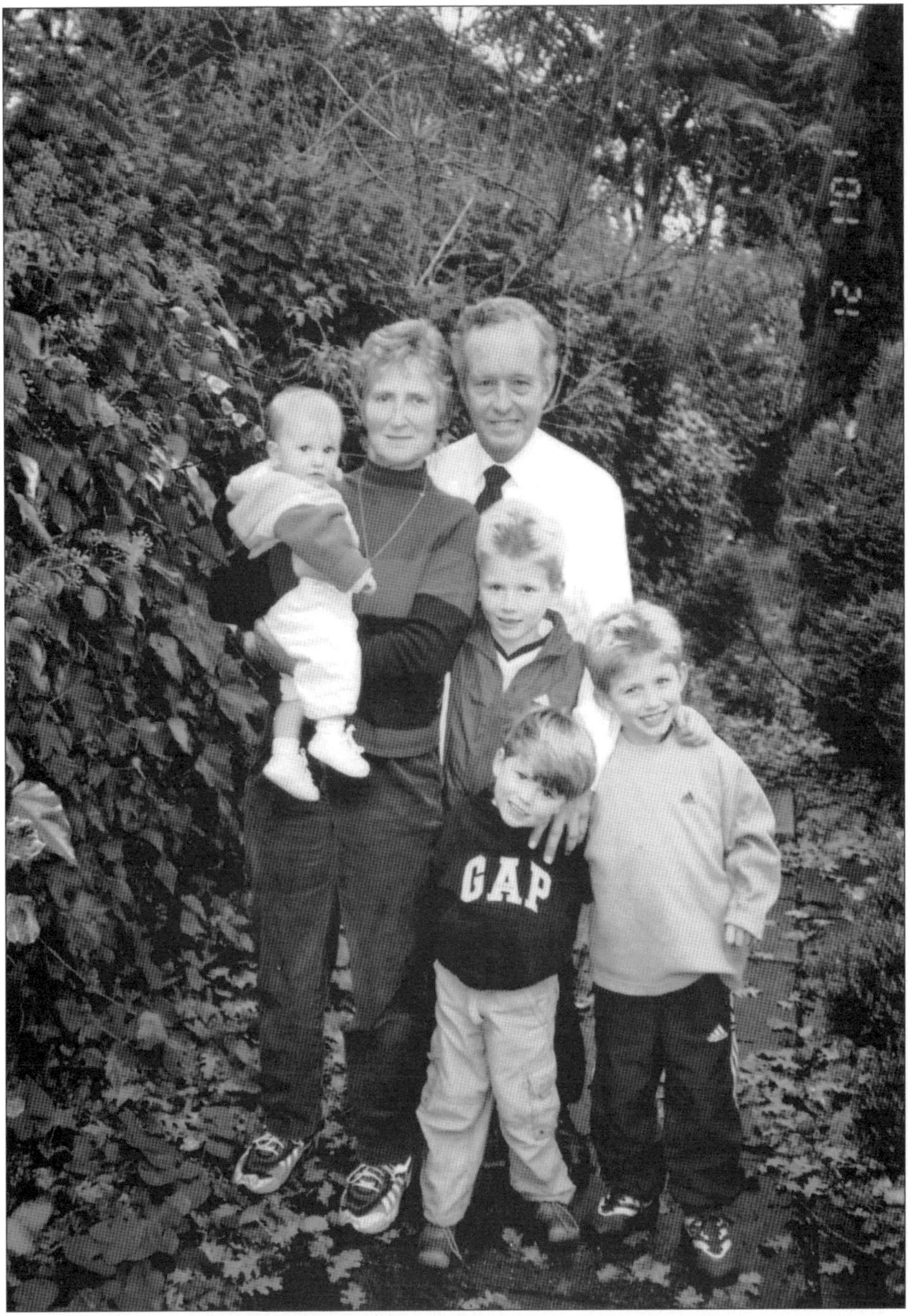

24. Author on 65th birthday, in back garden at home with wife Liz and from left to right: Chloe, Joseph, Morgan and William, 2001

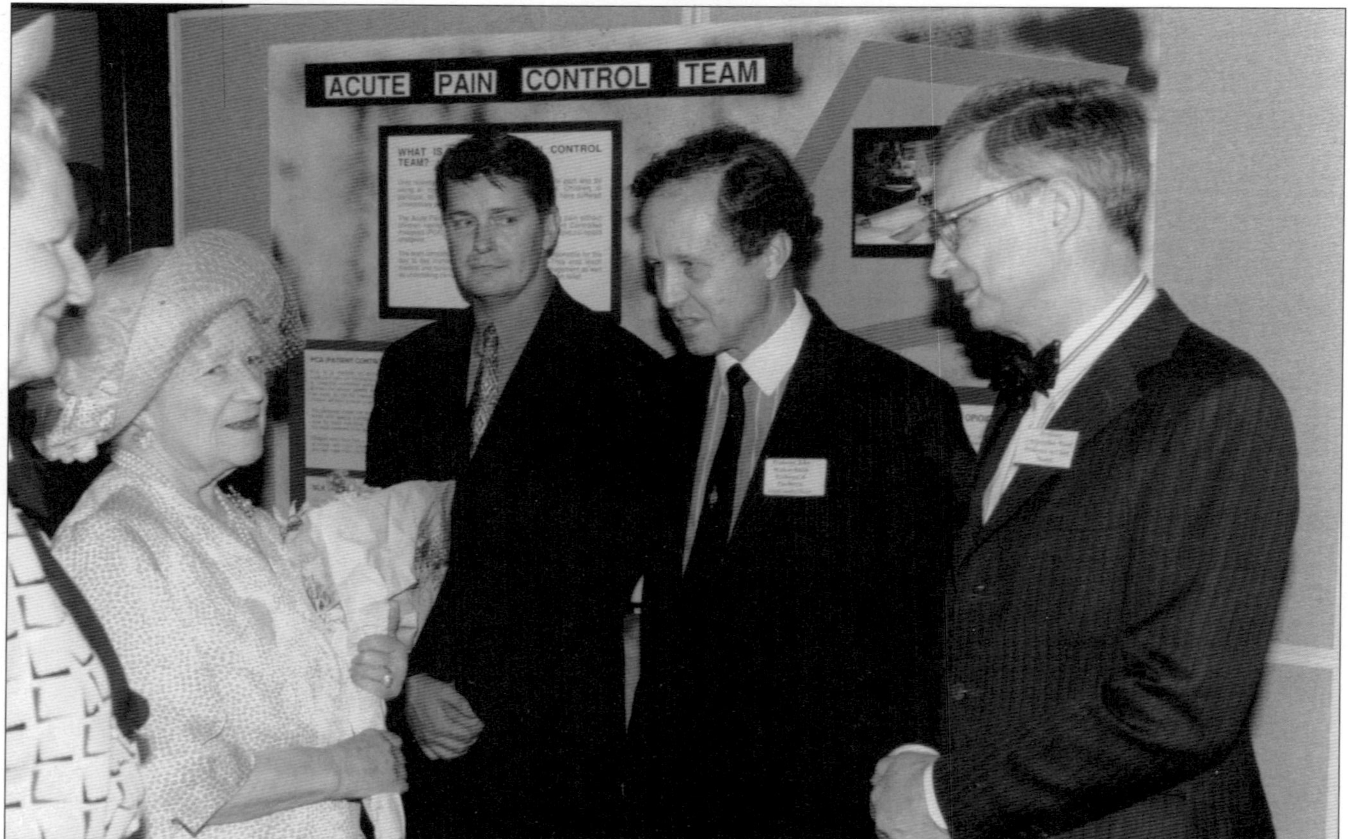

25. Visit of Queen Elizabeth the Queen Mother to Queen Elizabeth Hospital for Children for 125th anniversary of the hospital with Lady Riches on the left, an hospital administrator the Author and Professor Chris Wood, 1992

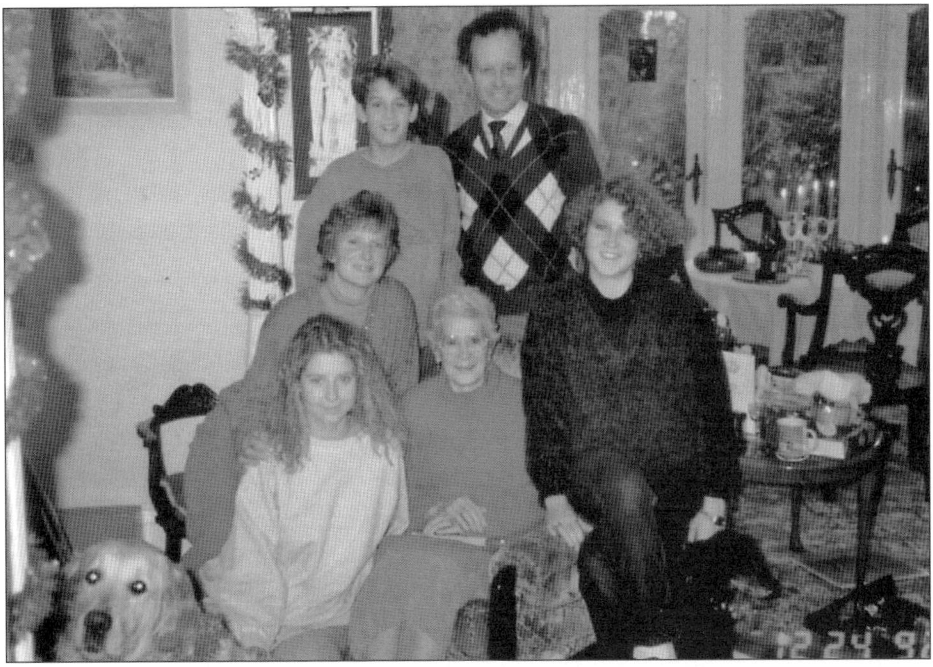

26. Family group at home of Author, from left to right: dog Louis, Laura, Liz, James, Mrs Isabelle Blaikie (wife's mother), Author and Louise, Christmas Eve 1992

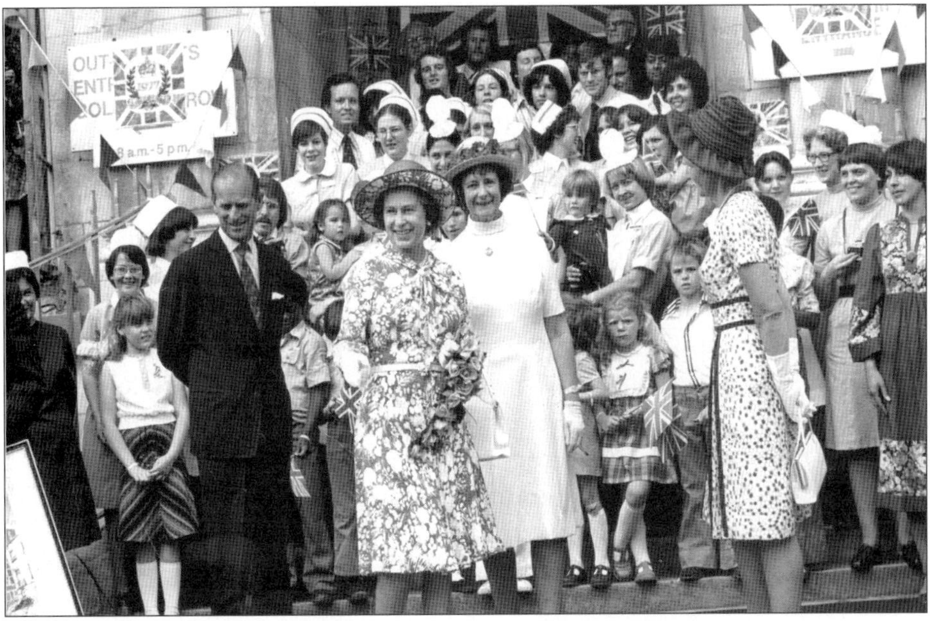

27. Visit of Queen Elizabeth II and Prince Phillip to entrance of Queen Elizabeth Hospital for Children on the occasion of the Queen's Silver Jubilee, with Mrs Audrey Callaghan, chairman of Board of Governors and Lady Riches plus patients and staff of the hospital, 1977

CHAPTER NINE

Specialist Paediatrician in Sydney, Planning the Future

THE NEXT FIVE YEARS were key years for me when the whole future shape of my life was decided. During the period 1967-1972, personally I married, had my first child, and my mother tragically and unexpectedly died six weeks later, professionally I obtained consultant status and decided that my future lay in London rather than Sydney.

On return to Sydney, I was appointed to the post of clinical supervisor (in reality, student supervisor) a half-time post combined with a temporary medical officer post in the Institute of Child Health which was also half-time, so making a full-time post overall. Graham Mortimer had vacated the supervisor post as he had returned to New Zealand. Rather astonishingly, I was appointed as an honorary associate physician, i.e. I was given honorary (i.e. consultant) status at the age of thirty years. I was pleased but worried whether I had enough experience. However in a relatively large department, I knew I had the benefit of supportive colleagues. I was to be a consultant for the next 33 years. However the next 5 years proved to be a period where planning for the future rather preoccupied me and I was pulled hither and thither. Before outlining my gastroenterology work I shall describe my changing status up till 1972 when I was appointed as staff physician in gastroenterology.

I had two offices, one for the clinical supervisor in the hospital adjacent to the main lecture theatre used for student teaching known as the Lorimer Dods theatre, the other was in the new ground floor laboratory in the newly completed Institute of Child Health building. This symbolized the continual tensions between the hospital and the Institute that I was to experience for the next five years. I was forever being pulled in two opposite directions.

The building of the new Institute of Child Health was a great triumph for Tom Stapleton, as at last he had proper teaching and laboratory facilities etc. The Institute was inaugurated on 12 May 1968 by Prince Philip, Duke of Edinburgh. I was very pleased to show him my laboratory and he was very interested to see intestinal villi looking down the dissecting microscope. Just over thirty years later I met him again at a reception given by the Britain Australia Society at St James's Palace with my wife Liz and son James who was just finishing at Bristol University. He was in good form and joked with James about getting on his bike! Back in Sydney it was quite a coup for Tom to have the Duke inaugurate his new building.

It is a remarkable and fortunate accident of my career that at each moment when I had a new beginning in the ICH in 1968, at QEHC in 1973 and at the Royal Free in 1995, I was given a brand new office in a newly built facility. This is always a tremendous boost to morale. It was for me a kind of renewal on each occasion.

A great advantage associated with the post of clinical supervisor was that there was a full time secretary for both the student work and my own secretarial needs. Eve Clark filled this position very ably. From the moment I achieved consultant status to have a good secretary was of key importance. In order to function adequately with all the growing demands made on one's time I quickly appreciated that a good secretary was a vital part of the professional team. I appreciated this even more as the years rolled by. This is especially important for an academic, with the double responsibility of service and university.

In my new life, I was pleased to be in charge of arrangements for the student course and being involved with medical undergraduates with quite a large teaching load. I liked teaching and I got on well with the students. I believe I have been an effective teacher despite no training whatever. I have had to learn as I have gone on. In addition I was happy to counsel students as need required, but for me this teaching post could not be a permanent position. This was not my life's work although it proved to give me invaluable experience for my future academic career. This position was but 'a step on the way', to give me employment as I built up gastroenterology on a part-time basis. The latter was of course a difficult task, but secretarial support for research paper writing etc. was invaluable help in its achievement. I was lucky to have Eve. I had no idea for how I long I wanted to be clinical supervisor. Tom Stapleton in conversation implied fairly indefinitely! I continued in fact till 1971.

My personal life now became of over-riding importance. I met my future wife Elizabeth Cantley Blaikie in 1968. In fact I met her in a complicated way in part via my medical connections. She had a Swiss flatmate who had a Swiss friend Willi Morgenthaler. Now I had met him through John Yu who had met him via some Hammersmith nurses who met him in Canada. So when Willi said he was going to Australia, they gave him an introduction to John Yu. So when Willi gave a fondue party he invited both Liz and me, there we met over a fondue bowl. Liz was a British migrant to Australia, she hailed from Edinburgh, Leith. She had come to Australia by sea, at the expense of the Australian government, apart from a fee of £12, provided she stayed two years. She had never been to England and was a staunch Scots patriot. When we were engaged my mother and father were delighted and dad especially appreciated the Scottish connection. It is not appropriate to go into details of my wedding at St Giles, Greenwich, my old parish church, suffice it to add that my dad generously gave us the gift of a return air ticket to have our honeymoon in Lucerne and then to go on to Edinburgh for me to meet Liz's mum, dad and family and also to go to Seaford to see Uncle Brian and Auntie Ethel. As I mentioned earlier, at the end of our honeymoon I was privileged to attend the European Society of Paediatric Gastroenterology meeting in the beautiful Swiss city of Interlaken between Lucerne and Edinburgh! In Interlaken we saw Charlotte Anderson and Michael Gracey from Australia, Beat Hadorn from Switzerland who had worked with Charlotte, and George Davidson from Canada amongst so many others who were to become my friends.

Returning now to my plans to develop gastroenterology, my personal focus was to undertake a MD based upon an analysis of the dissecting microscope appearances of the small intestine in children at post-mortem dying from both gastroenterological and non-gastroenterological causes. Looking back I am astonished that I was able to study as many as 116 child autopsies during the period 10 October 1967 to 11 August 1969. That so many children should have died in a children's hospital during this period of one year ten months shows how much we have advanced during the following thirty years. During my last five years at the Royal Free not one child died of a gastroenterological cause. Of course for this work to be a success, I had to have the support of Dr Douglas Reye and his department. This was generously given. David Shmerling, Alan Skyring and Charlotte Anderson gave me helpful advice and Tom Stapleton encouraged me throughout. The thesis was completed in 1970 and I was awarded the MD and attended the impressive degree conferring ceremony in the Great Hall of the University of Sydney in 1971.

Before that happy event, an even happier occasion was the birth of our firstborn Daughter Louise Juliette on 13/8/1970 in King George V Hospital. It was followed tragically six weeks later by my mother's death from a myocardial infarct. She died suddenly and unexpectedly within 24 hours.

This was a terrible loss for me.

In due time life had to go on and I continued developing the gastroenterology service. I was particularly indebted to the outstanding paediatric surgeon Arch Middleton who had a special interest in gastroenterological surgery. We established a joint gastroenterology/surgical outpatient consultation clinic, quite separate from my own gastroenterology outpatient clinic. This was quite invaluable to for my professional development and this clinic was a model for a similar one I was to establish with Vanessa Wright in future years at Queen Elizabeth Hospital for Children in London. I also shared consultant care of the gastroenteritis ward in rotation with an honorary, but I effectively made overall policy decisions for the ward. Dunlop ward, reserved for children with gastroenteritis, was 'down the hill' in the infectious disease block. This was geographically separate from the main hospital. This separate provision for children with infectious disease reflected the great concern in earlier years of the century concerning the risk of cross-infection within the hospital. In-patients with gastroenteritis were still very common at that time and children died even in hospital from dehydration due to gastroenteritis, despite modern intravenous fluid therapy.

The fact that viruses are one of the many infective causes of gastroenteritis had still not been discovered. Only three bacterial pathogens namely shigella, salmonella and enteropathogenic E.coli were recognized at that time as causes of infective gastroenteritis in children. These bacteria were found in the faeces on bacterial culture of about 25% of children with gastroenteritis requiring hospital admission. The rest of the children were diagnosed as non-bacterial gastroenteritis which was of quite unknown origin. I developed close links with David Dorman the hospital microbiologist and we did a study of the annual monthly admissions of children with gastroenteritis over the period 1961 to 1972. Interestingly, in 1964 there was for the very first time a winter peak in the number of admissions. This peak rose in that year to 949 children admitted, compared to 589 the previous year. Throughout this period (1967-1972) winter was the worst time for a surge in the number of admissions. I undertook a one year prospective study for 1970 of all gastroenteritis admissions. This was published in the Medical Journal of Australia in 1972. It confirmed the winter peak but also showed that children admitted as fee-paying as well as those who were not fee-paying (i.e. affluent versus non-affluent parents), still had a winter peak in admissions. This suggested that whatever agent was the cause of the gastroenteritis it was unlikely to be due to poor hygiene due to social deprivation. I stated that 'it must be assumed that the mere improvement in living standards will not lead automatically to a disappearance of gastroenteritis. Such measures may just result in a change in its aetiology (causation).' From Ruth Bishop at the Royal Children's Hospital in Melbourne in 1973 came the evidence that this winter peak was due to infection with a new and previously unknown virus, namely rotavirus. This virus was highly infectious and could spread from person to person very easily. This discovery was an historic break-through.

Gastroenteritis in children was to be one of the great interests of my life. I was to be consultant in charge of a gastroenteritis unit from 1967 to 1995 first at RAHC and then at QEHC. Looking back, our oral management of children with gastroenteritis at RAHC in the late sixties and early seventies was largely antediluvian. For oral therapy we used equal parts of sweetened condensed milk with equal parts of whey, whereas at QEHC when I arrived in 1973, a carefully formulated oral rehydration solution was being used and had been since 1952. In fact re-formulation followed later research with Michael Farthing some years in the future.

Another great interest now opened up, namely children with coeliac disease. I used the technique of gluten challenge following a period of gluten elimination related to serial changes in the small intestinal mucosa to make the diagnosis as I had been taught by David Shmerling, as soon as I returned to Sydney in 1967. This approach led me to recognize children with transient gluten intolerance. These were children, who when this diagnostic approach was used, did not have permanent gluten intolerance, i.e. coeliac disease. They had recovered from their gluten intolerance. All such children were under two years of age at onset of symptoms and gluten had been introduced very early into their diet. Publications also resulted from this work. Also an important study with Ken Kenrick of the Children's Medical Research Foundation (CMRF) of the serum immunoglobulin levels in children with coeliac disease was undertaken. We found elevated serum immunoglobulin A (IgA) levels especially in coeliac children under two years, which returned to normal on a gluten free diet. To my absolute delight this paper was published in *Gut*, my second paper in that prestigious journal.

All this publication lead to international recognition. As a direct result but quite 'out of the blue', I was delighted to be approached to answer a questionnaire concerning diagnostic criteria for coeliac disease being prepared by Jarmo Visakorpi of the new European Society of Paediatric Gastroenterology (founded in Paris in 1968) for their meeting to be held in Interlaken in 1969 on the Diagnostic Criteria for Coeliac Disease. So I was privileged to be party to the historic recommendations on diagnostic criteria for coeliac disease to be adopted in Interlaken. I also investigated a group of seven children with autism aged three to twelve years who had gastrointestinal symptoms to seek for evidence of coeliac disease. The study proved negative but little did I know that I would return to the issue of autistic children with bowel symptoms more than twenty years later at the Royal Free.

In 1970, the whole conception of Disease of the Small Bowel in Children was discussed in a paper I was invited to publish in the Postgraduate Medical Journal. This was followed by the publication of a Symposium on Disease of the Small Intestine in Children, which reported the proceedings of a meeting, convened in the Institute of Child Health in 1971. Diseases of the small intestine as an important area of paediatric gastroenterology were thus being recognized. Why was this? It related to the technological advance resulting from the increasing diagnostic use of small intestinal biopsy in children and the associated ability to assay the disaccharidases as mentioned earlier. As a result a number of paediatric centres internationally were coming to a consensus that there were a group of important diseases in children due to damage of the small intestinal mucosa from a variety of causes.

I also undertook some clinico-pathological studies. Liver disease was part of my remit unlike the future situation at QEHC. One of the most important case studies I undertook was in collaboration with Jeanette Blomfield of the CMRF. This concerned a child who tragically died from liver disease due to copper poisoning, from outback NSW. The farmhouse where he lived used water from a natural bore which was very acid (low pH). Tragically the house had had new copper pipes installed for drinking water. The acid water leached out the copper, and was present in the drinking water for the family in large amounts. This excess copper intake damaged the child's liver fatally. Copper assay of the water and of the child's organs, which was undertaken in the CMRF was key to this study. It was not published till 1973 in the *Archives of Disease of Childhood*, after I left Sydney, but it proved to be a very influential report in the long term for the understanding of Indian childhood cirrhosis. That disorder is related to excess copper intake from eating and drinking from copper vessels. In 1998 Beat Hadorn asked me to present a summary of the 1973 paper together with an account of the long-term outcome of its publication. This I did at the Emma-Thaler Symposium on Copper Associated Diseases in Children in Munich. I recalled how in 1979 six years after the paper was published Stuart Tanner asked me if Bernard Portmann and he could review the liver histology from the child who had died. I relayed this request to department of Pathology of RAHC who duly arranged for this to be done. Remarkably this review by Tanner and Portmann showed the changes present were indistinguishable from Indian Childhood Cirrhosis, thus providing strong supportive evidence that copper poisoning accounted for that illness. They published this observation with my collaboration in 1980. Immediately afterwards, our original paper of 1973, which had never been cited before their paper, began to be regularly cited in the medical literature with a peak number of citations occurring in 1996, twenty-five years later! I was reminded of the words of the poet Henry Wadsworth Longfellow in his poem '*The arrow and the song*'

> 'I shot an arrow in the air, it fell to earth I know not where.'

One of the fascinating things about publishing medical research results, one never knows if or when these may have unexpected positive outcomes. The report of the tragic death of a child from copper poisoning in Australia, contributed to the prevention of liver disease in Indian children.

I should perhaps mention at this point my long friendship and association with Beat Hadorn. I first had met him when he applied for, but withdrew from the senior laboratory post at the Institute of Child Health as I shall mention later in this chapter. He had been working with Charlotte Anderson in Melbourne on cystic fibrosis. We became immediate friends and met up again in Interlaken in 1969. Once I settled in London, we had regular contact with exchange of ideas and I visited his unit several times, and he mine. Finally I attended and reviewed transient gluten intolerance at his retirement meeting in 1999. He sang in the Great Hall at Barts at my retirement dinner in 2000. He has a marvellous voice and is also a talented painter, a man of many parts.

Another era of research developed unexpectedly strangely also involving copper. This concerned Menkes kinky hair syndrome which we showed was associated with copper malabsorption. It is a strange disorder diagnosed usually by an unusual kinky malformation of the hair visible on light microscopy and accompanied by severe mental retardation. Our efforts to treat children with this disorder by copper injections were disappointing. It later was discovered that there was a more general defect of copper transport throughout the body. As well as Jeanette Blomfield, or Brian Turner of the CMRF was a key player in this research. He was also to be a candidate for the post to which Peter Rowe was appointed. There were several publications from this work, showing that I had developed a very good collaborative role with the CMRF.

I also had four overseas research fellows who joined me during this period. First Tom Stapleton arranged for Jan Mangiwa and Pitono Soeparto from Indonesia and then there was Ramanand Kamath from Malaysia and Magdalena Araya a refugee with her husband from Allende's Chile. It was exciting developing research and training programmes for them and I was to continue contact with them for many years. I visited Pitono and Magdalena in their home countries many year later.

In 1968 I was fortunate to have my old friend George Soutter as the Professorial registrar. He had decided to settle in Australia in view of the uncertain situation in Rhodesia. How right he was. His wide breadth of paediatric knowledge was a great asset to us all.

Funding for the medical officer part of my post was not secure and so in 1970 Stapleton applied for me to have a Wellcome Clinical Research Fellowship to support my work on diseases of the small intestine. His application was successful and the Fellowship was awarded to me in 1971. This was my first connection with the Wellcome Trust, which was to continue intermittently over the years. I am very grateful for their considerable support over so many years. This Wellcome Fellowship gave me a full-time salary. Tom Stapleton was delighted and told me how prestigious it was but it did not cut much ice with my colleagues in Sydney. In fact the fellowship did not pay very much and it was of course for a finite period. I was quite unclear what the future might hold. In a way going back to holding a research fellowship whilst still having honorary (consultant) status, felt like a step backward rather than forward. A tenured post was now my clear goal. In fact I felt quite unsettled by this move. My own personal situation had now completely changed. By 1970 Liz and I had a baby Daughter Louise. So now for the first time, the size of my salary did matter very much to me, as well as future prospects. Tom found all this hard to understand.

Clearly my immediate goal was a senior lecturer position but because of the ever present uncertainty I was forced at this time into considering a tenured hospital staff position with some research opportunities, rather than a fully university position which seemed to be receding into the distant future, despite my success in publication in peer reviewed journals. My father had a phrase he liked to use 'O what a tangled web we weave'. The affairs of the Institute were web-like in their confusion to me at that time. Prof. Stapleton was adamant that a staff physician post in gastroenterology should not be advertised until university recognition, which he was seeking, was attached to the position. I had written in a letter to the university authorities that I wanted such a post with senior lecturer status. Stapleton persuaded me, for his own (unexplained) tactical reasons, that I should withdraw the letter which I did reluctantly. One of the hospital honoraries Don Hamilton came to see me quite shocked that I had done this. I felt I was a pawn in some high strategy game. So I told him I was indeed still interested in the post of staff physician in gastroenterology even without university recognition and I wrote a letter accordingly. This was in January 1972. I was in due course appointed to this newly created hospital post (without mention of university recognition) to Stapleton's chagrin. He felt I had let him down. I moved to a new office and was joined later by a band of staff physicians, appointed subsequently, including John Yu. An unfortunate by-product was I now had much reduced secretarial services, quite a blow as my research activities were blossoming. John Yu also moved over to the hospital, also with Stapleton's displeasure. It was all such a great pity, as I was grateful for all Tom had done for me in the past. Indeed I agreed to remain in charge of the gastroenterology laboratory in the Institute, continuing clinical research.

At this time Tom Stapleton was a bespectacled, balding man slightly stooped who spoke with an accent described in Australia as Oxford, associated in Britain with a Public School education. He would say things like 'Oh John, there has been the most frightful kerfuffle about...'. He then would regale me with the latest crisis in university or medical politics. He was not a man who fitted easily into the Australian scene but his intentions for the improvement of paediatrics in Sydney were of the highest.

Looking back at this period it was a time of considerable productivity in both development of the gastroenterological service, which was flourishing, and the production of a number of publications in peer reviewed journals. However medical politics overhung everything and even with a tenured post I felt quite unsure what the future held for my clinical research activities in the Institute.

A further problem for me was my great disappointment that I had no shared research interest with Peter Rowe who had eventually been appointed as Associate Professor. I liked Peter a great deal and he was clearly a high achiever but fundamental research along American lines unrelated to clinical issues was his clear focus. When Peter was appointed he was one of three initial candidates I mentioned above. The other two were first Beat Hadorn from Switzerland. After visiting to consider the post, when he saw the medical politics he withdrew. I sometimes think how different my life might have been if he had been appointed. I should probably have stayed permanently in Sydney. The unsuccessful candidate was Brian Turner who again was a clinical investigator but who was to die tragically young. There is no doubt that Peter Rowe's appointment has been very successful in the long term, but for me personally it was a clear signal that I should begin to look beyond the Institute.

At that time socializing at lunch was great fun. We usually all ate together informally with sandwiches etc. in the Institute tea room. We were often joined by Norma Porteous a dynamic psycho-analytically minded social worker who like Tom was a great advocate of Sigmund Freud. We therefore used to often have animated discussions about psycho-analysis, university politics, world politics, religion etc. The extraordinary visit to Sydney of L.B. Johnson, the first American President to visit Australia, was fiercely debated. The effusive words of the Australian Prime Minister Harold Holt 'All the way with LBJ!' divided us down the middle. We formed indeed a very diverse group with a broad spectrum from left to right and from atheism to evangelical Christianity. I was to miss all this very much when I left.

However in August 1972, I was sitting in the gastroenterology laboratory in the Institute of Child Health browsing through the *Lancet*, and I chanced upon the job advertisements section. I came across an advertisement for the post of consultant/senior lecturer in child health at St Bartholomew's Hospital (Barts) and Queen Elizabeth Hospital for Children (QEHC or Queens) in London. It arrested my attention immediately. I had very warm memories of Barts, as I have mentioned earlier. I was much aware of its time honoured reputation as one of the great traditional centres of British Medicine. Furthermore I was also very much aware of the distinguished department of adult gastroenterology lead by Tony Dawson with its interest in small bowel disorders. This was of course my own area of special interest, albeit in children. I had never visited Queens but was aware of its fine reputation in paediatrics.

The scene in Sydney in 1972 was still unsatisfactory for me as I have already outlined. Despite my tenured appointment as Staff Physician in Gastroenterology, I continued to have two positions, one in the hospital and one in the Institute, which was honorary. There was dual accountability to the respective authorities. This boiled down to John Yu who had become physician in charge of medicine in the hospital and Tom Stapleton in the Institute. There were already clear tensions between them both. A further source of tension for me related to Professor Stapleton's recently appointment of Peter Rowe to lead the Institute's research programme with his approach towards fundamental research, away from clinical or applied research. This seemed to me to be in conflict with my own task to create a new discipline, i.e. paediatric gastroenterology, with both a clinical and a research (academic) component. At that time despite the development of paediatric gastroenterology at the Royal Children's Hospital in Melbourne, led by Charlotte Anderson, I in Sydney felt very remote from the great centres of paediatrics and adult gastroenterology in the Northern Hemisphere. I had enormously benefited from my training in adult gastroenterology in London and later paediatric gastroenterology in Zurich. I had learnt so much more abroad than ever I had in Sydney. I had been really excited by visiting centres in Canada and the United States. The meeting of the European Society of Gastroenterology in Interlaken in 1969 had shown me the excitements and practical benefits of mixing with fellow enthusiasts for our new discipline, who, surprisingly, were often the same age as me. Ours was a young and emerging discipline. To have been present in 1969 at the historic meeting in Interlaken which laid down the diagnostic criteria for coeliac disease in childhood (later known as the ESPGHAN criteria) had been a great privilege and advantage for me right up to the present.

I admired Charlotte Anderson very much, but whilst being personally friendly, she had made me feel I was a rather junior rival to her research department. My junior status was undoubtedly true but she did nothing to encourage my lonely solo task at the RAHC. Indeed she had made one, rather patronizing, visit to my unit which had rather depressed me. Although she did offer good advice in relation to my MD later on and I was grateful for this. Little did I realize that she herself was to move to England some years in the future, in 1968. Looking back, my feelings also in part related to the traditional rivalry between Sydney and Melbourne. This in turn related to the long history of competition between these two cities, which had been capitals of two separate colonies until federation in 1901. At that time I am afraid that I myself would have much preferred to go to London or elsewhere overseas, than to go to Melbourne for training! Another general circumstance was the lack of any local paediatric gastroenterology professional fora in Australia. Sydney and Melbourne at that time were the only centres.

Although as already outlined I had established a new paediatric gastroenterology service at RAHC and begun an independent research programme, I felt professionally lonely and unsupported in my new discipline in Sydney. By contrast I had been very, very happy in London. At that point I looked on them as the happiest days of my professional life. I also felt that the tensions between the Institute and the hospital appeared irresolvable and would progressively sap my morale for years to come. I was also torn between the choice of being an organ specialist or an academic. I wanted to be both.

After much reflection that day, I went home and told my wife Liz that I thought I should apply for the job at Barts. She characteristically was very supporting and her advice was go for it! Within 24 hours I had sent in my application with my curriculum vitae by airmail. The application had itself been difficult. I did not know exactly what was required and John Yu, (appointed staff physician in paediatrics shortly after me) with his own knowledge of the UK scene, was practically helpful with this task. One immediate problem was to decide upon the names of three referees, to support my application.

I realized of course that I was very unlikely to get the post. By applying and failing I would very much weaken my position at the RAHC. So I decided therefore, to ask Sir Christopher Booth, my original mentor in gastroenterology at the Royal Postgraduate Medical School in London, and Professor Andrea Prader of Zurich to be referees. From Sydney I asked Professor Julian Katz, Professor of Child Psychiatry in the Institute of Child Health to act as referee. I had already consulted him about the wisdom of my decision to apply for the Barts job. He was most enthusiastic and felt it was a great career move for me and the right decision to take. He felt for my peace of mind I needed to leave RAHC. So John and Julian were the only local colleagues who were aware of my application.

Then came the wait. It was agonizingly long. Eventually I was astonished, but delighted, to get an airmail letter telling me that I had been invited to London for interview. I had of course to pay my own airfare. Time was short. First I had to be certain that I had a real chance of being appointed and that there was not some local favoured candidate, with the interview just a charade! There was a telephone number on the letterhead, for Dr Patrick Cox, physician in charge of the Department of Child Health at Barts. With some difficulty, involving several telephone calls, I managed at last to arrange a time when we could speak. He was characteristically blunt and straightforward. Yes I did have a real chance. I would not have been invited from Australia, with the air flight involved etc. If I had not been a serious candidate. There was no local favoured candidate. However it was by no means certain I would be appointed. All would depend upon the interview and appointments board!

So I booked my flight with Qantas and within a few days I was off to London. On the way we stopped over at Hong Kong, Delhi, Teheran and Vienna, a great contrast to the current single stop-over. It was a long, long flight. I finally arrived on a Saturday morning on a dull September day, staying at the President Hotel Russell Square. Patrick Cox came to pick me up and drove me to Barts. I felt a real glow of pleasure, anticipation and fear as we drove under (what seemed to me, to be) the hallowed portals of the Henry VIII gate, to park in the marvellous square with its beautiful fountain and trees. Years later I was to come across the poem by Sir John Betjeman on St Bartholomew's Hospital where he spoke of its fountain etc. being hallowed.

The ghost of Rahere still walks at Barts
It gives an impulse to generous hearts,
It looks on pain with a pitying eye,
It teaches us never to fear to die.
Eight hundred years of compassion and care

Have hallowed its fountain, stones and square.
Pray for us all as we near the gate,
St Barts the Less and St Barts the Great.

John Beijeman

This square with its fountain was to become the emotional centre of my professional life thereafter, even with the winter 2001 meeting of British Society of Paediatric Gastroenterology, Hepatology and Nutrition held at Barts.

My son was years later to be baptized in the church of St Bartholomew the Less within the hospital itself. Strangely early in 1973 my wife, daughter and I sat next to Sir John Betjeman at a service at St Paul's Cathedral. He at that time lived in Cloth Fair just opposite the church of St Bartholomew the Great. The ground floor of the house is now a quite expensive restaurant called Betjeman's where we have had occasionally some informal Bart's social occasions.

However going back to 1972, I must admit to disappointment at the poor physical state of the two children's wards, Kenton (top floor of the Lucas Block) and Lucas. They had been built in the early nineteenth century and had impressively tall windows but they looked archaic and not like any modern hospital. The consultant and secretarial offices were quite inadequate. The state of the children's outpatients was even worse, this time on the first floor of an eighteenth century block. It did however have one large clinic room with space for students where the new consultant would see patients. The new consultant was to succeed Dr Alfred White Franklin who had retired two years earlier and was to be notionally in charge of Kenton ward, whereas Dr Cox was in charge of Lucas ward. However Kenton ward seemed already to be largely full of child oncology patients cared for by Professor Jim Malpas. There did not appear to be much room for expanding to include paediatric gastroenterology patients. There were two other paediatric consultants at Barts, Prof. Chris Wood who did one outpatient clinic and had an occasional inpatient and Dr Geoff Udall who was a senior lecturer in developmental paediatrics but who did not have in-patients.

Patrick Cox arranged to have lunch at Simpson's on Strand, my favourite watering hole in London, with Professor Chris Wood joining us. They both jokingly reminded me that this was not the usual way consultants lunched. Still it was a most enjoyable meal. Whilst I was all too aware that my candidacy for the post was being probed I was also able to obtain valuable background information.

After lunch we drove to Queen Elizabeth Hospital for Children in Hackney

Road situated in Bethnal Green in the east end. There can be no disguising my shock when suddenly as we drove down Hackney Road, the grey building of the Hospital loomed up above us on a rather gloomy day and we drove down a grotty lane beside the hospital to the large parking area. What a depressing gloomy environment and what a contrast to sunny Sydney! Was I mad to be in London? However Chris took us into a modern newly built research block, the Haywards Building, at the back of the hospital. We went up in the lift to the fifth floor and visited the new academic department. This included an excellent library and the previously unoccupied and quite spacious office for the new position. This post was indeed a new creation, as was the academic department itself. It linked a new part time senior lecturer post at Queens with the part time position vacated by Dr White Franklin at Barts.

Chris Wood was a young man recently appointed from Bristol and I felt he would clearly be a less stressful colleague for me than Tom Stapleton.

We visited the entire building and I was impressed by the facilities. They were not luxurious but very satisfactory. I was especially pleased to see there was an electron microscope, although no electron microscopist had yet been appointed. I had been associated with electron microscopy of the small intestinal mucosa of children with coeliac disease in Sydney as the research fellow I was supervising, Dr Magdalena Araya, was doing this project.

By contrast the hospital itself proved to be in poor state of repair, although Professor Wood and the new appointee had restored some wards including Barclay ward, which housed the new Professorial Unit, which would be shared. Observation ward, where children with gastroenteritis and other infective diseases were admitted, however, had not been significantly changed since it had opened in 1948. However it did provide a separate cubicle for each child and there was room for a temporary bed to be put up for a mother in each. In its day it had in fact been a pioneer in design. Gastroenteritis was one of my major research interests so I was pleased to see these isolation facilities, which in fact were better than those in Sydney, despite the antique architecture.

After these visits I returned to my hotel to reflect. Should I withdraw and return home? Clearly much of the facilities at both hospitals were far inferior to anything we had at RAHC and indeed anything I had ever seen in Australia. Yet I was excited by the historic ambience of Barts and its aura of past achievements, for me an inspiration for the future. Both Patrick and Chris impressed me in their different ways. I thought they would be supportive colleagues.

My spirits rose on Monday morning, 11 September, when I met Tony

Dawson and saw his impressive gastroenterology laboratory, but more importantly his enthusiastic support for paediatric gastroenterology was most encouraging. It was also obvious that he was a man of high intellect with considerable leadership skills, a man of power and influence. He was a maker and a shaker in this world. I felt honoured to have the chance to work with him. He himself had been appointed as a general physician and had had to fight to create a department of gastroenterology. He made clear to me the enormity of the task of developing paediatric gastroenterology at Barts but he pointed out there would be opportunities for developing research both at Barts and Queens. He would give me his support if I were appointed. He would not be on the appointment committee, as the job advertisement was not asking for a paediatric gastroenterologist, so I would have to make the case to the appointments committee that a paediatric gastroenterologist would provide the best value both academically and clinically for the post.

In the late afternoon of Monday, I duly appeared at Barts and was taken to wait with the other candidates for interview in a smallish gloomy room on the ground floor of the Clerk's Wing. I was introduced as having just flown in from Australia. It was obvious that this information surprised and even dismayed the other candidates. There was at first a profound silence. Then there were some probing questions. I was astonished that the mother of one of the candidates was present. Was I really Australian, not just living there? When I said I was, this was again followed by an incredulous silence. I was of course familiar with the psychological warfare that is often waged when waiting for medical interview. In Australia there were at that time no interviews prior to appointment. I said as little as I could, but I hope gave as well as I got, when forced to speak. It was not a pleasant time. Resignedly I waited to be the last called for interview. Having a surname beginning with W made me all too familiar with the routine of usually being the last candidate, on a variety of occasions from school days onwards. At last the door opened. It was my turn to be led up the staircase into a grand, indeed beautiful, room, the Guild Room. This panelled room I had never seen before, but in future years it was to become very well known to me as a meeting room, culminating in 1994 with the drama of the visit of Sir David Hull for the Tomlinson Report which appeared to signal the end of Barts. The room was overlooked by a large and impressive portrait of the eighteenth century doctor, Percival Pott. It was however, dominated by a large rectangular table. Around it sat some very eminent figures. There was the Professor of Medicine, Professor Eric Scowen (a rather intimidating figure with large bald head, black horn-rimmed glasses with enigmatic eyes), Miss Turner (Administration) Dr Philip

Evans and Dr Martin Barrett of Great Ormond St, as well as the somewhat more familiar figures of Chris Wood and Patrick Cox. However there was no one there who I had known or had known me for more than two days. I was on my own.

The interview was gruelling and probing. I tried to make the case for paediatric specialties in general and paediatric gastroenterology in particular. I quoted the document published by the British Paediatric Association, 'Paediatrics in the Seventies', edited by Donald Court. My lack of training in neonatal medicine was referred to. I emphasized my proposed link with Dr Dawson and his team. Why did I want to leave the beauties of Sydney etc? I just did not know how I was doing.

After the conclusion of the interview, which seemed interminable, I was led back downstairs to wait. This time the candidates said little. We waited in melancholic agitation. The wait was not very long. The door suddenly opened 'Dr Walker-Smith, would you please accompany me?' I jumped up nervously and mounted the stairs with my heart beating fast. I entered the Guild Room. I was offered a seat once more, at the end of the long table. The lay chairman then, to my real amazement, offered me the post (subject to ratification by the Medical School at its next meeting.) I rapidly accepted. There were smiles and congratulations all around the table. My head spun. Yet for a moment I wondered if I was mad to accept. Would my wife and daughter be as happy in London as Sydney? I could see Patrick Cox looking at me quizzically. Maybe he could read this thought. Then with the congratulatory mood and the offer of a glass of wine, my spirits soared and I exulted in the most dramatic move in my professional life that I had ever undertaken or would ever undertake again. The talk was all then of where I should live, south or north of the Thames, when would I arrive, etc., etc. Practicalities and immediate farewells to my new colleagues followed rapidly and I dashed away to telephone the news to my wife Liz in Sydney and also to my dad who I knew would be so pleased but very sad to lose us.

Looking back now I realize it was Barts and Barts alone that drew me to London. Despite the problems I have mentioned earlier there was simply nowhere else in the UK that could have taken me away from all that I already had in Sydney. Years later, in 1995, it was this that made it so hard at first for me to accept the invitation to transfer to the Royal Free Hospital.

The next day I flew home to Sydney. On return I was inhibited about telling my colleagues what had happened until the medical school had ratified the committee decision. However the news leaked out. Understandably Tom Stapleton was both angry and hurt. He was almost unbelieving that I had actually been able to secure a consultant post at a great centre such as Barts without his help. I believe he had my welfare at heart but he under-estimated my abilities. He did not understand that I had to make my own decisions for my own life. I remain very grateful for all his help and support over the years. There was consternation in the hospital administration and the general manager was not pleased. After all I had only been appointed as staff physician earlier in the year and I had just created a new and successful department of Gastroenterology. Sadly my move did indeed upset some of my closest and most valued colleagues and allies such as the paediatric surgeon Archie Middleton and the radiologist Denby Bowdler, with whom I had worked so closely. I regretted this very much. Some of my own friends felt I had made a bad decision, others like Phil Thompson that I had made a very good one, but Liz and I were pleased by the prospect of a great adventure.

However it did seem to me to be vital that the new department of gastroenterology I had recently created at RAHC should continue with a good leader. I also had to consider the interests of my research fellow Dr Magdalena Araya who was inconvenienced by my departure and needed a supervisor for her research project. The obvious candidate it seemed to me was Dr Ramanand Karnath FRACP of Kuala Lumpur who had been a very successful research fellow with me. I knew him to be an outstanding clinician and I knew he would lead a clinical team very well. I telephoned him and he was very interested. Of course the job was not in my gift and Stapleton preferred Reub Dubois, an Australian who was then in Denver Colorado. Ultimately an appointment committee recommended Ramanand and he was duly appointed. My faith in him has been amply rewarded by his success in expanding the department over the years and his appointment as Associate Professor. In 1993 I was delighted for him to come to London and do my locum for three months whilst I was on sabbatical leave at the Wellcome Institute for the History of Medicine. Reub Dubois, also a very good colleague, was later appointed to the Institute.

In the end I was given a great send off from the hospital. My wife Liz, Daughter Louise and I duly sailed from Sydney in the MV *Britannis* of the Chandris Line in December 1972. It was my father who most regretted our departure and his sense of loss was so great that he could not bear to come to the ship for our farewell. Part of him was delighted we were settling in a land he loved so much, but a greater part regretted the loss of part of his family. He was to visit us in England several times but died in Canberra 26/2/1975 a few days before his two grand-daughters were born, our Laura in London and her Cousin Christine, Judith's daughter in Canberra. To my great regret I could not go out to Australia for his funeral because of our baby's imminent birth. The tyranny of distance is all too real on such family occasions. It is hard to have family in two countries on opposite sides of the world. In fact Liz and I with Louise and new baby Laura were able later to attend a wonderful memorial service held for dad at the Prince Alfred Hospital Chapel in Sydney. There was a large gathering of my entire family, dad's friends and colleagues and remarkably a number of his old patients. His favourite disciple Dr Lou Wheeler, one of his successors at Prince Alfred, gave a moving address appropriately the Presbyterian chaplain conducted the service. A plaque in his memory is there to this day. A reception was hosted by the hospital in the boardroom in the old Princes Block.

Returning to December 1972, we had farewelled my sister Judith and her cardiologist husband Howard Peak in Canberra a few days before we left Sydney. So at the wharf to wish us farewell was my Auntie Lella (as ever) and my dear Cousin Joan Buswell and one of my oldest friends Phil Thompson with his wife. It was a poignant moment, as the coloured streamers connecting us to the shore broke signalling my permanent move away from the land of my birth and my journey back to the land of my ancestors.

However it was not long before Liz and I were excited to be travelling on our great adventure. We had chosen to travel the old fashioned long way by sea rather than by air to have a holiday after all the exertions of 1972. For me it was an appropriately long break to signal the end of my old life and the beginning of a new one.

By 1972 the number of ships travelling to and fro between Britain and Australia had dramatically reduced from earlier times. However it was still possible to make the traditional voyage, which is no longer the case (other than a modern cruise, for part of the journey which is still possible). In fact the Chandris Line, a Greek shipping company, was one of the last shipping lines to provide such a service. The ship appeared full and interestingly had on board many English migrants to Australia, who had been disillusioned by Australia, and were returning home. These are what Australians call the whinging poms! We shared a table throughout the voyage with two young cockneys returning to London.

Our memorable voyage took us via Wellington in New Zealand, then on to Tahiti with its beautiful beaches of back volcanic sand, and so to the Panama Canal with a stop at Panama City. We were able to make brief visits to each. Then we called at the Dutch island colony of Curacao in the West Indies, sampling some of the delicious local liqueur and then on to the Atlantic Ocean. We had fine weather up till then, but bad weather arrived in the North Atlantic. This led us to miss our planned visit to the Azores. As we approached England the weather got very much worse. Alarmingly the ship developed a noticeable list to starboard in mountainous seas with twenty-foot waves. The ship's company disturbingly 'split' between the officers and the crew with frank hostility expressed openly between them. We learnt that the Officers supported the 'Colonels' who by a coup d'etat had taken over the government in Athens. We were advised even more alarmingly to wear our life jackets. Fortunately the weather eventually abated and the ship regained its balance and we arrived at Southampton, albeit 36 hours late. This meant when we duly arrived late at the Charing Cross Hotel, our booking had been cancelled, as the shipping company had not informed the hotel of our delayed arrival. After some haggling a room was found. The next night my two year-old Daughter Louise had a bad attack of croup. I almost first arrived at Barts as a parent of a sick child. Fortunately after placing her in the bathroom amidst all the steam generated by turning on the hot water taps, she recovered fairly quickly.

We duly arrived the next day, at the Barts Hospital flat arranged for us, on the ground floor of a block of flats in Charterhouse Square. A whole new future lay ahead of us.

Had we made the right move?

CHAPTER TEN

Young Academic in London, Fighting the Corner

OUR ARRIVAL AT OUR hospital flat in Charterhouse Square was not the most propitious. It had only one bedroom. This we needed for Louise. Then there was one large living room where Liz and I both lived and slept. Worst of all, most things were covered with a dusting of what looked like soot. There had been some delay in our arrival after my appointment, the previous September. So the flat had been ready for us for some time, but had not been recently cleaned. This was not a good start, but the neighbourhood delighted us. We were right in the heart of the city close to St Paul's Cathedral and only five minutes from Barts. It was a great luxury to live so close to where I worked. Although I also was to work at Queen Elizabeth Hospital for Children (QEHC or Queens) in Hackney Road, that was only a fifteen-minute bus ride away. I had a warm welcome from Patrick Cox on my first day at Barts hospital and he showed me the ropes. He and his wife very soon asked us for Sunday lunch, the first of many happy visits to their home. Louise had the joyful experience of catching frogs in their garden pond for the first time in her life. This was to become a passion for her. Next day, I visited Queens and was delighted to find I had been given a fine brand new and large office on the fifth floor of the Hayward building, with interesting views over London. Chris Wood and my first clinical lecturer Malcolm Boyce gave me a very warm welcome. I was glad I had come.

Later in the week, I met Tony Dawson again at Barts and also had a warm welcome from him, and this was accompanied by an offer of access to his laboratory. He was to become my only mentor and role model at Barts. He was a wise man with very sound clinical judgement, an outstanding doctor. He was white haired and quite tall but walked with a marked limp, owing to a long-standing disability of one leg. This was never mentioned. The half lens glasses he wore were in the style popularized by Sir Alec Douglas-Home, and these added to his aura of distinction. I attended regularly at the adult weekly activities of his department namely, the weekly gastroenterology clinical meeting, the radiology/gastroenterology meeting and the journal club at Friday lunchtime, for most weeks until I left Barts 22 years later. This close link with adult colleagues was immensely valuable to my professional development and also for my younger colleagues. Tony Dawson very soon invited Liz and me to their home for dinner, the first of many occasions.

Tony Dawson's example concerning the best way to run a research department was a very great help to me. One example was his requirement that any presentation to be made at any national or international, medical or scientific meeting, by a member of the department, should be rehearsed in advance. I adopted this practice for my own unit. He would assemble the whole department with a 'three line whip', the department member, at whatever level of seniority, would make the conventional ten minute presentation. Then from all and sundry, there would be fierce, but constructive, criticism. This included criticism of the visual aids used. In those days these were projected photographic slides. The Medical Illustration Department staff prepared graphs and typed statements, which were then photographed by the staff of the Photographic Department. This was a time consuming business. Often Tony Dawson during the rehearsal would insist that the unfortunate presenter would have to change most of the slides. This often meant grovelling to illustration and photographic staff, beseeching them to find time to make the revisions, because of the meeting deadline. Tony Dawson was oblivious to such practicalities, but demanded that the alterations etc. must be made. What a difference there is now in the twenty-first century in the age of the computer. The use of Power Point with computer prepared presentations has almost become the 'norm'. With this system, alterations to 'slides' can now be made in minutes. Visual aids for presentations since the late nineties have been transformed. Going back to the seventies to Tony Dawson, sometimes there would be second and even third rehearsals. Now Tony had been known on occasion to contradict himself at a second rehearsal, saying the exact reverse of what he had said before, as we are all prone to do on occasion. Once an intrepid junior doctor recorded his words and confronted Dr Dawson, when he re-played his words, after Tony had contradicted himself This was a *cause célèbre* amongst the junior doctors. Tony did have a very grand demeanour with his white hair and elegant manner of speech. He was a real 'figure' in the Victorian model, despite his devotion to science and the modern world. I am enormously in his debt and I mourned his passing in 1997.

Several days after I arrived in London, I had an astonishing telephone call at Barts from an immigration officer telling me that the stamp in my passport which had given me the right of indefinite entry to the UK was incorrect. I should send my passport to him for alteration to a limited stay! I discussed this with the hospital administration and was firmly advised not to send my passport anywhere. I was most disconcerted, as I had sold everything I owned in Australia and I had just taken up a permanent position in London. I did however have great faith in British democracy so I wrote a letter each to the Prime Minister Edward Heath and to the leader of the Opposition Harold Wilson explaining my plight. As an Australian I always felt it best to go to the top. So I took the tube to Westminster and walked to the entrance to Parliament and gave my letters to the policeman I encountered there and he kindly passed them on. This action produced a furore of activity and within days I had an apology from the immigration officer and I was told that my passport had in fact been correctly stamped. This boosted my respect for British democracy but I had expected nothing less.

I must now try and explain the complex post to which I had been appointed. It was a joint academic and NHS position on two sites. My position was in the local jargon, an A plus B appointment. I had dual status as a senior lecturer of the University of London within the Joint Academic Department of Child Health of the Medical School of St Bartholomew's Hospital and the Medical School of the London Hospital (this academic department was situated at Queen Elizabeth Hospital for Children in the east end of London at Hackney Rd) and as a NHS consultant paediatrician at St Bartholomew's Hospital situated in the heart of the city of London. As I said I had been appointed to a very complex post, on the verge of being unworkable, but I was determined to make it work. Furthermore my salary came from two sources the Medical School of St Bartholomew's Hospital and the National Health Service, with two superannuating schemes! Sadly the finance department of the medical school did not draw my attention for this dual need for superannuation for many many months. This dual salary also caused a problem for me, when the building society, from which I was later on to seek a mortgage, only consulted the medical school, for a confidential enquiry about the size of my salary. I nearly failed to get the mortgage! This difficult, dual salary came to an end some years later, when I was promoted to Readership, when my salary entirely came from the medical school. So the whole thing was not an easy business.

The new Joint Academic Department of Child Health situated at Queen Elizabeth hospital for Children, established in 1972 (at the time of my interview in September 1972 Prof. Wood was just taking up his position), found itself in a very complex situation. In the 1960s it had become apparent that the education of undergraduates in paediatrics in London was lamentably poor. London University had not kept pace with the academic achievements of paediatricians elsewhere in the United Kingdom. A British Paediatric Association report on this matter (Jackson Report) coincided with the Todd Commission, which investigated the future structure of the medical schools of the University of London. By serendipity I had met Lord Todd at a barbecue given by Professor Bob Walsh in their home in Epping, a suburb of Sydney, in 1971 and chatted about his schemes for London University. Little did I imagine that I would be working in London myself so soon and that I would be trying to work in the scenario he had recommended.

Despite a great deal of hostility, the Todd Commission recommended pairing of Medical Schools to 'achieve economy of resources and to enhance academic function' (how I hate such phrases, which experience has taught me are not true!). The first such joint department in London was ours! Little did I know that these schemes of jointness and mergers were to extend and develop and become a perpetual feature and distraction, overshadowing my entire future academic career. I grew to hate the word 'joint' it was all so unrealistic and impractical.

Yet, in practice for us, in 1973 this pairing meant that the students of both Barts and the London did have the advantage of being educated in the second largest children's unit in London at Queen Elizabeth Hospital for Children. It was a marvellous teaching resource. However the situation was even more complex as QEHC was administered jointly with Great Ormond St Hospital (GOS) to form the Hospitals for Sick Children. This in turn was part of the British Postgraduate Medical Federation. For most of my subsequent career in the department there were perpetual problems between the staff of these two hospitals linked together, in what clearly proved to be an unhappy marriage. Prof. John Soothill expressed the view that the greater (i.e. GOS) would always parasitize the less i.e. (QEHC).

The consequences of all these linkages were that undergraduate and postgraduate institutions were integrated for teaching undergraduates. So this meant that the staffs of the Institute of Child Health as well of Great Ormond St were to take a small share in teaching undergraduates and indeed a share of patient care at Hackney Road. So the undergraduates were to be taught by these post-graduate staff members plus the staff of Barts, the London and QEHC! It seemed to me from day one, that organization of all these interactions was an administrative or bureaucratic nightmare for teaching, patient care and research. Although it had to be admitted that the whole concept did have its visionary dimension and opened up the possibility of a remarkable centre for paediatrics. However the administrative resources were never given to pull all these institutions together on four geographic sites, some way apart from each other. Travel in London's heavy traffic or by inefficient and unreliable public transport lead to many unexpected problems. Furthermore the local loyalties of the staff of the individual institutions meant there was a great deal of time lost in petty squabbles in the numerous and proliferating committees concerning the role of these institutions per se in the medical schools themselves. Academic paediatrics never had the influence that the other 'big hitters' such as medicine and surgery had in the medical schools of Barts and the London, until near the end when Lesley Rees was Dean of Barts. It was only in her time that the importance of paediatrics came to the top of the academic agenda of the medical schools. There was perpetual tension and sometimes frank hostility between GOS and QEHC at several levels including doctors, nurses and laboratory staff. Ultimately, after much pain, some years later, following the recommendation of the Tomlinson Report in 1993, the whole system was abandoned. But this will be discussed later.

Returning now to my personal situation in 1973, professionally I had a dual role with my clinical and research activities at Queen Elizabeth Hospital being confined to gastroenterology, whereas at Barts I practised both general paediatrics and paediatric gastroenterology, with the expectation I would develop a research programme on both sites. Paediatric gastroenterology had to be developed entirely from scratch at Barts, as it had not previously existed there. Although as already discussed above, there was a very distinguished adult gastroenterology department lead by Tony Dawson. By contrast although gastroenterology in children had already existed in practice at Queen Elizabeth Hospital for Children from the time of Dr Winifred Young in the 1950s it had been a part of general paediatrics, rather than a specialism in its own right. Her theme had been to foster clinical research rather than found a new discipline within paediatrics. When I arrived Dr Brian Wharton had some interest in this area, he ran an efficient coeliac disease follow-up clinic, although his chief interest was in nutrition. In this small world of paediatrics, I had previously met Brian at the Colloquium on Protein Calorie Malnutrition in Cambridge in 1967, as I mentioned in Chapter 8. He shared the care of the Observation Ward at QEHC, where most cases of infective gastroenteritis were admitted, with the Academic Department of Child Health, lead by Professor Wood. Upon my arrival Chris passed his share of Observation ward, as far as children with gastroenteritis was concerned, to me.

Later during 1973, when Brian Wharton moved on to Birmingham, I became the consultant in charge of all children admitted to hospital with gastroenteritis to Observation ward, which pleased me very much. This was a continuum of one of my most important roles at RAHC.

What were my goals on arrival in January 1973? First was to create a major national and international centre for paediatric gastroenterology at Barts/Queens and second in due course to be appointed to a chair in paediatric gastroenterology. I could only envisage my senior lecturer position as a staging post to a professorial appointment. My ultimate hope at that time, rather than a goal, was to have a separate academic department of paediatric gastroenterology. Above all, I sought academic and clinical recognition of paediatric gastroenterology as a significant specialty of paediatrics, which would lead to improved care of children with gastroenterological disorders,. Overall, these were more ambitious goals than I had set myself in Sydney. This was because I believed that with the assistance of such outstanding colleagues, as those at Barts particularly it was possible to construct a major international centre. I had moved into bigger league than the RAHC.

It took me twelve years to achieve the goal of a personal chair. It was a long hard battle, fighting for recognition, fighting the corner. I often felt it was easier to get recognition internationally than it was locally amongst the paediatric staff and also in the Medical College of Barts. Tony Dawson took a key role in each of my promotions, first to reader, then to professor within the Medical of St Bartholomew's Hospital.

He was very influential in both the college and hospital as a leading physician.

In those days the Council Meeting of Barts Medical College was held in the Guild Room, a wonderful eighteenth century room at Barts dominated by a contemporary portrait of the eighteenth century physician Dr Percival Pott. It is adjacent to the Great Hall. The Dean chaired the meetings which were very formal but grand occasions dominated by senior establishment figures. Paediatrics was a minor matter for these great people! The meeting was always followed by a meeting of the Barts Council, the assembly of the NHS consultants at the Hospital.

In relation to the Medical College, i.e. School, I had very little contact with the Deans until the appointment some years later of Dr Lesley Rees. Dr Jim Malpas was the Dean when I was appointed. I knew Jim well, not as Dean, but through his involvement with paediatric oncology. However Professor Reggie Shooter quickly succeeded him, followed in due course by Dr Ian Kelsy-Fry, radiologist. Neither initiated any visit to my service either at Barts or QEHC, but I did invite Reggie myself to one of our lectures on gastrointestinal infection, as he was interested in Public Health. To Australian eyes, he appeared quintessentially English. He was a laconic man who spoke with an upper class accent. He gave me the impression that it was an effort to speak at all, yet he was very kind to me, in the very limited contact we had. Similarly with Ian Kelsy-Fry, although I did have one clash with him at a committee meeting concerning the clinical lecturer post which rotated to my firm at QEHC each year. I pointed out that the post was so loaded with additional clinical tasks such as covering casualty, working frequently at nights and weekends and organizing the student course that there was little time for research. So I thought the post in reality was hardly academic. The Dean clearly felt it very bad form to make such a point at an open committee. However I had raised this question in the past with Chris Wood, so often without outcome, that I raised the matter in front of the Dean.

Actually I valued the clinical lecturer post very much. Mary Harrison was my second clinical lecturer and she contributed notably to our research programme in cow's milk allergy. The clinical lecturers were mostly trainees in general paediatrics who wanted some experience in gastroenterology. So they spent one of their three years with me, one with Chris Wood and one variably elsewhere. Sadly most of them did not go on to become academics. I felt this was a sad waste of academic positions. As the years went on, I worked hard to change this post into a true academic training post for paediatric gastroenterology per se. I met great resistance from several quarters and wasted a lot of energy. It proved to be impossible until I achieved a separate department. It was ironic that the only truly academic post for which I was responsible for a junior doctor was the CICRA funded research fellowship at Barts i.e. a soft money funded post.

However I did successfully arrange for the clinical lecturer post to rotate for one year to Sydney. The clinical lecturer at QEHC swapped jobs for one year with a registrar from RAHC, thus extending the post by one year. Chris Wood enthusiastically backed this exchange and it was a great success and immensely popular with both English and Australian junior doctors. The rotation broadened the horizons of both. In fact three English trainees on the scheme Paul Hutchins, David Isaacs and Andrew Cotterill have settled in Sydney (Paul and David) and Brisbane (Andrew). John Mitchell from Australia has settled in England. Alan Phillips has described the impact these young Australians had upon the hospital, in the following words 'What a breath of fresh air this brought to the department! Strong-hearted, straightforward, highly intelligent young clinicians, who gave back at least as much as they took from the experience, they raised standards in the department and gave impetus to research. It also gave the home team lecturer the opportunity to experience the Australian system, and the delights of outback doctoring by plane.'

I have been fortunate to live in a peaceful environment for most of my life, but three times in my early days of life at Barts, this peace was shattered by Irish terrorism. The first came in 1973 whilst we were living in Charterhouse Square when the Irish Republican Army (IRA) exploded a car bomb outside the Old Bailey Law Courts not far from the hospital. The force of the blast was such that some windows in Barts blew in, but the hospital was mainly involved by receiving the injured in the casualty department. Fortunately no one was immediately killed, but one person subsequently died of a heart attack, said to be related to the event. I was at Queen Elizabeth Hospital. I was given the cryptic message 'The IRA have blown up the Old Bailey, come back to Barts'. I immediately took the bus back as quickly as possible, very concerned as to just where my wife Liz and Daughter Louise were, when the bomb went off. Liz had been outside the Barbican Tube station and had heard the bomb go off Louise was in fact with the family of Anthony Newman-Taylor, Tony Dawson's houseman at Barts, who lived in the same block of flats as we did. Fortunately they were both all right, but in Bart's casualty there were people with terrible glass wounds from the shattering of the huge windows of the Old Bailey. Fortunately I did not have anything to do as there were no children involved.

However when the next similar occasion occurred in July 1974, children were involved. The IRA had then exploded a bomb in the basement gallery of the White Tower of the Tower of London. The casualties were brought to Barts. There were two child casualties a German boy with severe facial injuries and a New Zealand boy Dafydd Hunter who had his right leg blown off below the knee. Dafydd's mother had very severe arm injuries as well. The family were tourists who had only been in the country for one day and were sightseeing in the Tower of London. Our paediatric registrar on duty was Rossi Shepherd from Brisbane. He was eventually some years later to become Professor of Paediatric Gastroenterology in Brisbane, a lifetime friend. He dealt admirably with the paediatric aspects of what was essentially a surgical emergency. Next day I saw the children in the ward, where all the bomb victims were being nursed. I shall never forget that terrible smell of burnt flesh, which was still there. It was frightful to see these innocent victims of brutal terror. I can use Dafydd's name ethically as it appeared in the press. Indeed wonderfully three years later in March 1977 we read in the *Daily Mirror* of Dafydd's triumph over his bomb blast injury with a front-page picture of

Dafydd jumping for joy with his two brothers using his artificial limb. He had been with us for many months in Kenton Ward.

Barts experienced a third blow from Irish terror when our Professor of Medical Oncology, Gordon Hamilton-Fairley was blown up and killed instantly as an innocent bystander in Holland Park near his home in 1975. In my view there is no cause existing which can ever possibly justify such wholesale terror with murder and maiming of innocents as I have just described. Post September 11, there is probably now general agreement with this statement, but it has seemed to me that this has not always been the consensus. What do the terrorists themselves who did these deeds and also those who supported them financially feel they achieved by a death such as that of Gordon Hamilton-Fairley? We, who knew him, know what the medical community lost. Gordon was a generous kind doctor of Australian origin of immense ability. There is a memorial to him in the crypt of St Paul's Cathedral. It is inscribed 'Gordon Hamilton-Fairley DM FRCP, First Professor of Medical Oncology 1930-1975 killed by a terrorist bomb. It matters not how a man dies but how he lives.' He is in good company. He is in a niche which also commemorates Sir Alexander Fleming, the discoverer of penicillin and Sir Henry Wellcome (his plague says 'patron of medical research and history').

These three events were the darkest of my career.

Going back to 1973, at a personal level it was a high priority to find a home to settle in. We were eager to get a place of our own, although we had made several good friends in our time in the flats at Charterhouse Square. Notably there was Ashley and Kathleen Mowatt, both Scots from Aberdeen. Ashley was a research fellow with Tony Dawson and is now a gastroenterologist in Aberdeen. We became lifelong friends and I have visited his unit in Scotland. We also had become friends with Dick Ellis an anaesthetist at Barts and his wife Liz. They lived in Chingford. My old friend Colin Barnes from Hammersmith was a rheumatologist at the London. He lived in Buckhurst Hill. Both Dick and Colin encouraged us to buy a house east of, London, which would be convenient for both Queens and Bart's hospitals and had the joys of being close to Epping Forest. Now we were determined to live in a house.and manner similar to our life in Australia, i.e. house with a garden. So we did need to move to the other suburbs. After a good deal of travail, Liz found a delightful but relatively small, albeit four bedroomed house in Fitzgerald Road, Wanstead, backing onto part of Epping Forest. It took absolutely ages to arrange a mortgage but we eventually did. It was an ideal place to start our life in England. We were close to the Central Line of the underground railway and thus convenient for both hospitals. We became parishioners at Christ Church Wanstead and became good friends with Rev. Paul Bowen and his doctor wife Elizabeth. Paul was later to baptize our Daughter Laura and marry our eldest Daughter Louise to Paul Letchford. We have been friends ever since and Liz and I visit them each Christmas in their retirement home in Canterbury.

Later because of the schools for our children, we moved further out to Woodford Green. We finally settled in 1981 in our quite large house with its extensive and beautiful garden and its four-hundred-year-old oak tree. While describing family matters, it should be recorded that our family was completed by the birth of our second Daughter Laura who was born in 1975 and our son James, born in 1978. So we needed our large house for the expanded family.

In this Chapter from now on, I shall not be taking a chronological approach, as this would be too restrictive, but range over some of the major issues over this twelve-year period, 1973-1985.

First I want to discuss some of the practical arrangements I faced on arrival and how I dealt with these at the two hospitals.

One of the first questions I had to address in London as a young academic (at QEHC) and consultant paediatrician (at Barts) was 'What should I wear at work?' In Sydney the honoraries (consultant paediatricians) had worn a suit but academics a long white coat. In both hospitals in London most paediatric consultants at that time, on the two sites, academic or NHS, wore white coats to do ward rounds or outpatient clinics, while academics wore white coats all the time. In the 1970s all junior doctors at both hospitals wore long white coats, the same as consultants and all medical students wore short white coats. By the time I left QEHC in 1995, received wisdom had changed and I was unusual in still wearing a white coat, although consultants at Barts still wore white coats. So when we moved to the Royal Free Hospital I abandoned the white coat and wore the suit my teachers in Sydney had worn! However whatever the current fashion has dictated, I have believed and continue to believe that the doctor should look the part and be recognizable to the child as to whom he or she is. I have made it clear to all the junior doctors on my ward round or in outpatients (i.e. where patients are involved) doctors should wear a tie. A few young doctors have ignored this advice on several occasions, as I have used no sanctions to ensure my views are fulfilled. During the 1990s most young paediatricians became convinced that white coats frightened children so junior paediatric doctors in the London hospitals have universally abandoned these. I have not been convinced of any hard evidence for this. This usage is a great contrast to the continent where almost invariably white coats are worn by all medicos. I wonder in what way, if any, the children cared for by doctors without white coats have benefited? My reason for favouring white coats is that children need to know the individual role of the confusing band of adults standing round them in the hospital. Especially when they are gravely ill they need to know who is the doctor. For me it is a question of knowledge and authority rather than status per se.

Throughout my career as a consultant from 1973 to 2000 I conducted formal consultant ward rounds accompanied by junior doctors, nursing staff, a dietician, and a social worker and variably with medical students, twice a week at each hospital. This meant four consultant rounds a week when there were two hospitals involved. I continued this practice after the move to the Royal Free Hospital in 1995 until my retirement in 2000. This traditional way of proceeding is efficient for decision making, continuity of care and above all for communication about decisions, for all those concerned in the multi-disciplinary care team. This team approach has been for me a vital part of paediatric practice from the 1970s. It is also a first rate vehicle for teaching. At Barts, from the beginning, each Monday Patrick Cox and I did joint rounds, which I found immensely helpful. He was a very good clinician with a special knowledge of neurology. When he retired I continued this with his successor Kate Costeloe, until she moved on to Homerton. At Queens I did not do joint consultant rounds until my first gastroenterological colleague Nigel Meadows was appointed in 1992, joined by Simon Murch in 1995. When we all transferred to the Royal Free with the appointment of Mike Thomson, the three consultants Simon Murch, Mike Thomson and myself did joint post-graduate rounds each Monday afternoon. I have found this a rewarding practice. It is great for communication and for one's continuing need to learn from one's own colleagues both young and old.

I learnt from J.G. Scadding at the Brompton the virtue of once a week doing a 'preliminary ward round', whilst sitting down in an office adjacent to the ward with each patient's notes before the true round. I adopted this practice for the Monday ward round from 1973 at Queens and at Royal Free from our transfer in 1995 for our joint consultant post-graduate round. Every case was discussed in advance in depth and any matters which were best not discussed in front of the child, could be dealt with in advance. Also important social or non-medical issues could be raised confidentially. Confidentiality was always very important to me and I made it clear to all those present, despite the size of the group, that what they heard about patients both medical and personal was completely confidential. Consultants have been accused of playing God. Traditional ward rounds such as I have described have been claimed to facilitate this. For me, I believe this was not so. Children and indeed the modern parent with all their queries etc. would not permit this, nor would the alert, highly motivated and often critical young doctor. I always encouraged parents to be present at the ward round and I involved the older children themselves in all decisions as far as possible. The junior doctors were asked to give a resume of the child's history at the bedside, i.e. in front of child and usually the parent, as a way of ensuring accuracy. As well, it was a logical way to begin the doctor-patient dialogue and to discuss the plan of action for each child patient. The input of nurses both senior and junior was vital. In paediatric gastroenterology the input of the dietitian was an essential part of care.

Earlier my general goals were outlined. I now need to describe the immediate tasks that needed to be undertaken. When I began at Barts/QEHC my initial mandate was to develop paediatric gastroenterology at both sites. At Barts I did this by commencing a small bowel biopsy service, which I performed myself. At Queens Dr Mary Rossiter, who was a research fellow with Brian Wharton, already performed small bowel biopsy very efficiently. She was to go fairly soon to Oxford for further training. Mary was a great asset to me, in helping me consolidate the paediatric gastroenterology service at QEHC and provide continuity. She is an extremely lively person and I have had on-going links with her ever since. She became the medical adviser to Crohn's in Childhood Research Appeal (CICRA), which she continues. After Brian Wharton left, I arranged a weekly gastroenterology outpatient clinic on the first floor of the Hayward Building. I tried to get the other consultants to ask me to see all the gastroenterological patients and ideally hand them over to my care. The general paediatricians eventually did so, if a bit reluctantly, but Chris Wood usually retained the gastroenterology patients but sought my opinion. His thinking was that the professor of paediatrics should care for all types of patient. He was a very good all round clinician. We in fact shared Barclay Ward as the professorial unit but we did not do joint ward rounds. We did it once and clearly it was not a practical arrangement.

At that time at QEHC there was some resistance to the whole conception of specialization in paediatrics. My senior colleagues Dr Tony Jackson (also at the London), Dr Bernard Laurence and Dr Roderick Brown were upholders of general paediatrics. The one exception was Dr Margaret Mearns who had an international reputation in cystic fibrosis. Although several years later there was the welcome appointment of Dr Martin Savage as a paediatric endocrinologist, a fellow specialist and ally, but back in 1973 this meant I had to fight to secure recognition for gastroenterology specialization within my own hospital. As there were several children with coeliac disease aged less than a year we were performing biopsies of the small intestine even in infancy. I was also convinced that in the younger age group particularly there were other causes of small intestinal mucosa damage causing chronic diarrhoea as well as coeliac disease (including damage as a sequel to gastroenteritis), especially in infancy. This performance of small intestinal biopsies in infants under a year, raised hostility in some of the above quarters. However we came to show by biopsy that cow's milk protein could severely damage the small intestine of infants causing chronic diarrhoea and failure to thrive, often as a sequel to gastroenteritis, and that as a result of this investigation, effective therapy could be undertaken. So eventually the hostility disappeared.

Tony Dawson strongly supported me in the stand I had taken concerning the importance of small intestinal biopsy in children. I believed that children deserved accurate diagnosis and indeed that clinical research was a vital concern to determine just what was the cause of the chronic diarrhoea and malnutrition, which was at that time such an important clinical problem. In a foreword he wrote to my book *Diseases of the Small Intestine* published in 1975, he wrote 'With the increasing awareness of the importance of social factors in the practice of medicine it is sometimes becoming fashionable to decry some of the sort of research which has made this monograph possible but I am sure parents of affected children will be grateful that it has been undertaken in time and that clinicians are making full use of it.' This is I believe so true.

This is an example of the kind of support I received from him. Another joint activity was the so-called Combined Gastroenterology Meeting, which had been commenced before I arrived in London. This was a tripartite meeting linking gastroenterology in adults at Barts with gastroenterology in children both at QEHC and at GOS. Tony Dawson, Brian Wharton and John Harries respectively were the founding fathers. It was to be a rigorous forum for young researchers and clinicians in which to participate. Criticism was tough and mostly constructive. These meetings occurred three times a year at each hospital in turn. They continue today. They were followed by a meal together and so a strong esprit de corps was built up amongst us all. Exciting things were happening in gastroenterology in London. I had never experienced anything so dynamic and forward-looking in Sydney.

A key event for me in the development of academic paediatric gastroenterology at QEHC was the appointment of an electron microscopist, Alan Phillips. I had developed a good relationship with the pathologist Dr Norman France. He was pleased that small intestinal biopsy had developed as an essential diagnostic technique. A new electron microscope had been installed in the department of pathology from the opening of the new Hayward Building, a great credit to the vision of those who equipped the new building. At first a part-time technician had only used it a little. Norman and I agreed it was essential that a properly qualified full time electron microscopist should be appointed. I persuaded him to include electron microscopy of small intestinal tissue as a key part of the job description. Years later this was an important factor in the transfer of the electron microscope unit to my own department. We appointed a very talented young scientist Alan Phillips to this post in 1975. This was a landmark appointment for me. Alan was young and very youthful in his manner at that time, but with clear determination and vision. It has been a privilege to observe his maturation and development as a scientist over many years.

Since working at Hammersmith I had had the view that it is essential for clinicians undertaking clinical research to work closely with basic scientists to ensure the highest standards and to keep abreast of scientific developments. I had hoped this could have occurred in the Institute of Child Health in Sydney but Peter Rowe felt that his agenda was to work in an area of fundamental science not related to gastroenterology. With Alan's appointment there was now a very talented young man of great potential who would be a major scientific collaborator in the field of small intestinal mucosa damage in children. This was to be my principal area of research for the next almost thirty years. Later he was formally to transfer to my department at QEHC. Alan at first focused upon electron microscopy as a technique to investigate the structure of the small intestinal mucosa but was quickly to be also concerned with electron microscope recognition of viral particles in the diarrhoeal stools of children with acute gastroenteritis. Now this may not sound exciting but it was. Quite dramatically for the first time in the early seventies the electron microscope was able to reveal with its vast powers of magnification that there were viruses in the stools of many children with acute non-bacterial gastroenteritis. Until then more than 70% of the children I had seen admitted at RAHC and QEHC with gastroenteritis had all infectious disease of unknown origin, i.e. without any of the bacterial pathogens then known to cause diarrhoea found in their stools. Then, in Melbourne, Ruth Bishop observed with the electron microscope a small round virus in the epithelial cells of the small intestinal mucosa taken by biopsy from children with acute gastroenteritis. Quite soon it became clear that this virus could also be identified in the stools in a routine way using the electron microscope. The virus in question looked like a motor car wheel and was called the rota (Latin for wheel) virus. In fact it was not the first virus to be found in the stools, that had been Norwalk-like virus which had been first identified in winter vomiting disease. As the experience of the Royal Marines in Afghanistan reveal in 2002, it can occur in hot dry environments as well. This virus obtained its name after the town of Norwalk, Ohio USA where it was first identified in an outbreak of non-bacterial gastroenteritis. All this was a technological breakthrough. We were able to participate in this research on site because we had the immense good fortune to have an electron microscope on site at QEHC. For the first time we were able to us it as a research tool following Alan's appointment.

In fact earlier, Ross Shepherd in 1975 was able to be first author on a report in the *Lancet* of the clinical findings of children in Observation Ward with gastroenteritis who had rota virus identified in their diarrhoeal stools by Dr Dick Bird, electron microscopist at the London School of Hygiene and Tropical Medicine. We had sent him stool samples before Alan's appointment. It was through Dick Bird that I first met Professor Arie Zuckerman, to discuss our results concerning rota virus. Little did I know that 20 years later we would be together at the Royal Free Hospital where he was to become Dean.

Later Alan Phillips was to study the way in which enteropathogenic Escherichia coli bacteria (an important bacterial cause of infantile gastroenteritis, especially in the developing world) attached themselves to the epithelium of the small intestinal mucosa and so damaged it. He had observed in 1978 that a child who had recently been in India had severe small intestinal mucosal damage and had bacteria adhering to the surface. We asked Dr Margot Shiner to look at the electron micrographs as she was a great expert on the small intestinal mucosa and its electron microscopy. When she was shown them she stated they showed 'Nothing of interest'. Sadly we allowed ourselves to accept this opinion, although I did show the picture at an international meeting in Barcelona in 1979 where it created much interest. Others were to be the first to publish these appearances. However Alan was ultimately to be concerned with which precise molecule accounted for this bacterial attachment.

Alan's general scientific interests knowledge of statistics and especially his willingness to train young doctors in research techniques lead him ultimately to become a pivotal member of the department, giving continuity over many years. He is the classical team player often putting the interests of other members of the team before his own. I had the honour to supervise his PhD and then to recommend his promotion as senior lecturer on our transfer to the Royal Free in 1995 and finally as reader shortly before my retirement. Subsequently, after my retirement he was appointed to a personal chair. It has been a privilege to observe his career development over all the years. Furthermore in the times of strife which were to come in the future in 1992, associated with the Tomlinson report, his steadfast personal loyalty I shall never forget. He early on received international recognition. He joined European Society for Paediatric Gastroenterology and Nutrition (ESPGAN) in 1979 as its youngest member. He has been a very active member ever since leading to many international invitations. He is now treasurer in ESPGHAN.

From the outset of my career in paediatric gastroenterology in Sydney it was clear that this branch of medicine was rooted in clinical science and that it was essential for any long-term research programme for a clinical investigator to work closely with a scientist. So Alan turned out to be the ideal candidate for this role. We were to work together for the next 28 years. I am extraordinarily lucky to have had such a capable and loyal colleague. The academic achievements at QEHC in paediatric gastroenterology are in large measure centred upon Alan and his work.

I tried to get one of the surgeons at QEHC to consider doing a joint surgical/gastroenterological clinic as I had conducted with Arch Middleton at RAHC but this was not agreed. I had to await Miss Vanessa Wright's appointment some years later. She is a real star with remarkable surgical talents in the tiniest babies and she had a special interest in gastroenterology. She soon established a good rapport, especially as she had had Australian experience working in Melbourne with the distinguished paediatric surgeon Helen Noblett. So a joint clinic was established, which I regularly conducted with her till I left in 1995. It was not possible sadly to develop a joint surgical clinic at the Royal Free. At Barts I worked with the adult surgeons who had most experience of Crohn's disease, when that disease became an increasing part of my practice at the end of the seventies. Most children who required surgery were over the age of ten years. Mr Ian Todd was the surgeon I worked with most often until he retired. He was later to be President of the Royal College of Surgeons and was knighted.

I also tried to develop liaison with the psychiatrists as I had had previously in Sydney. At Barts, Tony Dawson had recruited an outstanding young psychiatrist Dr Gerald Libby but his interests were confined to adults, however some years later Dr Terry Bruce, an outstanding child psychiatrist, was appointed at Barts who was particularly interested in the emotional aspects of chronic disease such as Crohn's Disease. His help was invaluable in helping children to cope with their illness.

At QEHC with Mary Rossiter's departure I was fortunate for the Heinz Fellowship to be continued so I was able to appoint my first research fellow Dr Anne Kilby. This was a key appointment to get clinical research under way at QEHC. Anne played an invaluable role in this and made important contributions especially in relation to cow's milk allergy. She was succeeded by Dr Peter Manuel who was funded by Queen Elizabeth Research Appeal Trust. The main research theme of both these fellows was cow's milk allergy. as initiated by Mary Harrison. We were also deeply involved in applying the Interlaken diagnostic criteria to our children with coeliac disease (see Chapter 13). Coeliac disease was always a major interest. The research was expanded with Alan Phillips to look at the problem of post-enteritis chronic diarrhoea in infancy, including the role that cow's milk protein allergy might have in causing persistent small intestinal mucosal damage in such children. I originally was a sceptic that cow's milk could damage the small intestinal mucosa, but using the technique of serial biopsies related to challenge, as we were using in coeliac disease, it clearly existed.

Alan, working with the department of microbiology lead by Dr Liz Price at QEHC and with the first rate technical support of Steve Rice now was able to identify stool viruses with the electron microscope as a routine diagnostic service. Not only viruses such as rota virus and small round viruses which were Norwalk-like could be identified but others as well, such as calici virus, adeno virus and astro virus in the diarrhoeal stools of children with gastroenteritis, using the electron microscope to diagnose their presence. I however experienced some personal hostility from Professor Alistair Dudgeon at the ICH because I directly involved junior staff in microbiology such as Steve Rice in our research without consulting him. Dr Hisham Nazer, a research fellow from Jordan, made a particular study of another 'new' virus called astro virus because it looked like a star on electron microscopy. It was an exciting time, recognizing the clinical features of these 'new' virus infections in the children themselves. It was a time when research in the laboratory could be rapidly translated into patient benefit. Rapid viral diagnosis opened a whole new way of efficiently and accurately diagnosing acute diarrhoea in hospital patients. The practical advantage was that patients who were at risk of infecting others could be rapidly identified and isolated. Alan later found viruses within the small intestinal mucosal epithelium on electron microscopy and had evidence that some cases of post-enteritis chronic diarrhoea were due to secondary infection with viruses or bacteria, which were different from the original infectious agent, i.e. had been acquired in hospital. This was an exciting time resulting in a number of publications and presentations at national and international meetings.

I used my old connection with Dr Pitono Soeparto of Indonesia who had been my research fellow at RAHC to arrange for Peter Manuel to undertake a research project concerning chronic diarrhoea in infants as a sequel to gastroenteritis in Surabja in Java. Peter showed, using serial small intestinal biopsies related to cow's milk elimination and challenge, that cow's milk allergy was an important cause of chronic diarrhoea in bottle fed infants in Indonesia.

Dr Colin Campbell, also funded by Queen Elizabeth Research Appeal Trust to continue this work, followed him as research fellow. However Colin also helped me with the care and research concerning the rapidly expanding chronic inflammatory bowel disease (CIBD) work at Barts. I wanted to try and pull together my unit on two sites as until Colin's appointment I was the only person who did any gastroenterology on both sites, so I arranged for him to do some research at Barts. There he undertook an important piece of research investigating the diagnostic value of a blood test, which measured the amount of circulating C-reactive protein. He clearly established its diagnostic value in children with Crohn's disease, where it was increased. When after completion of his fellowship he moved on, Queen Elizabeth Research Appeal Trust was not keen to continue to fund research off site at Barts. So we needed to develop a Barts fellowship. When the parents of my child patients at Barts heard that the work that the research work Colin had begun was to cease, they were quite dismayed. Remarkably, they resolved to raise money to continue and indeed expand the research at Barts. At that time no other research in this field was occurring specifically in children in the UK. As a result of this, Crohn's in Childhood Research Appeal (CICRA) was founded. However I am racing ahead and what was happening at Barts needs now to be recalled.

At Barts I was not happy with the idea of just duplicating what we did at QEHC, e.g, small bowel biopsy. I was perplexed what to do for the best. However events were to determine what should be done. From 1975 we began to see at Barts increasing numbers of children with chronic inflammatory bowel disease, particularly Crohn's disease, which was most surprising. At first these were older children aged between 13 to 16 years referred by Dr Tony Dawson, but passed on to me by him because of their age. A very good diagnostic team for inflammatory bowel disease was developing at Barts.

First, a great improvement in barium radiology had occurred. Dr Clive Bartram, the radiologist, had developed an improved diagnostic service for barium follow through X-ray examinations. I met him each week in the most valued gastroenterology/radiology meeting I mentioned earlier. The most frequently affected part of the bowel in Crohn's disease as found at that time was the terminal ileum (i.e. lower end of the small intestine). It takes some time for the barium to reach the terminal ileum after oral indigestion. The radiologist views the passage of the barium as it advances and takes X-ray pictures as may be necessary for documentation. The ileum can be difficult to recognize except by experienced experts. Non-experts can make an incorrect diagnosis of Crohn's disease because of swelling of lymph glands in the terminal ileum, a disorder known as ileal lymphoid nodular hyperplasia. Clive used a technique of acceleration (using a drug) and compression (applying pressure to the abdomen with the protectively gloved hand of the radiologist) to produce very fine images of the small intestine speedily i.e. whilst the radiologist was still present. Using the drug metaclopromide to produce acceleration of the barium, it was then practical for the radiologist, to be able to see the barium enter the ileum during the screening process. Without acceleration it might take some hours. Then unsatisfactory X-rays of the abdomen would have be taken hours later. This acceleration approach enormously increased the accuracy of X-ray diagnosis of Crohn's disease. This technique is only available in special centres.

Second a revolution had occurred in endoscopy. The limited technique of sigmoidoscopy which I had used at Prince Alfred was replaced in the mid-seventies by flexible total colonoscopy, based on fibreoptics. This was a British invention but was commercially exploited by the Japanese. Dr Christopher Williams an expert colonoscopist had been appointed with some sessional time at Barts, although principally at St Marks Hospital. He began to use a system of fibre-optic colonoscopy with a video camera attached to the colonoscope for investigation of children. This had transformed endoscopy both diagnostically and educationally as observers could be present at colonoscopy and see exactly what the endoscopist was seeing. This could be videoed and individual photographs taken as a record and as a souvenir gift to the child (Christopher Williams's idea). This technique also enabled small biopsies of the lining mucosa to be taken from the large bowel (the colon). Most remarkably of all not only could the whole colon now be examined but also Christopher had developed the skill to enter the terminal ileum (lower end of the small bowel) from the colon, via the ileo-caecal valve, a very difficult technique. This really was a diagnostic revolution. For the first time a tissue diagnosis could be made of Crohn's disease of the ileum, which had hitherto been based entirely on radiology. Radiology is after all is only a technique which produces pictures! Endoscopic biopsy is a technique which actually produces tissue, which can be looked at under the microscope for accurate diagnosis. In the seventies this was quite an innovative concept for paediatricians. The appointment of Christopher Williams was a great boost to me at a personal level. He is a tall humorous outgoing man who was a great success with the children and their parents. He was also a great support personally to me and I used to attend part of his endoscopy list every week from 1978 till our transfer to the Royal Free in 1995. He trained a number of future leaders of paediatric gastroenterology in the technique of paediatric colonoscopy, including entry to the ileum, for practice at 'home', Sonny Chong, Ian Sanderson and Simon Murch, and 'abroad' Christian Braegger (Zurich).

Some may ask why did I not take on training in fibreoptic colonoscopy myself? Well as I mentioned earlier I had severed my ulnar nerve in my left wrist aged 14 years, and have been left with a partial palsy of third to fifth fingers of my left hand which made holding the endoscope difficult. In fact being both an academic and a clinician I was so busy in my career that I believe this was a good practical decision, quite apart from this disability.

Third, the endoscopic revolution most importantly provided diagnostic biopsy material for our pathological experts. Eventually we were privileged to have Professor Gerry Slavin and Dr Paolo Domizio to examine this tissue.

So it was from 1978 there were increasing numbers of children referred directly to me at Barts with suspected chronic inflammatory bowel disease, instead of via adult gastroenterology, who could benefit from the above diagnostic expertise. The children were getting younger down to the age of five years. So for this reason Christopher Williams established a paediatric colonoscopy diagnostic service at Barts, quite distinct from the adult service. This was a landmark development for paediatric gastroenterology at Barts and for my own career.

I was now able to make a decision to rationalize the paediatric gastroenterology service and associated research between the two hospitals. Small intestinal biopsy was stopped at Barts and centred at QEHC. All children with coeliac disease were transferred there as well as all infants with chronic diarrhoea. The paediatric colonoscopy service was centred at Barts, and any children referred to QEHC with suspect chronic inflammatory bowel disease were transferred to Barts. A paediatric inflammatory bowel disease outpatient clinic was established there. The focus for the clinical research programme at Barts I decided was to be Crohn's disease in children. Then, as I mentioned earlier, we had the extraordinary good fortune for the parents of our children, to band together to form the Crohn's in Childhood Research Appeal (CICRA) to support this work following Colin Campbell's departure. In 1979 CICRA made a commitment to fund a research fellowship in Crohn's disease in children at Barts. This CICRA fellowship was to continue after our transfer to the Royal Free and the last CICRA fellow was Dr Rob Heuschkel who concluded his fellowship in 1999. Little did I realize at the beginning that this fellowship was to continue for a remarkable 21 years. What a wonderful continuity it has given to our work. Remarkably, one parent, Mrs Margaret Lee, OBE, has remained actively involved with CICRA from the outset right up to my retirement. One great benefit, unforeseen at the beginning, was that the appointment of a CICRA fellow would be a great boost for the NHS and indeed a great saving for the NHS. We could not have developed the service for children with inflammatory bowel disease without this private funding. Furthermore the CICRA fellowship was for some years one of very few training posts for paediatric gastroenterology in the United Kingdom. Seven consultants currently in post in 2002 were trained in this way. It could be argued that it would have been very difficult for them to obtain adequate training in paediatric gastroenterology, without the CICRA fellowship. The first CICRA fellow was Dr John Douglas from the RAHC in Sydney. This appointment was a pivotal moment in my career.

CICRA however was to support our research in other ways as well. They gave a remarkable commitment to laboratory research. In 1982 Dr Tony Dawson, who gave his strong backing to CICRA, suggested that I put in a bid for research laboratory space, which was being built for Barts by the special trustees in St Bartholomew's Close. CICRA strongly backed this proposal and wanted to support research in the new laboratory. I was successful in this bid but there was some unpleasantness as Professor Wood also had made a bid for research space. This puzzled me as he already had laboratory space in the Hayward's Building to which I had only limited access. As a compromise, it was suggested that he and I should share the laboratory allotted to me. I was deeply embarrassed by this as I could not in good conscience agree. However after consulting with Tony Dawson to seek his advice, I stated publicly that I could not agree to share the laboratory and that paediatric gastroenterology, which in my view was an expanding discipline, would indeed need all the space allocated to me. In fact my wishes prevailed, due no doubt to Tony Dawson's support. Chris Wood sadly was both angry and upset. This led to quite a big rift between him and me but it reflects an historic contest between general and specialist paediatrics. It took a while for the rift to heal but heal it did. Yet it reinforced my resolution to secure a separate department in due course.

The new St Bartholomew's Centre for Clinical Research, including our laboratory, was opened by Princess Alexandra on 25 November in 1982. It was a gala day for us all. The Princess and her husband Angus Ogilvie spent some time in our Paediatric Gastroenterology Laboratory and expressed great interest in all that they saw. Sonny Chong our CICRA research fellow was a very enthusiastic guide. Dr Robert Dourmashkin had come to begin research in the new laboratory, supported by the Medical Research Council and with the backing of my old mentor Chris Booth now the director of the CRC at Northwick Park. The MRC provided much of the new equipment. However CICRA made a commitment to provide equipment and unusually to provide running expenses for the laboratory. This was a wonderful and very practical gesture. What is clear from all this was that all the funding for staff equipment etc. came from non-exchequer funds i.e. soft money.

Bob Dourmashkin established a very successful foetal organ culture system in the laboratory. Dr Tom MacDonald succeeded him in due course, a research scientist who had joined the laboratory as a research fellow having been working in industry in the USA. I was delighted to have him join us. I had first met him some years earlier while he was a PhD student with Dr Ann Ferguson, a gastroenterologist in Edinburgh I held in high regard. He immediately began work in gut immunology. He was at first funded by a CICRA fellowship for one year. He then was appointed to a Welcome Senior Lectureship for five years. He was to be one of the most important colleagues of my career, but I shall discuss him and his research programme etc. in more detail in the next Chapter. Dr Lisa Lipson from Canada succeeded Sonny Chong. They were both very capable research fellows. In turn Dr Ian Sanderson followed them. He was destined to become later on Professor of Paediatric Gastroenterology at Barts but within the new combined school of Queen Mary College.

A key aspect of the consultant life is to take an active interest in young trainees and endeavour to support them in obtaining in due course a consultant post. Such interest in my case continues life long and I have been most interested to keep in touch and follow their subsequent progress. This is the role of the mentor.

From Sydney, I kept in touch with Pitono Soeparto from Surabaja until his retirement. I visited Indonesia twice and saw him there. He visited me once at Queens. I have mentioned how I arranged Peter Manuel to work with him. Both Magadalena Araya and I have visited each other's units in Santiago and London. I have visited my successor at RAHC, Ramanand Kamath, many times. I have been impressed by his work in expanding the department since I left RAHC. I was very grateful that he was able to do a locum for me for three months in London in 1993, during my history of medicine sabbatical.

One of my overseas fellows, Dr Hisham Nazer, a Palestinian doctor, invited me to Amman after his return there as a consultant. Later he was to move to Riyadh in Saudi Arabia where he had been appointed as a paediatric gastroenterologist at King Faisal Hospital and he also invited me to visit him there. It was very interesting to visit both countries. In Amman I was travelling with Dr Alex Mowatt and we were both shocked to visit a Palestinian refugee camp and meet a family who had been refugees since 1948 when they had left their original home in what is now Israel.

Four house physicians at QEHC, Paul Hutchins, Ian Sanderson, Warren Hyer and Robert Heuschkel, during my consultant career came back as registrars/fellows, all have had remarkably successful careers to date and are all consultants now.

Paul Hutchins contributed to our research on oral rehydration solutions and post-enteritis diarrhoea but changed over to developmental paediatrics and currently is a consultant at RAHC in developmental medicine. Ian Sanderson uniquely first came to see me as a Barts medical student to discuss his interest in paediatric gastroenterology. It was clear to me ab initio that he was a young man of considerable talent and quiet determination. He would go far. In due course he was to be my houseman at QEHC, CICRA fellow at Barts and later registrar at QEHC as part of a rotation with GOS. He then spent some years doing significant research with Allan Walker in Boston. Finally he was appointed to the re-created chair of paediatric gastroenterology in 1998 at Barts, three years after our transfer to the Royal Free Hospital. Warren Hyer was houseman at QEHC, another young man of talent and determination. He was later to be clinical lecturer at Barts (my last) and now is a consultant paediatrician at Northwick Park, collaborating with Christopher Williams at St Marks in the field of intestinal polyposis. Rob Heuschkel was houseman at QEHC. His clinical skills and determination to succeed were clear at that time. He was later to be CICRA fellow jointly at the Royal Free and Barts (my last CICRA fellow) and in 2002 was appointed consultant paediatric gastroenterologist at the Royal Free with a major interest in chronic inflammatory bowel disease. He later moved on to Addenbrooke's Hospital in Cambridge and established a new department of paediatric gastroenterology. These were four exceptional young men and in my retirement nothing gives me greater satisfaction than to see how successful they have been in medicine and what all asset they are to sick children and the wider paediatric community.

We had many visitors now to the department, the most notable was Allan Walker of Boston. He had come to London to lecture at the Hammersmith and I met him on a visit to Barts and we immediately got on very well together. He was to play a most important part in my professional life right up to the present. He is principally interested in the gut as an immunological organ. He made the very important observation that food antigens can be absorbed in increased amounts when the small intestinal mucosa is damaged leading to immunological sensitization to the ingested food. He has been based at both

Boston Childrens' Hospital and Massachusetts General Hospital for many years within Harvard Medical School where he holds a tenured chair. He is the leading internationally recognized figure in Paediatric Gastroenterology in the United States. He was a successor of Harry Schwachmann whom I had visited in Boston in 1967. I have made since many visits to see him in Boston and vice versa.

He and I established a most important mutual exchange programme for our respective trainees. Each would send a trainee to the other's department for one month. The first from London was Ian Sanderson who later on was to spend some years in Boston with Allan before returning to Barts in 1998 as I mentioned earlier. The first from USA was Barry Wershil, now an important investigator in paediatric gastroenterology in USA. Fifteen young Americans over the years rotated through my department. This was great for transatlantic friendship and academic exchange of knowledge. The last CICRA fellow Rob Heuschkel also spent a longer period in Boston to his great benefit.

In the early eighties we were lucky to have another young scientist collaborate with us. This was Joe Unsworth a PhD student with Dr John Holborrow at the Royal London who was doing a research project in coeliac disease. He gave us an 'entrée' to an interesting world of humeral immunology, especially in relation to antibodies to gliadin and other foods. This serendipitously was to lead us to a new disorder or syndrome. We had a most difficult clinical problem, a child with all the features of coeliac disease, including a flat small intestinal mucosa (as in untreated coeliac disease) but he did not get better on a gluten-free diet. He needed intravenous parenteral nutrition to keep him alive. I asked Joe to look for any unusual antibody in his blood and he discovered the child had an antibody against his own small intestinal mucosa, an autoimmune antibody. This means an antibody which attacks one of the body's own tissues. From this we coined the term autoimmune enteropathy. Enteropathy means pathology of the enteron i.e. the small intestine. This was a new syndrome. Joe to his great credit after successfully passing his PhD then took on medicine and is now a consultant immunologist in Bristol. I also had a very useful collaboration with Dr Michael Dillon (later professor of Paediatric Nephrology) of GOS/QEHC over many years, concerning the above child's renal problems, as he also had an antibody against kidney structures. The investigation of this child was a classical example of the modern team approach to research and treatment.

We were attracting a steady stream of overseas fellows for training and research from many different countries, Chile, Venezuela, Switzerland, Israel, The Sudan, Spain, Greece and Jordan as well as the Commonwealth. Many of these are now leaders in paediatric gastroenterology in their own countries. It was all very exciting. I relished the cosmopolitan unit we had become.

Yet I also rejoiced in the traditional life at Barts. The two hospitals were so different. QEHC, a children's hospital serving a deprived multicultural and multi-racial community in east London, and Barts a general hospital mostly caring for referrals, right up to date with the latest technology but basking in its ancient traditions. I shall describe something of QEHC's history in the next Chapter as we were to celebrate its 125th anniversary in 1992. However here something of Barts' history and traditions will be described. These added immeasurably to the quality of life of the staff both medical and nursing and so influenced the quality of patient care.

Remarkably in 1973 shortly after our arrival we were able to participate in the 850th anniversary celebrations and notably took part in a banquet in the Great Hall modelled upon King Henry VIII's coronation banquet with us all in appropriate period costume. The Royal Hospital of St Bartholomew had been founded in 1123 by the monk Rahere. Whilst on pilgrimage to Rome, so it is told, he fell ill. Fearful of death he prayed for recovery in the Church of St Bartholomew where the bones of the apostle lie. This is situated on the Isola Tiberina, an island in the River Tiber. Priests from the island of Cos the home of Hippocrates, Father of Medicine had settled there in antiquity. He vowed that if he recovered, he would found a hospital in London. He duly did and on his way home had a vision of St Bartholomew who bade him found both a church and a hospital in Smithfield. King Henry I gave the hospital its first royal charter. There is thus a kind of 'apostolic succession' from the ancient origins of western medicine on Cos to the Isola Tiberina in Rome and then to Barts in London. Then it might be added the 'succession' from Barts went around the world. When I was a child in Sydney I had heard Barts described as the Mother Hospital of the Empire! On the foundation stone laid on July 6 1904 by Edward VII of new buildings at Barts the inscription concludes with the words 'through the increase of knowledge of the medical art here attained to the alleviation of human suffering throughout the world.' It is this international ethos of Barts that I have very much appreciated.

Returning to Rahere's time, Henry I established an ecclesiastical foundation under the rule of St Augustine of Hippo. The monks were known as the Augustinian or Austin canons. Rahere died in 1144, and his tomb which dates from the fifteenth century wonderfully survives intact, despite the destruction of the nave etc. which occurred during the reign of Henry VIII at the time of the reformation. A service is held in the Church of St Bartholomew the Great each year, which I have often attended, when his memory is recalled in a simple but moving ceremony, when a junior nurse places a red rose on his tomb. The hospital was suppressed with all religious houses by Henry VIII but re-founded by him on 13 January 1547 after pressure by the mayor and 'commonality' of London. From that time physicians and surgeons were appointed to replace the monks. In the late eighteenth and early nineteenth century medical students were taught and eventually the medical college established. From 18th to 21st centuries many distinguished doctors have practiced at Barts. It is not appropriate to list them here, but they provide a great source of inspiration to the present day staff.

The traditions of Barts are still honoured each year in a ceremony called View Day when the hospital is on show. In days past, the Board of Governors used to process around the hospital. Nowadays the Lord Mayor of London visits. The consultant staff usually wear morning dress on this occasion and encourage their family to visit the hospital. I did this most years from 1973 to 1995. It was always both a memorable and enjoyable occasion. In the early years, my wife and children used always to accompany me and once my sister and family from Australia too. It was a great occasion for all the family. On our first view day our Daughter Louise covered her face with chocolate and generously the then Clerk to the Governors, (administrator) Mr Goody took us up to his beautiful flat above the Guild Room to wash her face. Sadly his post and the ancient Board of Governors were abolished in the first of the many reorganizations of the Health Service that occurred during my career.

Each Christmas Day from 1973 till 1994 I took my children into Barts for the arrival of Father Christmas, one of the junior doctors appropriately disguised. They each received a fine present after all the sick children and their siblings had received theirs. In the early years there were many children still in hospital but in the latter years only the most severe cases. However this visit with a preliminary visit to Queens remain with me and my children as key memories of Christmas. The ward sisters Jackie Clark (Sister Kenton) and Maggie Bates (Sister Lucas), in the seventies put great significance upon the maintenance of such traditions and senior and junior doctors alike would usually gather in the childrens' wards each Christmas morning with their own families. The two sisters liked to be called by their ward names in the old Barts tradition, symbolizing their complete commitment to the children and their care. They belong to an ethos of nursing now long gone.

Eventually in October 1979, I was appointed a reader in paediatric gastroenterology, which thankfully at last gave me one salary from one source. Then finally in September 1985, after what seemed a long six years, I at last was appointed to a personal chair. It seemed a long, long time. By then I had over 120 publications in peer reviewed journals and we had a clinical research programme on two sites. At QEHC we had focused on gastroenteritis, post-enteritis diarrhoea, food allergy with a particular interest in cow's milk allergy and coeliac disease, all problems chiefly of the small intestine. Then at Barts we had established a research laboratory focusing upon chronic inflammatory bowel disease in children and Crohn's disease in particular. My own research interests were morphological which means the shape or structure of the small intestinal mucosa when studied microscopically, but Alan Phillips and Tom MacDonald were the key players in our laboratory research programmes on the two sites.

However before I go on to discuss events after my professorial appointment, I think it is important to put the development of paediatric gastroenterology into a wider context. This will be discussed in the next Chapter.

CHAPTER ELEVEN

Recognition for Paediatric Gastroenterology, Specialism in Medicine

AT THE MOMENT when I at last achieved full academic recognition, by my appointment to a chair of paediatric gastroenterology in the University of London, it is appropriate to pause and to consider how this appointment related more generally to the recognition of paediatric gastroenterology as a legitimate specialism in medicine in the wider world and elsewhere in Britain, and also how my own career was interwoven with this development. First I should discuss the more general point concerning why I wanted to be a specialist rather than a generalist, and to go further even to study a specialism within a specialty (paediatrics). It is because the subject matter of medicine is so vast and boundless. As Prof. Blackburn told us in Med IV, to try and master all the factual material of modern medicine would be like trying to learn the telephone book by heart. I selected a paediatric specialty and an area within it, namely disorders of the small intestine, so that it might indeed be achievable to become an expert in the field. This could be described as elitist, well so be it.

How do medical specialisms arise? This is a difficult question to answer, but could simplistically be summarized as through urgent clinical need. As a generalization it would be true to say that the development of paediatric specialties and organ specialties in particular has been remarkably slower than the development of specialties in general or adult medicine. For example national societies of gastroenterology were established first in Germany in 1895 and then the United States in the 1897. By contrast the first paediatric gastroenterology society, the European Society for Paediatric Gastroenterology, did not come into being until 1968, more than seventy years later.

In 1995 the British Paediatric Association (BPA) looked at the issue of the need for paediatric specialties in their document 'Tertiary Services for Young People'. They pointed out that before specialist services developed children were treated mainly by general paediatricians, adult specialists or by a combination of both. The results of treatment for some children and babies with life threatening diseases were often poor with high levels of morbidity and mortality. The outlook for these children had changed dramatically with the development of a specialist to co-ordinate an expert hospital based multidisciplinary team and also to liaise with local consultant paediatricians, primary care providers and community services. So this role of co-ordinating a multidisciplinary team was suggested to be the first feature for the development of a paediatric specialty. Indeed for my own practice of paediatric gastroenterology from my time at RAHC, a multi-disciplinary team had been at the heart of our service provision. However in my view nothing would have happened without the second feature listed by the BPA leading to the appearance of paediatric specialties. This was the development of new techniques and therapies specifically for children, not for little adults. The principal example for paediatric gastroenterology was the development of the technique for safe and effective small intestinal biopsy. This technological advance in my view, was the major factor for the development of paediatric gastroenterology in Europe and Australia, with a particular focus upon coeliac disease, where biopsy is central to diagnosis. In the United States the focus was perhaps more upon the development of liver biopsy and the trickle down effect of several other adult gastroenterological techniques and approaches, to the management of children.

The development of parenteral nutrition, i.e. giving an individual all their requirements intravenously, i.e. by a tiny plastic tube in the patient's veins, was also of central importance for the development of the discipline. From 1969 onwards, this therapeutic technique had a big impact on paediatrics as a whole and especially for infants with life threatening chronic diarrhoea which had become intractable, i.e. resistant to all therapies. Remarkably children who otherwise would have died were now being kept alive by this technique. These children could then be investigated and the cause of their diarrhoea discovered. As a result hitherto unknown diseases were described for the first time. Sometimes, but sadly not always effective therapeutic strategies could be developed. An example of this is autoimmune enteropathy mentioned in the last Chapter. For those children where no therapy specific for the disease has yet been developed, small intestinal transplantation would become a practical option in the nineties. I became an external assessor of the first small intestinal transport programme at Birmingham Children's Hospital from 1997 to 2000.

Again as this is an autobiography, it is not appropriate here to give a full history of the development of this specialty. This has been covered in a joint article, written with Allan Walker, entitled History of Paediatric Gastroenterology and published in 2002 in *Pediatric Research*. However it is important to make some general observations concerning the long British tradition of hostility towards the whole notion of specialization and to paediatrics in particular. The distinguished Barts physician Dr Samuel Gee provides an example of this going back to the end of the nineteenth century. Although he largely cared for adults he also looked after children at Barts as well as at Great Ormond St Hospital where he had also been appointed as an honorary physician. This was normal practice at that time. He vehemently-opposed the whole notion of specialization. He wrote that there were two names he abhorred, the name of a specialist and the name of a consultant! How he would disapprove of me. He was a very influential figure and his views were listened to. He vehemently opposed the whole conception of paediatrics both in lectures and in his writings. Yet he is famous for giving the first description of coeliac disease in children in 1888. In fact he gave a reminder that the ancient Greek physician Aretaeus the Cappadocian had first described the Coeliac Affection in antiquity but in adults. Gee was the first to describe the disorder in children. Gee was also the first to describe cyclical vomiting in children. So it is ironic that whilst he made a great contribution to knowledge of children's disease and gastroenterological ones in particular he opposed the development of the specialty of paediatrics.

Yet there were distinguished physicians who took an opposite position. One was another Bart's consultant Sir Archibald Garrod. He is now regarded as the father of biochemical genetics. He gave a lecture in 1899 to medical students at Barts in which he said the time had come to regard the diseases of children as a special branch of medicine. In due course he was to found the Department of Child Health at Barts in 1904. He was the first Physician in charge of Diseases of Children at Barts and I was to be the last. At RAHC there was a similar situation with physicians largely concerned with adults being appointed ab initio, until in the first decades of the century when Dr Lindsay Dey and Dr Margaret Harpel were appointed. Just before the war there were only four full-time paediatricians on the staff of RAHC, including Margaret Harper and Kate Winning. At QEHC Dr Helen Mackay was the first full-time paediatrician to be appointed in 1919. She was a remarkable woman and continued on the staff till 1959. She became the first woman Fellow of the Royal College of Physicians of London in 1934. The first woman President of the College Professor Dame Margaret Turner Warwick came to a dinner at QEHC in 1992 to celebrate the 125th Anniversary of the Hospital. On the occasion of the celebratory dinner, she also honoured the memory of Helen

Mackay. It is clear that women paediatricians were important pioneers at both RAHC and QEHC.

So in Britain and Australia, although children's hospitals had been founded in nineteenth century, the development of paediatrics was really a twentieth century phenomenon. Gradually paediatricians were appointed in London to care for children at GOS, QEHC and Barts itself rather than adult physicians, but it was not until the establishment of the Health Service in 1948 that the need for appointment of paediatricians everywhere for the care of children, became universal in the United Kingdom. Interestingly these same general paediatricians have often in turn themselves resisted the development of the paediatric specialties. As I pointed out in an earlier Chapter the Netherlands, Finland, Switzerland, Australia and the United States were ahead of Britain in the early sixties when the specialty began to appear internationally. Although there were individuals making contributions to knowledge of gastroenterological disease in children such as Dr Winifred Young at QEHC, they did not seek for recognition of a paediatric specialty.

I believe there are seven criteria which when fulfilled indicate that a paediatric specialty has become fully recognized as a legitimate medical specialty. These are:

1. A body of child patients who require grouping together for specialist medical care.

2. Special diagnostic techniques and therapies of complexity requiring training and skill to perform.

3. Consultants (specialists in the discipline), appointed full or part-time.

4. Academic appointments are made in the discipline.

5. Medical textbooks and specialist journals are published.

6. International and national professional bodies are established.

7. Training programmes in the discipline are developed.

In Britain by the end of the seventies all these criteria had been met, except the seventh, which was not established till the nineties. Assisted by Dr Deirdre Kelly, I and she developed a training programme which was ultimately approved by the Royal College of Paediatrics and Child Health and became the basis of the European training programme for ESPGHAN. We visited a number of leading centres for paediatric gastroenterology in England and Wales and reviewed their training programmes for the college.

Looking back, for paediatric gastroenterology, it was really the creation of the European Society of Paediatric Gastroenterology in Paris in 1968, which was of pivotal importance for the formal recognition of the specialty internationally. This was the first society for the discipline in the world. It was followed by the North American Society of Pediatric Gastroenterology (later NASPGN) in 1973. It is of interest that these were both international societies. It was to be several years before the national societies appeared in Europe and around the world. This related to the small number of emerging specialists in each country, so at first they could gain strength by banding together internationally.

For Britain a major landmark for the development of paediatric gastro-enterology was the foundation of the British Paediatric Gastroenterology Group, on 19 September 1974, at a meeting of the British Society of Gastroenterology (BSG) in Birmingham. The first convenor of the group was Dr Sandy McNeish, senior lecturer in Birmingham at the time. Charlotte Anderson, who had moved from Melbourne to become Professor of Paediatrics in Birmingham in 1968 and the British Paediatric Association (BPA) itself, supported this move. Indeed the principal annual meetings of the group were subsequently held at the time of the annual BPA meetings, until it became a society. In 1986 the British Society of Paediatric Gastroenterology was formally established with strict criteria for membership, and also a paediatric section of the British Society of Gastroenterology in the same year. This section had a rather uncontrolled membership and included adult gastroenterologists.

Over the years I have attended most of these paediatric gastroenterology meetings held in association with the BPA and since 1996 with its successor, the Royal College of Paediatrics and Child Health. These meetings are held annually each year in the spring, most often at the University of York. The society in recent years has become the British Society of Paediatric Gastroenterology, Hepatology and Nutrition (BSPGHAN).

The University of York is an ideal place to host such medical meetings. It is situated around a small lake with modern, indeed somewhat ugly, largely concrete buildings, which however are very functional. It is an attractive environment largely due to the lake with its wild birds, ducks, geese etc. and green surroundings. We stay in the students' accommodation, which is rather spartan, but satisfactory.

The principal purpose of these meetings of BSPGHAN is to present short 10 minute research papers (clinical or scientific) and to hear one or two guest lectures, which review important topics. In the early years there were quite often professional tensions at these meetings. In the seventies there were really only three paediatric gastroenterology teams in the United Kingdom, all led by academics who had been appointed to paediatric positions rather than to specialty posts. These were Dr (later Professor) John Harries at Great Ormond St Hospital (GOS) and Institute of Child Health (ICH), Dr Sandy McNeish (later Professor at Leicester and then Birmingham) and myself at St Bartholomew's Hospital and Queen Elizabeth Hospital for Children as senior lecturer in Child Health. Tragically John Harries died young in 1983 and Dr Peter Milla (later Professor) in due course succeeded him. John was a dynamic, albeit short of stature, Welshman. He was a rugby player and had a fine voice. He had a great talent for clinical research, the paediatric gastroenterology community was diminished by his untimely death.

There were variable rivalries between the three gastroenterological groups, which have gradually diminished over the years. These rivalries centred really upon professional recognition in a new and at first often unrecognised specialism. Looking back this competition centred probably on power and the desire to be the leading group in the newly emerging discipline. However the three principals remained personal friends throughout, despite inter-personal tensions at times. I had great respect for Sandy and John. Hot issues of rivalry centred upon the numbers of papers presented by each group and their quality, composition etc. when presented by the junior doctors. There was tough peer pressure. Sometimes an issue leading to controversy concerned what was perceived as mean-spirited questions asked during the discussion time after a presentation.

Nevertheless for a time there was a kind of triumvirate, which was able to shape policy in the early days of the group and to define its relationship with both the BPA and the BSG. Although other centres such as Manchester appeared, where Dr Victor Miller had been appointed as the first full time NHS paediatric gastroenterology consultant post. A major issue was to endeavour to ensure that the president of the British Society of Paediatric Gastroenterology and the chairman of the Paediatric Section of the British Society of Gastroenterology were one and the same person, to avoid unnecessary rivalry between the two.

There was, and is, another major group and that is the King's College Paediatric Hepatology Group lead by Dr Alex (later Professor) Mowatt (brother of my friend Ashley in Aberdeen). However although that group from the outset presented papers at the conference, it was not so concerned by the medical politics of the group. In later years hepatology became a major aspect of the specialty with the name hepatology being added to the title of the Society. Professor Meili-Vergani succeeded Alex Mowatt after his untimely death and Dr Deirdre Kelly (later Professor) developed a second major hepatology unit at Birmingham. Deirdre had been a very successful registrar on my firm at QEHC. She came to us highly recommended by Sheila Sherlock. Deirdre and I have been friends ever since. The hepatology interest was also recognized when Dr (later Professor) Stuart Tanner succeeded me as third and last convenor of BPGG before it became the British Society of Paediatric Gastroenterology and Nutrition.

I was greatly honoured to be elected first President of British Society of Paediatric Gastroenterology in 1986, but by then gastroenterology had expanded well beyond the original groups and a council was elected reflecting this. Ian Sanderson was the trainee representative at the first council and he was to become President himself in 2001.

The York meetings were also important occasions for young trainees to job-hunt and for trainers to assess what the market was like for good trainees. Also these were occasions for the development of friendships across the whole country and beyond and so later they became occasions for reunions for old friends. This social aspect was consolidated in the 1990s when an annual dinner hosted by Mead Johnson Nutritionals was arranged in the Merchant Adventurers Hall, in the city of York. This became the annual social highlight of paediatric gastroenterology in the UK. These occasions have lead to a reduction in old tensions within the Society and today it is remarkably free of such inter-personal rivalries.

The University of York is situated just outside the city of York, but far enough away to require a taxi, bus or car to travel into the city. The city itself is marvellous, with its ancient medieval city wall, with the green grass-covered slopes leading up to the walls, covered in daffodils when we have visited in spring. The Merchant Adventurers Hall where the annual dinner was and continues to be held each year is a superb medieval monument in a quite remarkable state of preservation. It was built between 1357 and 1361 from local oak trees. The Merchant Adventurers traded with all the ports of northern Europe and had great powers of patronage in the city of York.

An annual photograph of the BSPGHAN members present in the Hall has become a wonderful souvenir of the meeting, a record of the growth and changing Dramatis Personae of Paediatric Gastroenterology in the United Kingdom.

Of course the greatest building in York is the Minster itself. Its great white/grey (colour depending on the light) mass, towers above the city. This can be seen distantly to advantage, on a hill adjacent to the University. It has a small paediatric gastroenterology connection too. When the new roof was built, following the fire in the vault of the of the south transept, children from all over the United Kingdom designed six new bosses, as arranged by *Blue Peter* of the BBC. One shows a dehydrated baby drinking a cup of oral rehydration solution. This is most appropriate as the discovery of oral rehydration therapy was one of the landmarks of the twentieth century.

For me, the Minster is a very special place for a number of reasons. First my father had an etching of the Five Sisters windows in his rooms in Macquarie St Sydney throughout his career, which I now have. These windows are slender lancets more than 50 feet high filled with glass of an almost abstract design. He also had a souvenir plate of the Minster at home. Dad had worked in Harrogate and had admired the Minster very much on visits to York. Another connection for me is that the towers of Sydney's St Andrew's Cathedral are architecturally modelled on York Minster. The Minster is a wonderful and very spiritual place which I always visit whenever I am in York. I enjoy being able to mix professional and historical interests together.

Returning to the theme of development of a paediatric specialty, the role of textbooks and journals needs to be mentioned. I was very excited in 1973, not long after I had arrived in London, to be approached by Pitman Medical Publishing Ltd. to write a comprehensive text on Paediatric Gastroenterology. At that time, only one text in the English language existed, namely *Pediatric Clinical Gastroenterology* by Silverman, Hoy and Cozzeto from North America, published in 1971. I was told that Charlotte (Charlo) Anderson had been invited to write a comprehensive text by Blackwells. I felt quite unable to take on such a large task, not wishing to compete with Charlo who was more than ten years my professional senior. However I did feel that my own particular theme of *Diseases of the Small Intestine in Childhood* deserved a small text, to draw attention to this group of diseases in children. It also allowed me to publish, in a review manner much of the work with which I had been concerned at RAHC and QEHC I highlighted gastroenteritis and its complications which was surprisingly not covered in any detail by Charlo, I discovered after publication. Also with such a busy job I could only take on a modest text. I completed the monograph in July 1974 and it was duly published in 1975, at about the same time as the text Paediatric Gastroenterology edited by Charlotte Anderson and Valerie Burke. These were the two first textbooks in this discipline to be published in England.

Writing a book in those days was a practical chore. I did not type then, so I hired a typist to type my handwritten text. It was quite difficult subsequently to make any alterations. What a contrast this is to the modern world of word processors/PCs used for this autobiography. The book reviews took quite a time to appear, but I was pleased with them when they did.

The book was a success and gave my whole career and future professional life an important boost. It and the subsequent editions made me known internationally and led to many invitations abroad. Foreign language editions appeared in German and Portuguese (for Brazil). Reflecting the rapid advances in the field, the second edition appeared in 1979, the third in 1988 and in 1999 the fourth edition with Simon Murch after a longer interval. I was very pleased to have Simon join me with his 'up to date' knowledge, especially of gut immunology. It was a great boost to have him as co-author. Furthermore, the text for the first time had colour illustrations and was so much bigger than the first edition, 412 large format pages compared to 260 small format pages.

Good reviews continued for the Second Edition. I was so pleased to read the following in the American journal *Gastroenterology*:

> This new text is a delight. Written in a flowing, easy style, it is extremely readable and one immediately feels the author's ease and enjoyment of his field. If the small bowel could be given a personality the author has done so.

Best of all, the fourth edition was highly commended by the Society of Authors.

The publisher with whom I dealt for the third and fourth editions was John Harrison. We have become long-term friends. He was with Butterworths for the third edition and then moved on to Blackwells when he was keen to publish the *Journal of Pediatric Gastroenterology and Nutrition*, and then he had his own publishing house, Isis Medical Media by the Fourth Edition. It was a great asset to have his personal involvement throughout. He later sold Isis Medical Media, which ultimately was taken over by Martin Dunitz, its present publisher. John now has a new publishing house, Bladon Medical Publishing Limited.

In fact he had first been involved with another book published by Butterworths in 1983. Dr John Apley had approached me in 1977 to contribute to the *Postgraduate Paediatrics* series published by Butterworths for trainee paediatricians, established paediatricians and general practitioners. I felt unable to undertake this large task alone. So this time I invited two co-authors to join me, my colleagues and friends, from Canada, Dick Hamilton and from USA, Allan Walker. It was natural to turn to these two colleagues as I felt I must have native English speakers and I believed they were the leading figures in the subject in their respective countries. More importantly this book led on to the principal and largest text in the subject Pediatric Gastrointestinal disease with the three of us as co-editors plus Peter Durie of Canada and John Watkins of USA. Allan Walker was the leader of this group. The first edition appeared in 1991. A third edition was published in 2000 by BC Decker of Canada after we had all met at the Silver Lake, in New Hampshire for its planning.

All these texts have helped the development of the discipline and also my own personal development. So medical publishing has played both a major part in my life and pari passu knowledge concerning paediatric gastroenterology has hugely expanded. The increased size of the texts over the years makes this point very clear.

Turning now to the role of journals, only one journal has appeared in this discipline, namely the *Journal of Pediatric Gastroenterology and Nutrition,* which was first published in 1983 with Emi Lebenthal (American and Israeli) as editor in chief and Ettore Rossi of Berne as its associate editor. Initially it was very much Emi's own initiative that had started the journal. It was taken over by the two societies as their official journal in 1991. I was elected by ESPGAN council to be the ESPGAN editor from 1995-2000 and in 1996 my old friend Allan Walker was elected to be NASPGN editor from 1996-2001. It was a great delight for me and also quite efficient for the two of us to work together, knowing each other as well as we did. Alan Phillips acted as my deputy and was a great help in the day-to-day practicalities liaising with Terry Lichay our administrative assistant. Ian Sanderson helped in liaison between the North American and European offices.

Finally in my judgement the greatest accolade that may be given to a paediatric specialty is University recognition. The University of London has played a very important role in this regard. It has recognized a total of five chairs in paediatric gastroenterology. Harries (the first chair), myself, Sanderson, Milla and Alan Phillips, and and two in paediatric hepatology. Mowatt and Meili-Vergani. The university has also recognized the Academic Department of Paediatric Gastroenterology at the Medical College of St Bartholomew's Hospital in 1986 and its translation as the University Department of Paediatric Gastroenterology to the Royal Free School of Medicine in 1995, continuing at UCL till 2000. Then it lost its independence and became a centre for paediatric gastroenterology. The University also recognized a re-creation of the Academic department of Paediatric Gastroenterology at the new combined Barts and London medical school in 1997 which has now merged with adult gastroenterology. This now is headed by Professor Ian Sanderson.

Unfortunately, this academic momentum has ceased in the United Kingdom. At the time of writing (2012) Ian Sanderson is the only occupant of a chair of paediatric gastroenterology in England. Neither my chair nor Peter Milla's chair were replaced upon retirement. This relates to the perception that professors should now have a larger basic research interest, than was the case in my time.

CHAPTER TWELVE

A Chair in London, Perpetual Change

I WAS DELIGHTED to be appointed at last on 1 April 1985 to a personal chair of Paediatric Gastroenterology. I believe it was a landmark for the new specialty as well as for me personally. Yet I still had one remaining goal, the achievement of an independent department. This in fact took three more years to achieve. Understandably, Chris Wood was not keen on the idea, as its creation would result in a reduction in the size of his own department. The Academic Department of Paediatric Gastroenterology was however duly established on 1 August 1988, however I did not secure an independent lecturer post till September 1993 when Dr Simon Murch was appointed as clinical lecturer in paediatric gastroenterology. For the first time the lecturer post did not rotate through other disciplines.

Once the independent academic department was established, I thought all would be straightforward and I could steadily move towards my retirement in 2002, pursuing our research goals etc. However this was not to be. Very soon we were to be in a period of considerable turbulence with mergers, closures etc. leading ultimately to the transfer of my department to the Royal Free Hospital. However I am racing ahead. I must first state that as I go on to discuss this 15 year period 1985-2000, and to mention people who are still in active practice, I shall be circumspect and brief in my comments concerning them and more recent events.

The mid-eighties was a period of great change for me. Suddenly, to my great surprise I found myself in the ranks of the most senior consultants. It did not seem long since I had been the youngest consultant at Barts and enduring a sarcastic comment about my youthful appearance when I first entered the consultants' dining room at Barts in 1973. First my senior paediatric colleague at Bart's, Patrick Cox, retired unexpectedly early in 1984. Whilst I missed both his wisdom and friendship, there followed in due course the very welcome appointment of Dr Kate Costeloe, a neonatal 'star' (consultant neonatologist) in January 1985 as his successor, after an interregnum. This was very ably filled by Roderick Brown, who had recently retired from QEHC. At first Kate was also a general paediatrician at Barts but her main task was to establish the neonatal care service at the new Homerton Hospital following the transfer of the obstetric and associated neonatal services from Barts. In addition to Roderick, the other two senior consultants at QEHC Tony Jackson and Bernard Laurence also retired in the early eighties.

Most notably of all my great mentor in gastroenterology at Barts, Tony Dawson decided to retire early without any advance discussion with his colleagues, at the age of 57 years, on 18 July 1986. For me, this was a considerable disappointment and it marked the end of an era. I missed him.

However as one set of doors closed, others door opened, albeit in a different direction. Tom MacDonald established a notable research programme in our laboratory and he rapidly advanced from a CICRA research fellowship to Wellcome Senior Lecturer and then on to a Readership in Gut Immunology. In 1992 he was appointed Professor of Mucosal Immunology. From the mid-eighties Tom was a major player in my professional life. I had first met him many years earlier, whilst he had been working for his PhD in Edinburgh. Then I met him in the train on the way to a research meeting at the Mendip Hotel at Blagden near Bristol. We both were attending a meeting on 'Immune response to food antigens before and during weaning', organized by the University of Bristol Department of Veterinary Medicine with whom we were doing some collaborative research in November 1984. At that time he was working for industry in the USA with Merck Sharp and Dohme Research Laboratories, but was keen to return to the UK. He was wearing an astrakhan coat and at that time he wore his hair long. He looked for all the world like the pop star Rod Stewart, a fellow Scot. Tom is a Scot of Scots. It proved to be a notable meeting for Tom as he met there his future wife, Jo Spencer, from University College London, a fellow immunologist. They were to do some notable collaborative research together after Tom came to our laboratory at Barts. One result was a seminal paper concerned the way the T-lymphocytes or T-cells within the small intestinal mucosa, when activated (in various ways) caused mucosal abnormality similar to that found in children with untreated coeliac disease.

The eighties were a successful time both for publication and for bringing in financial resources. It would be boring if too much financial detail were included but suffice it to say that in the financial year 1986/7 paediatric gastroenterology at Barts/Queens brought in £110,557 administered by the Medical College of Barts and £23,508 administered elsewhere. CICRA, followed by the Wellcome Trust, were the biggest contributors, with various other sources of soft money funding including the Queen Elizabeth Research Appeal Trust.

The eighties were a time for developing closer links with surgical colleagues at Barts. One of the great assets of the service at Barts was our access to the superb surgical team lead by Mr William Shand who had succeeded Sir Ian Todd. He was an expert in the surgical treatment of Crohn's disease and also a great Barts patriot and delightful colleague. This need for surgery gradually built up as the years went by as we learnt that quite a number of children with chronic Crohn's disease needed surgical removal of diseased bowel so that they could fulfil their growth potential and have a normal puberty. Dr Martin Savage played a key role in defining the most opportune time for surgery to permit normal growth, i.e. before puberty is complete.

At Barts by 1990 it had become clear, after a long interregnum, that Michael Farthing was Tony Dawson's heir from a clinical research perspective, and he was appointed to a Chair of Gastroenterology, the first at Barts. Tony, although a very distinguished clinical researcher had never sought academic status. He had felt his title of physician at St Bartholomew's Hospital was the greatest recognition he wanted. Tony also became physician to the Royal Household and was knighted in due course. Clearly by 1990 things had changed and a professional appointment to facilitate gastroenterological research at Barts had become essential. I had seen Michael grow in stature first as a young research fellow, then as consultant and finally as professor. He always had an air of youth and enthusiasm about him which carried his colleagues forward. It was he to whom I personally handed over the care of my young patients with chronic inflammatory bowel disease as they moved from childhood to adolescence. These hand-over clinics were so important. I was pleased to see the look of relief and anticipation on their faces when I introduced the young people to him.

He has a gift for working with young adults and seems able very easily to identity with their needs and problems. In 2000 he moved on to the post of Dean of the Faculty of Medicine in the University of Glasgow.

Working together we undertook a major research programme concerning the use of a low sodium low osmolality oral rehydration solution for children with acute gastroenteritis in the United Kingdom. This was a joint laboratory and clinical study, whose outcome influenced ESPGAN'S recommendations for the composition of oral rehydration solutions for the children of Europe. From my team notable investigators in this study were Elizabeth Elliott from RAHC, Sydney and Roque Ferriera from Lisbon. Liz achieved an MD whilst she was with us and is now a distinguished academic in paediatric gastroenterology in the University of Sydney at RAHC, whereas Roque has changed careers and ultimately left medicine to have an equally distinguished career in business in Portugal. Michael also helped with the supervision of PhD studies for two Commonwealth 'Medical' Scholars from Bangladesh A.F.M. Salim and Mamoun Shahrier. Salim has returned to Bangladesh offered a spell as a medical officer in Brunei. Whereas Mamoun has settled in the USA as an adult gastroenterologist.

In 1990 my life took a new direction when I was elected chairman of the senior staff at QEHC and appointed chairman of the Hospital Management Team (HMT) for three years. This team was a triumvirate where I joined the Director of Nursing Services Miss Olga Kurtianyk and a succession of unit administrators. Judith Banfield filled this post in 1992. This was my first and only experience as a medical administrator it was an interesting and testing time. It was a time of considerable concern by QEHC staff that GOS was progressively asset stripping the laboratories of the hospital. Progressively histopathology, bacteriology and virology were being rationalized to GOS/ Institute of Child Health (ICH).

This was also the time when hospital trust status was being considered by the NHS as a whole and so the HMT decided to explore the issue of trust status for QEHC as a separate entity or merged with Barts. This was not happily received, as might be imagined by the Board of Governors of the Hospitals for Sick Children whose meetings at GOS I now attended as an observer. Dr Ken Grant CEO of City and Hackney Health Authority was very positive but warned me that if QEHC joined City and Hackney it risked being closed down. How prophetic he was! In 1998 the event after extensive consultation the HMT decided to it was best to stay with GOS. However closer academic links between the Institute of Child Health and the medical colleges of Barts and the London were planned. I had the great responsibility of chairing several meetings of the three deans in the boardroom at Queens. These discussions were all to be aborted by the recommendations of the Tomlinson Report.

The most enjoyable thing about the post of chairman of HMT was contributing to the organization of the 125th anniversary year of the hospital. The hospital had been founded in 1867 as the North-Eastern Hospital for Children by the Quaker sisters Ellen and Mary Phillips in the wake of the London cholera epidemic of 1866. Ellen had nursed children with cholera in the London Hospital. The awful sights she saw at that time were seared on her memory during that terrible summer of 1866. These memories led both sisters to seek to practically help the deprived sick children of East London. They were assisted by Dr Alexander Fox. He had emigrated to New Zealand but had returned to study medicine at the London Hospital. There he met Ellen, fell in love with her and in due course, married her. Later Alexander and Ellen were to return to New Zealand, partly because Ellen had become seriously ill with a lung abscess. Interestingly this connection with New Zealand was never forgotten and was recalled in May 1982 when the centenary of the first cargo of frozen lamb brought from New Zealand to Britain in the Dunedin was commemorated. The New Zealand High Commissioner visited the hospital and frozen New Zealand meat was given as a gift to mark the event, to patients and staff alike. The hospital thrived during the latter part of the nineteenth century. In 1908 it was honoured by the name 'The Queen's Hospital for Children', with permission of Queen Alexandra. In 1942 the hospital was amalgamated with the Princess Elizabeth of York Hospital at Shadwell. It was then re-named the Queen Elizabeth Hospital for Children. The Queen and her husband King George VI took great interest in the hospital. Their Daughter Princess Elizabeth, the future Elizabeth II, made her first speech in public there in 1944 to the Annual Court of Governors as President of the Hospital. The event was recorded on film. She was to return several times, most notably to open the new Hayward Research Building in 1972. It was this building together with the advent of the Academic Department of Child Health, housed within it from its inauguration, that made the last twenty-six years of the hospital's life so productive in clinical research terms. It also provided a transfusion of vigour and vitality into the patient service provided by its modern laboratories which had dual role responsibilities for research and routine service. All this was to be cut off and destroyed by the Tomlinson Report, a tragic blow to the good care of the sick children of East London. Although the laboratory base had already been considerably weakened in the latter days by GOS, 'rationalizing' histopathology and microbiology to their site in West London. Perhaps this regrettable policy, which I had opposed as chairman of HMT, made the hospital ripe for closure.

As chairman of the HMT, I was able to catalyse a book edited by Jules Kosky entitled *Queen Elizabeth Hospital for Children, 125 Years of Achievement.* This was a multi-author text providing an important insight into the care of children in east London over this period. Judith Banfield and Jules Kosky wrote in their Chapter on 'The Hospital Today' as follows:

> Queen Elizabeth Hospital has a development plan for a new V-shaped building to be built on the present car park further along Goldsmith's Row behind the Hayward Building, designed to blend with the style of surrounding residential buildings, it is planned to contain a new Accident and Emergency Department,

> a new Outpatients, and a new Operating Theatre Suite. There will also be room for a new Medical Records Department and other patient services.
>
> The future of the Queen Elizabeth Hospital for Children is assuredly a bright one, full of unshakeable hope in its future ability to provide and improve on its care for the children of the East End. In the surrounding area, the number of births was higher than had been prognosticated by over 500 for the last year, a trend directly contrary to most other areas. The future we are always told is in the hands of our children.The Queen Elizabeth Hospital has shown by its past and present record that the future health and happiness of those children lies to great extent in its care.

Tomlinson in his report and the government acting on his advice ensured that this vision was destroyed. We did not have any inkling of this, as our celebratory year of 1992 began. Indeed looking back, for me early 1992, with the notable celebrations for the 125th anniversary of the foundation of the Queen Elizabeth Hospital for Children, was a peak in my career.

The central event of the celebration in 1992 was a children's party attended by Queen Elizabeth the Queen Mother, the patron of the hospital, who had visited the hospital so often during her long life. As well as the local schoolchildren my son James and some friends from Chigwell school were also able to attend this celebratory party. Then there was the inauguration of a scientific and historic exhibition by the Lord Mayor of London. Alan Phillips had done an enormous amount of work to produce the exhibition which demonstrated the hospital's remarkable history serving the deprived children of the east end since 1867 and also its contemporary research activities. Little did we realize at the time that lamentably the hospital would only survive another six years. After the inauguration of the scientific exhibition, the medical, scientific and nursing officers wearing academic dress, processed with the Lord Mayor from the hospital to the nearby St Peter's Church of England for a remarkable multi-faith religious service. A Jewish rabbi and a Moslem iman joined representatives of the Christian churches (Roman Catholic, Greek Orthodox, Salvation Army, United Reform Church and the Church of England). This symbolized the truly remarkable multicultural and multiracial community, which the hospital served. At that time, quite often more than half of our child patients were of ethnic origins outside Britain.

At this point it is important to emphasize the multiracial aspect of the hospital which was so valuable. In my earlier years at the hospital, quite a number of the child patients had been born in the Indian sub-continent, especially from the region of Sylhet in Bangladesh, but as time went on, with immigration controls, most were born in the United Kingdom. The east end of London has a remarkable tradition of receiving newcomers to this country. This is symbolized by a building in Brick Lane which was built as a protestant church for the Hugenot refugees from religious persecution in France in the eighteenth century. In 1890 it became a Jewish synagogue and then in the 1970s it became a mosque, as it remains today. So it reflects the three great immigrations to this part of London over two centuries.

Most Bangladeshi families seek to take their children born in this country back to their ancestral homeland before their children are two years old, so that their elderly grandparents who have remained in Bangladesh can see them. Often as a result the children acquire gastrointestinal infection during their visits followed by chronic diarrhoea and malnutrition, which usually last several months. Some such children returned to this country gravely ill and came to QEHC. One of my clinical lecturers Paul Hutchins wrote a paper describing this as 'Travellers diarrhoea with a vengeance'. The plight of such children significantly stimulated the research programme that Alan Phillips undertook over many years and he continues today at a more basic or molecular level concerning the infective bacterium Enteropathogenic E.coli, one significant cause of this problem. It was this experience with children with chronic diarrhoea and malnutrition that stimulated me to initiate in 1986 the Commonwealth Conferences on Chronic Diarrhoea and Malnutrition which lead ultimately to the foundation of the Commonwealth Association of Paediatric Gastroenterology and Nutrition (CAPGAN). It was a huge privilege to be involved in these problems, which are so important in the developing world.

However the most bizarre event of the 125th anniversary celebrations was the extraordinary visit of the American pop star Michael Jackson, on 29 July 1992. I wrote at the time 'He flitted in and out of the hospital like a bird. He did not like bright lights and constantly was adjusting his dark glasses and twisting a long forelock of his black hair'. He fingered the gold chain worn around the neck of the local mayor who greeted him in the foyer of the hospital. Michael Jackson asked the mayor if he could buy it! I escorted him to see a gravely ill older child patient who was delighted to see him, but he seemed more concerned to be photographed with the patient and he had very little to say. I thanked him and shook his hand, which was small and soft and almost seemed to melt in my grip. He was escorted through the hospital by enormous bodyguards. Indeed, as was reported in the Daily Mirror 'excited youngsters were unable to see him behind a phalanx of security guards and camera crew - including his own video unit.' In fact as reported there were more tears than cheers from the children and the whole visit ended after 15 minutes. What had been conceived by the general manager as good publicity for the hospital turned into a media circus with children being pushed aside by overzealous guards.

It became clear later in 1992 following the Tomlinson report, which is discussed in Chapter 14, that all was to change. The future dramatically became quite uncertain. The optimism of the 125th anniversary turned overnight to profound pessimism. Yet the day-to-day life of my own paediatric gastroenterology department had to continue. Indeed with the appointment of Simon Murch as clinical lecturer in 1993 a whole new direction in clinical research, i.e. patient related research began, which focused upon the gut as an immunological organ in clinical situations in individual patients with rare disorders and also with food allergy and Crohn's disease. How gastrointestinal immunological defects produced the symptoms and signs of disease in the children themselves was investigated. This programme expanded when Simon was appointed as senior lecturer with consultant status in March 1995 and this expansion continued following the transfer of the department to the Royal Free in September 1995, utilizing our new fully equipped laboratory.

Simon is immensely talented with a great capacity for original ideas based upon the latest developments in international research. I had first met him professionally at Barts in 1988 when he was clinical lecturer. It was a difficult time when we had temporarily to move out of our own ward to Rees Mogg ward, whilst it was being refurbished. He was very helpful in picking up the pieces. After this he began a laboratory base research study involving immunological aspects of lung disease in neonates supervised by Tom MacDonald with the collaboration of Kate Costeloe in our laboratory at Barts. He did remarkably well and achieved his PhD. He however gradually moved over from neonatology to his lifetime principal interest, i.e. gut immunology. So he changed his career ambition to be a paediatric gastroenterologist rather than a neonatologist. This in due course led on to his appointment as my first full time clinical lecturer in paediatric gastroenterology. He in addition has a great capacity to be a very caring doctor who closely involves himself in the individual child patient's problems. In addition he has a well-developed sense of humour with a literary dimension. As an example of this a quotation follows from our Fourth Edition:

> A variety of tissue-specific factors... rather splendid names such as 'winged helix'... derives from the appearance of these transcription factors when bound to DNA. Other names appear less pure in their provenance, and, when not fearsome acronyms to shame immunologists, suggest a predilection for

> B-movies and cartoons, over the novels of Jane Austen... perhaps as educational standards continue to rise (politicians continue to affirm that this is the case) Darcy transcription factor may yet make its appearance.

Despite the personal trauma for me and my colleagues and patients and their parents, the transfer to the Royal Free occurred with remarkably little disruption of the clinical service or the research programme. Some ongoing collaboration occurred with Barts via the CICRA fellows John Fell and Rob Heuschkel. We received a very warm welcome from all and sundry when we arrived at the Royal Free. Our 200 new department and modernized ward (Malcolm ward) were all we could have hoped for. It provided for the first time in my career the ideal set-up in terms of physical facilities for child patients, their parents and staff both medical and nursing. There was ample opportunity for both parents to 'live in' with very sick children. The facilities were comparable to those of a good hotel. What a contrast to the ward facilities I had observed at Barts and Queens when I had first arrived for interview in 1972, quite a revolution in quality. What a contrast in practice to those limited visiting hours I had encountered in Zurich in 1967. What a challenge this excellent provision for service and research represented for us all. Would we be able to live up to the high expectations of our new colleagues? Whether we did or not do so, is for others to judge. However the move was a wonderful renewal for us all and despite the pains and regrets of leaving Barts and Queens a whole new world opened up.

A very significant addition to the consultant staff at the Royal Free, was Mike Thomson who was appointed at the young age of 32 years. He had had a good deal of his training in Brisbane Australia, notably in endoscopy. I had first met him when he had attended our post-graduate course at Barts. He was clearly a young man of talent, ambition and drive so I was delighted when he was appointed. Mike in fact led further developments in service provision after our arrival, most importantly he led the move to develop facilities on the ward itself for endoscopy in a side room, where general anaesthesia could be given. For children and their parents this was a huge advantage. As a consequence no long journey in the lift and along corridors to the endoscopy suite was now necessary. The endoscopic work rapidly expanded till by 2000 we had three endoscopy sessions each week. For me one sad by-product of this was the abandonment of the Crosby capsule for small intestinal biopsy. I was persuaded by Mike Thomson that all such biopsies should now be performed as an endoscopic procedure under general anaesthesia. This was of course more expensive and cumbersome but it did mean that we also were able to look at the oesophagus and stomach in every patient with some important and unexpected diagnoses such as infection with helicobacter pylori being made, which could be treated effectively. Mike also believed it was a safer procedure than the Crosby capsule biopsy and avoided the heavy sedation necessary for a few children. However I had myself invariably over many years found Crosby capsule biopsy to be very safe indeed. Endoscopic biopsy also avoided the occasional failure to obtain a biopsy which occurred when the Crosby capsule failed to 'fire'. Other units in Europe such as those in Finland still use the Crosby capsule biopsy but in the USA its use has virtually disappeared. For me it had personally been the most notable technological advance of my career. So its departure was a great change for me and perhaps a signal to prepare for retirement. Sir James Paget, the distinguished nineteenth century physician, is reported to have said that as men grow old and wish for rest they dislike the changes which come from increased knowledge. I hope that is not seen as my position for I have tried with optimism and enthusiasm to embrace new advances as they occurred. Whilst I see myself as a conservative in general outlook on life in matters of medicine I should like to be thought of as a radical.

Alan Phillips and Simon Murch both set up important research programmes in our new laboratory. The facilities for research which we had previously had been on two sites at Barts and Queens. These were now united on one site. Our electron microscopes from QEHC were transferred with us, although the Royal Free had to purchase them, which did not appear fair to me! This move was most appropriate as the Wolfson family trust and other benefactors at QEHC had specifically made donations for its purchase for gastrointestinal research by my team. At this point the issue of research funding must be mentioned. Part of our funding was grants from research bodies and trusts and part from commercial firms mostly pharmaceutical firms and infant nutrition enterprises, as well as from individual donations as mentioned above. The firms included Nestlé, Cow and Gate, Milupa, Nutricia and Scientific Hospital Supplies (SHS). Controversy has surrounded the acceptance of funds from some of these in relation to the issue of promotion of infant feeding formulae, i.e. bottle feeding rather than the much preferred breast feeding. I firmly endorse breast feeding as the ideal and have done so throughout my career. However in our research over the years two key collaborations with such firms have developed in relation to special feeding formulae required for treatment. The first has been the development of a special feeding formula Modulin with Nestlé as enteral feeding for the treatment of older children with Crohn's disease, and the second has been the use of a special amino acid formula for babies with severe food allergy i.e. Neocate produced by SHS.

I have felt it right to accept research funds from these companies because there were no strings attached and we were free to present and publish the data. The Nestle company has been the object of a boycott by some workers in the field, especially from developing communities, but societies such as ESPGHAN have felt it right to accept funding from the company for the annual council meeting in Vevey, for many years. I am especially grateful to Dr Franck Arnaud-Battandier of Nestlé in Paris, who contributed importantly. to our research on enteral feeding, also to Mr. Graham Coates of SHS who facilitated research in Zambia with Dr Beatrice Amadi.

At the Royal Free I was impressed by the leadership of Martin Else as GEO in the hospital and Arie Zuckerman as Dean in the Medical School. Both gave me great support. The controversies related to MMR are discussed separately in Chapter 15. Apart from these my five years at the Royal Free were a good time with the steady development and consolidation of our expertise in paediatric gastroenterology both in the research laboratory and in the clinical care of children. Three separate thematic consultant led outpatients clinics were established for the better care of children, a Paediatric Inflammatory Bowel Disease Clinic led by me, a Food allergy and Coeliac Disease Clinic led by Simon Murch and Nutrition and Upper Gastrointestinal Clinic led by Mike Thomson. This thematic approach enabled the support teams of dieticians etc. as well as the nursing staff to be more focused and to produce a service of greater quality.

Another specialty clinic was the joint growth inflammatory bowel disease clinic I ran jointly with Professor Martin Savage, paediatric endocrinologist at Barts, who graciously continued attending the clinic after we had transferred to the Royal Free. The collaboration with Martin was invaluable as he taught me so much about growth and how it was impaired in chronic inflammatory bowel disease. I also valued his friendship and sage counsel over many years.

The role of the supporting team over the years must now be mentioned. Nursing staff were of key importance. Over my career there were dramatic changes in the nursing staff. When I arrived at Barts the ward sister had a job for 'life' but by the time I had retired, this had changed to the sisters only spending two to three years in a particular ward. This had great implications for continuity of care and indeed tradition. The development of specialist nursing sisters to assist the ward sister was however a great advance. The multi-disciplinary team became increasingly a vital part of our work Also of key importance were the dieticians. Their specialized knowledge of the many specific types of diet and feeding formulae of therapeutic importance to children with gastrointestinal disorders played a vital part in the care provided.

One dietician I must mention is Mrs Christine Carter of QEHC/GOS whose knowledge, care and devotion to her calling was remarkable. We missed her when we transferred and it took some time to develop the excellent dietetic services we eventually had at the Royal Free. From 1973 to my retirement I was able to secure a paediatric dietician interested in gastroenterology to attend my ward round and outpatient clinic. This enormously facilitated both patient care but also clinical research, as dietary therapy is so central to paediatric gastroenterology.

The vital necessity of good secretarial support services must also be mentioned. I could not have functioned over the years Without the help of personal secretarial support which for most of my career was outstanding. At the Royal Free it began on a high note with Victoria Milson and finished on an equally high note with Debbie England who was my last secretary.

One immense area has not been covered in this autobiography that is the story of the child patients themselves and their parents. This I cannot discuss for reasons of confidentiality but this excludes a huge area of my life as much of my time was actually spent with the children and their parents. One boy I can illustrate in a photograph as he gave his permission to be photographed as a news item, as our first patient in the new department at the Royal Free, having transferred with us from Barts Hospital. I do want to pay tribute to so many incredibly brave children I have encountered over the years, very especially those fighting Crohn's disease, an embarrassing diarrhoeal disease which often at first evokes unkind lavatorial jokes rather than sympathy from other children and even adults, including school teachers. I also must pay tribute to their parents. Through CICRA I have kept in contact with a number of them and I have been greatly impressed by their devotion and dogged determination to better the quality of their children's lives. One of the things most appreciated by retired doctors is news of the success of their former child patients in adult life. As I was writing this Chapter I was delighted to hear from a parent concerning her son, a patient of mine at Barts who had been gravely ill with Crohn's disease, who had just graduated in medicine. It is remarkable how many of my former patients with Crohn's disease have become successful doctors both general practitioners and consultants. I also must pay particular tribute to those parents labouring to care for the gravely disturbed children with autism who often display aggressive destructive behaviour. It is very humbling for professionals to see this devotion.

I have much appreciated the many many medical students who over the years have passed through my hands. I feel it a great honour to have taught them. I really enjoyed teaching and I am pleased to be still teaching them the history of medicine. I especially appreciated the feedback from my weekly tutorial groups I conducted in my office at QEHC from 1973-1995, When I meet former students years later it is fascinating to learn what they have done and how they look back on their student days. They also taught me a great deal over the years by their general insight and helped me to try and cross the generational age gap.

As I come to the end of my professional life, I am afraid a sour note must be sounded by yet another, merger, this time of the medical school to which I had just newly bonded to form the Royal Free and University College London School of Medicine, whose administrative base was off site at University College London (UCL). The subsequent decline in staff morale in some quarters was quite obvious. However by the time of my retirement many adjustments had been made and new relationships I forged yet I remain a sceptic concerning the value of this merger and all the other mergers in London, but it was a far less emotive, merger than the Barts London merger.

In more general terms looking back over the last five years of the twentieth century it has become clear to historians that there was a major paradigm shift in medical research away from classical patho-physiology and classical genetics towards molecular biology (although molecular genetics to some extent reconciles the two approaches). Put in more lay terms scientific medicine had really come of age and disease could often be viewed as the consequences of a defect at the level of individual molecules in the body. The success of the human genome project and the associated leap in technology, has set the scene for successful gene therapy in the twenty-first century of hitherto incurable chronic diseases, probably on a large scale. So now in the first decade of the twenty-first century is a time of optimism for continuing medical progress based upon the continuing advances in technology. The United States has taken the lead in rapidly recognizing the continuing importance of such technological progress by its policy on research funding. Paradoxically delivery of care may often be defective in America under their system of insurance but American dominance in medical laboratory research becomes ever clearer. Yet Britain has made a greater contribution than her population or size would indicate to medical research and she follows the American lead in this direction. The Wellcome Trust has played a large role in funding in the UK. In both countries what the historians are calling the 'molecularization' of medicine is now moving forward rapidly. In addition the highly competitive nature of American research is rapidly spreading to Britain. In our own experience we have seen the value of the molecular approach. Tom MacDonald, and Simon Murch in the Paediatric Gastroenterology Laboratory were able to show that excess production of the molecule, tumour necrosis factor alpha was of key importance in the production of the inflammation of the wall of the bowel in Crohn's disease and was associated with impaired growth. Investigators largely in the Netherlands were able to take this observation forward and produce a drug called a therapeutic monoclonal antibody which acted against this molecule.

Reflecting these developments, new Medical Professors at University College London are now required to be skilled both in the techniques of molecular biology and also be able to attract very large sums of money as research grants. So it was a great disappointment to me that my chair of paediatric gastroenterology was frozen upon my retirement, as a result of this revolution in policy for professorial appointments.

This decision coupled with the ending of the autonomy and indeed the very existence of the University Department of Paediatric Gastroenterology did cast shadows over my retirement. My former department was merged with all the other paediatric departments on the two sites of the Royal Free and University College Hospitals to form a unitary University Department of Paediatrics and Child Health. This ironically was the very situation that I had escaped from at QEHC and Barts in 1988, which so sadly was restored on my retirement at the Royal Free, the cycles of history!

I favour the traditional university department and this concept was intact in the University Department of Paediatric Gastroenterology at the moment of my retirement. This conception is now being challenged in the university. Centralization is the present trend and there is a push in some quarters to create ephemeral research teams and abolish the traditional departments. The permanency of university departments is in my view a focus for loyalty and stability, not qualities admired so much in the current frenetic times.

The Festschrift arranged by Alan Phillips at the Royal Free Hospital to mark my retirement and the dinner in the Great Hall at Barts arranged by Ian Sanderson and the subsequent publication as a supplement of the *Journal of Pediatric Gastroenterology and Nutrition* in 2002, edited by Alan, crowned my career. I was delighted and honoured that so many of my former trainees, colleagues and friends, even from as far afield as Australia, USA, Canada and Singapore joined me and my family in a celebration of paediatric gastroenterology, recognizing what had been achieved but recognizing how much more needed to be done both for cure and prevention of gastrointestinal disease in children. There is no possible room for complacency.

Reflections in 2002

As I now come to an end of the chronological account of my life up to the time of my retirement, I wish to briefly take stock of my forty years in clinical practice from graduation in 1960 to retirement in 2000.

It was a time of sentiment when I graduated in Sydney. Sentiment was then a powerful force in Australian society. At a political level, our Prime Minister Sir Robert Menzies believed in the everlasting unity of the British world, as a major determinant of Australian government policy. At a personal level, my father spent the greater part of his professional life working in an honorary capacity.

It was a time of cynicism when I retired in London. At a political level much of the media perceived British government policy as a question of 'spin' rather than conviction. At a personal level, enlightened self-interest was the major motivation for many of my colleagues but by no means all. There is a paradox here. By leaving Sydney and coming to London I had naively hoped to preserve sentiment and to avoid cynicism. This was not to be, as the rise of cynicism has been the inexorable reality throughout the former worldwide British community.

Our move to London was the most dramatic and unexpected decision I ever took. The seed was planted in London between 1962 and 1964, it germinated with the disappointment of my return to Prince Alfred and came to fruition and harvest with unexpected opportunity to work at Barts that presented itself in 1972. Reflecting now I believe that part of my reason for moving was my wish that I, my children and future grandchildren should remain British. I could see that the era of Australian Britons such as me and my family was coming to an end. Just before our departure a vivid pointer of the unwelcome direction in which Australia was moving came in December 1972 with the election to power of Gough Whitlam. My reflections on these matters and Anglo-Australia are outlined in Chapter 17.

I retain a real love for Sydney, the city of my birth. It is with real excitement that I return every two or three years, but our home now is in the garden suburb of Woodford Green, close to Epping Forest and on the edge of what for me is the greatest metropolis in the world, London. However I and my family will always be pulled hither and thither by our dual loyalties to the two cities and what now sadly are two completely separate and distinct nations.

2002-2012

After my retirement the shadows over my former department proved to be greater than I could ever have foreseen. First the two most senior colleagues Simon Murch and Mike Thomson in due course availed themselves of job opportunities elsewhere, Simon to a chair of Paediatrics at University of Warwick and Mike to a consultant post in Sheffield. I was delighted when

Rob Heuschkel, my former CICRA fellow was appointed as a consultant. He expanded and developed the Paediatric Inflammatory Bowel Disease Clinic. However he too chose to move on, to Addenbrooke's Hospital in Cambridge. There he has created from scratch, an outstanding new centre for paediatric gastroenterology. He also recruited Franco Torrente, from the Royal Free. His wife Camilla joined Rob's team as a third paediatric gastroenterologist. Research developed in epigenetics with Matt Zilbauer as Lecturer.

The twentieth annual course in paediatric gastroenterology was held at the Royal Free for the last time in 2010. It then transferred to Cambridge in 2011 as a new Masterclass in Paediatric Gastroenterology.

In 2009 Alan Phillips retired and to my great sadness the paediatric gastroenterology laboratory was closed, at the Royal Free Hospital. Alan however had fulfilled in every way my expectations, at the time of my retirement. His many achievements were recognized by the University College London. He was awarded a personal chair. He chose the title of Professor of Paediatric Gastroenterology because his major research interest lay within this field, although he was not a clinician.

CHAPTER THIRTEEN

Paediatric Gastroenterology, International Connections and World Travel

APART FROM THE obvious pleasure of visiting new countries and also renewing old friendships in distant lands how can an academic doctor justify world travel? Although the question might be posed another way, how can an academic justify staying at home? In my view the academic purposes of foreign travel may be summarized as follows:

1 To attend international conferences such as the annual meeting of ESPGAN (later ESPGHAN) both to learn about and to contribute to the current state of the art and perhaps most importantly of all to meet other researchers face to face.

2. To visit, a centre to develop joint research plans and to raise finance for research.

3. To undertake lecture tours especially in less developed centres. This could be called the missionary function for the discipline of paediatric gastroenterology. In the 1970s I did this quite often but with the spread of knowledge and expertise and appearance of text books etc., this has become much less important, so that more recently lecture trips abroad are more about exchanging information, i.e. these have become occasions for bilateral exchange of ideas.

Over the past 35 years I have visited professionally every country in western Europe except Luxemburg, most countries of eastern Europe, Israel and many Arab countries of the Gulf and the Middle East, many countries of the Far East, especially Commonwealth countries such as India Pakistan, Brunei, Singapore and Malaysia but also Taiwan and Thailand. There have been many visits to North America since 1967 and more recently increasing trips to South America, to Venezuela, Brazil, Chile and Argentina. What a privilege it has been to meet so many colleagues and to make friends around the world. I feel as if I am a citizen of a country called Paediatric Gastroenterology. I believe I have now met most of the members of our community around the world.

Perhaps the most memorable I have ever attended was the second annual meeting of the newly formed European Society of Paediatric gastroenterology in Interlaken, Switzerland in 1968. This meeting produced very influential recommendations for diagnostic criteria for coeliac disease (the Interlaken or the ESPGAN criteria). These criteria emphasize the central importance of small intestinal biopsy (or diagnosis of coeliac disease and the need for several, i.e. serial biopsies taken at the time of diagnosis, after recovery of the child all a gluten-free diet, after return to a normal gluten containing diet, showing relapse of the abnormality. When this has been done then a gluten-free diet is recommended for life, as coeliac disease is a disorder of permanent gluten intolerance. This complex approach was recommended as it was considered that in this age group there was also a disorder of transient or temporary gluten intolerance.

I was privileged to join two working parties held to follow-up and to modify these criteria first in Zurich in 1978 and then in Paris In 1989. Paris was an especially important meeting as we decided, based on further research, to step back from the need for three serial biopsies in older children but kept this recommendation for children who first had symptoms under the age of two years because in that age group there are many other causes of small intestinal mucosli abnormality. We also recommended a new blood test which was available to screen for the disease. In Paris it was an honour for me to join with my old teacher from Zurich, David Shmerling, Jarmo Visakorpi (one of the great pioneers of coeliac disease from Finland) and Stefano Guandalini from Naples who at that time was a rising star in our discipline, as well as our host Jacques Schmitz of Paris who by then was an old friend. For me making international friendships across Europe has been one of the great values of the ESPGHAN meetings over the past 33 years.

In Interlaken in 1969 I was accompanied by my wife, as it occurred just after our honeymoon in Lucerne. At that time I little thought that I myself would ever become a member of the European Society, yet once I settled in Britain in 1973. I did so and I have attended every annual meeting each year since, up to and including Taormina, Sicily in 2002. I have been very lucky to have had a published abstract at every meeting from 1973-2002. I was honoured to be elected secretary from 1988 to 1991, under the presidency first of Salvatore Auricchio of Naples and then Birgitte Strandvik of Stockholm. The society appointed me ESPGHAN editor of the journal of *Pediatric Gastroenterology and Nutrition* from 1995-2000.

In 1979 with John Harries of GOS as co-host, the annual meeting was arranged in London at the Royal College of Physicians and Barts. Then in 1990 I was sole host as an emergency for a meeting organized at Barts with enormous help from Alan Phillips and Tom MacDonald a well as the rest of my department.

So ESPGHAN has played a very important part in my professional life and also in my personal life, as I was able to make so many friends of colleagues in Europe and beyond at these meetings. However, predictably there were often tensions. The medical politics of ESPGHAN is quite fierce with not so much national rivalries (although these can play a part on occasion) but personal rivalries, there sometimes being conflict between people from the same country. During my tenure as secretary two contentious things happened. First there was the issue of who should publish the *Journal of Pediatric Gastroenterology and Nutrition* once the two societies ESPGAN and NASPGN took over the journal in 1990 from the first editor/founder Emi Lebenthal. Basically it came down to a decision in the end between the existing publishers Raven Press of America or Blackwells press of Oxford. The president Birgitte Strandvik preferred Raven Press, and I, the secretary, preferred Blackwells. The argument swung back and forth at the annual council meeting in Vevey, Switzerland, and was finely balanced. I wanted to refer the matter to the annual general meeting of the society. Although Birgitte and I were friends, I felt it right that we should have honest differences, but this was not to be.

Now in my opinion the council and its officers which run ESPGHAN function in practice as a self-perpetuating oligarchy, as occurs so often in many medical societies. Ex-presidents for ever after appear to have a major influence. This was made so clear to me at the time of this argument, when Sandy McNeish, an ex-President but with no office at the time, wrote to me quite unsolicited in April 1990 and told me if I chose to reveal my dissension from the Raven/Blackwell decision at the AGM he was afraid that this would mean my resignation as secretary. It was his opinion that the council should run like a cabinet, taking collective responsibility for decisions. He told me that he would be very unhappy if I chose to act like Michael Heseltine! His advice was to support the majority decision and the President. This advice was offered in good faith but it effectively silenced me. Raven Press won the day.

The second contentious matter was the site of the annual meeting due to be held in Jerusalem that year, which was the year of the First Gulf War. The Israelis naturally were unhappy to give up the meeting. It was quite a blow for my Israeli friends, especially Serem Freier and David Branski. I offered to hold the meeting in London as an emergency at very short notice, supported by my colleagues. The ESPGAN council decided to accept this option. The meeting was a great success.

The annual dinner was held in the Great Hall of St Bartholomew's Hospital. The hall was designed by the great architect James Gibbs and was built between 1730 and 1732. The hall is a remarkable place to have a formal dinner. Many are the dinners I have attended there. Numerous plaques are around its walls commemorating the benefactors of the hospital. The hospital was always free for the sick poor from its foundation. At the dinner for ESPGAN in 1991 as a part of my welcome I said:

> As you came up the stairs you will have seen the wonderful two paintings by William Hogarth, the one of the Good Samaritan and the other of Jesus healing the sick by the pool of Bethesda. You will have in front of you the article that I wrote about the Pool of Bethesda in Jerusalem with Allan Walker. In fact I have been able to visit Jerusalem twice, once in 1964 when the city was divided - I had to pass through the Mandelbaum Gate to go from one half to the other - and then in 1987 when the city was re-united. We all show sympathy for our Israeli guests and hope that we will be able to meet again in Jerusalem at some time in the future.

The annual meeting was in fact later held in Jerusalem in 1995. It was a great success but I do remember the misgivings many of us felt, when we saw young Israelis walking triumphantly, waving Israeli flags, along the Via Dolorosa through the Christian and Moslem quarters on Jerusalem Day, which commemorated the Israeli Victory in the old city. Yet I also had a wonderful experience when visiting once more the Church of the Holy Sepulchre at dusk, with Peter Sullivan. We had the great privilege to be the only ones at the time to visit the tiny shrine of the resurrection. In the background we could hear the singing of the Armenian liturgy. It was a powerful moment.

Just to say a little more about the pool of Bethesda and Hogarth's painting. There is good evidence that the site of the pool of Bethesda that I visited in 1987 with Allan Walker is indeed the true site of the pool depicted by Hogarth. What one can see is a very deep and wide pit within an extensive archeological site adjacent to the fine crusader church of St Anne. To me this is Jerusalem's most beautiful church. Its bare simplicity, symbolic perhaps of northern Europe, with its lofty grey stone arches and tall columns form a stark contrast to the complexity and ornamentation of the churches of Jerusalem typical of the eastern rites of the church. Through the centuries the Pool of Bethesda has been regarded as a place of healing by the Jews, Romans, and Christians (Byzantine and Crusader). A place of healing is fine symbolism for Barts. Hogarth took the opportunity to use the patients at the time of painting as models. Thus this painting provides an astonishing record of the time. Over the years opinions have changed about the diagnoses of the original patients but whichever these may be, this is an amazing visual record of eighteenth century individuals.

Returning to ESPGHAN itself, this European connection had two practical outcomes for me, in as much as it has meant, first that I have attended the annual meeting of ESPGHAN, each year in a different European city, the three exceptions being the joint meetings which I attended in America, in New York and Houston, jointly with NASPGN and in Boston, held as part of the First World Congress of Paediatric Gastroenterology, Hepatology and Nutrition, second, it meant, as a result of the contacts made, that I received a number of invitations to lecture in European cities and beyond.

Perhaps the most notable of these was the invitation from Giacomo Banchini to lecture regularly in Parma from 1983 with my French colleague Jean Navarro, concluding in November 2001. This lead to a joint personal initiative with Stefano Guandalini to create a series of British-Italian meetings every three or four years beginning in Parma followed by Cambridge, Naples, Oxford with Lucca in 2003. Overall Britain and Italy have been perhaps the two leading countries in research in paediatric gastroenterology in Europe over the years. Despite the temperamental differences between the two peoples there is a remarkable meeting of minds at these meetings and the Italians with their ever present good humour make us all laugh, following these meetings several young Italians decided to come to London for training in my department and over the years more Italians have been trained than any other national group from Europe. These have included Dr Paolo Lionetti, Dr Elizabette Fabiani, Dr Stefania Castellanata, Dr Silvia Salvatore and Dr Franco Torrente.

Parma, and Italy herself, have perhaps made a greater impact upon me than all the other European places that I have visited over the past thirty years as a medical visitor. Parma is a remarkable city. It seemed to me when I first visited in 1983 that it was a place where the human spirit had blossomed and flowered over many centuries providing a rich harvest. The city, which has produced such painters as the incomparable Correggio and musicians such as Verdi and Toscanini, must have something about it which stimulates and inspires the human spirit. Perhaps it is the perfect harmony around the medieval square at the heart of Parma with the truly remarkable baptistery, towered cathedral and Bishop's palace. The subtle shades of brown and yellow intermingle and contrast creating a feeling of security and strength. The interior of the baptistery conceived and executed by Benedetto Altemani is remarkable both for its galleries rising up to the distant roof and for the Romanesque figures, especially those of spring and winter, so alive and vibrant. I have only seen comparable beauty in the great Romanesque figures on the doors of Chartres cathedral in France. However it is the interior of the dome of the cathedral or duomo which is the most remarkable. It is frescoed brilliantly, perhaps transcendently by Correggio between 1527 and 1534 and illustrates the Assumption of the Virgin into heaven. It provides a truly remarkable exercise in the technique of perspective with countless figures apparently ascending to heaven with her, in a mass of faces, limbs, feet and flowing robes. The intensity of modern electric light illumination enables us now to appreciate this great work of religious art with a greater brilliance than perhaps at any time since that of Correggio himself.

Much of Parma is painted in a colour known as Parma yellow. This was the inspiration of the still remembered and still admired Grand-Duchess of Parma, Maria-Luigi, better known internationally as Marie-Louise. Empress of France, Napoleon's second wife, an Austrian Hapsburg. Her memory is still alive and well in Parma, in a series of beautiful buildings, including the Theatre Royal. My host in Parma has usually been the paediatric gastroenterologist Giacomo Banchini, a muscular athletic man devoted to rugby, an outstanding host with a vivacious and charming wife Cosetta.

Another part of Italy I have visited often is Naples and the beautiful craggy Isle of Capri where I have attended several conferences but we also have had two family holidays, once as the guest of my old friend Professor Salvatore Auricchio in his holiday house in Anacapri, away from the tourists. He and his colleague/rival Professor Amido Rubino have made Naples one of the great world centres of Paediatric Gastroenterology, training many of the leading Italian figures in the discipline.

I cannot fail to mention the wonderful city of Rome where I have visited more often as a tourist/pilgrim than as a professional. H.V. Morton's travel book has added enormously to my enjoyment of that incomparable city. My son James joined me once on a medical visit when we stayed in the centre near the Pantheon, an unforgettable visit.

The larger international meetings such as those of paediatrics and gastroenterology can be difficult occasions both to make contact with colleagues and friends or indeed gain much benefit. In recent years I have only attended such large occasions if I was making a personal presentation. In 1971 I did however attend an international paediatric meeting which was very valuable for me, after I had taken up my position at RAHC in Sydney. It was XIII International Congress for Paediatrics held in Vienna, that great capital city of the former Austro-Hungarian Monarchy. I have always been interested in the Hapsburgs so it was a great to visit this great historic city for the first time. The meeting was held in the winter palace itself. I was able to consolidate the contacts I had made in Interlaken with other paediatric gastroenterologists. It may have contributed to my later decision to settle in England with its proximity to Europe.

In 1984 Sandy McNeish and I co-hosted an international meeting on 'Diarrhoea and Malnutrition in the Children of the Commonwealth' at the Royal Commonwealth Society and St Bartholomew's Hospital London, which proved to be the first of a series. Sandy advocated a successful strategy of giving the meeting a clear structure. An important book of the proceedings of the meeting resulted which we edited. All this led on to close contact with colleagues in developing nations of the Commonwealth and ultimately to the foundation of the Commonwealth Association of Paediatric Gastroenterology and Nutrition (CAPGAN) in Hong Kong in 1994 at the initiative of Peter Sullivan. He was the organizer of the third commonwealth conference in childhood in Hong Kong. Before that one of the key players in pursuing the initiative begun in London in 1984 was Dr Santosh Mittal who was to be the host of the second Commonwealth Conference in New Delhi in 1991. Earlier I had been his guest in India in 1985. Thus I have twice visited that extraordinary nation which captivated my interest from early childhood, but it was the first visit which was so memorable and I kept a diary of my days there and this will now be quoted from:

> How does one describe the indescribable? First impressions are fraught with the risk of hasty judgements and superficial value judgements. Nevertheless they have an immediacy a brilliance, a clarity all their own when perceptions are crisp, clear and intense. I had been apprehensive about arriving at Delhi airport, fearing crowds and chaos. In this event through the good offices of my secretary's brother I was met and shepherded rapidly through customs and passport control. The Commonwealth rates a separate gate! Whilst awaiting the car outside the airport I had the first opportunity to experience India. At 4.30 a.m. it was surprisingly cold on a crisp clear and intensively dark night. My first impression was of tall young men standing around eager to encourage new arrivals into their taxis. A number had large tartan blankets wrapped around them looking for all the world like eighteenth century Scots wrapped in plaids.

> In the afternoon I was taken to Maulana Azad Medical school... and toured the wards with Santosh Mittal. Some of these wards were 50 years old and the golden jubilee of the hospital will be celebrated next year. The hospital was

> originally Irwin College named after the Viceroy at that time.
>
> How can one describe the wards? The darkness and cave-like feel is the first impression. Row upon row of beds in a long Florence Nightingale ward with very little in the way of obvious ventilation and a smell of stale urine. The ward was rather cold and several radiators were there to heat the ward. In the first bed (two babies at each end), each with meningitis and being given intravenous antibiotics. Then there was bed after bed with very sick children sometimes with mothers in their bed too. Fathers, mothers and other family members were here, there and everywhere. It seemed like a visit to an eighteenth-century ward. At the end was a girl with rheumatic cholera full blown! This is still not an uncommon disorder apparently in India today. All was squalid and the whole environment seemed dirty. I suppose this is inevitable with so many of the general public encouraged to be in the ward.
>
> Despite this the medical care seemed excellent and the laboratory back up was very good apparently with sophisticated techniques such as CT scan being readily available. The hospital is being gradually rebuilt.

I understand this is now complete. I had very warm hospitality from Santosh and his family and he took me on a sightseeing tour of the city. To quote again:

> A girl of no more than seven to eight years carrying a baby in her arms of about nine months of age to engender sympathy for girls of money was begging amongst the cars at the traffic lights. How can a modern society and how can paediatricians especially tolerate such horror? Santosh says that institutional care would be worse, making them all criminals. Surely a church organization at least can do something?

Later I visited the All India Institute of Medical Sciences which was very impressive, if somewhat spartan, but with much high technology. I met Dr Raj Bhan, a very energetic man, leading a dynamic research group into the problems of chronic infantile diarrhoea. He and his colleagues took me to the Imperial Hotel for lunch. It was so like the Raffles hotel of Singapore that I had a sense of déjà vu. On the way back from the Imperial Hotel we suddenly came upon the Rajpath and I shall continue from my diary.

> On the right was the India Gate or War Memorial Arch of the First World War and on the left the Secretariat buildings. I was immediately seized by the beauty of the scene, the majestic buildings were not overpowering but nonetheless magnificent in their strength and confidence. Everywhere there was a sense of

> space and strength. We drove up to the left along the Rajpath to the gate of what is now the President's Palace formerly the Viceroy's House... The great ornate gate to the palace is flanked on each side by a horseman with a lance in brilliant uniform with a scarlet turban. The air was misty with a light heat haze. The scene was magnificent. The architecture and general planning is quite superb. Nostalgia and regret swept over me for the days of the Empire that are gone. Somehow here not in London, is symbolized the apotheosis of Empire. A lump came to my throat and all I could think were Kipling's words, echoing around my head, '. . . Is one with Nineveh and Tyre . . .' not desolate as is Nineveh today, but a living monument to the glory and magnificence of the British Empire (or as some would say the Raj) and its greatest legacy Indian democracy now flourishing. My companions chattering away were quite unaware of the strong emotion that suddenly swept over me.

The Viceroy's House, now the Presidential Palace, was designed by Sir Edwin Lutyens, together with much of Imperial New Delhi. It is an architectural masterpiece. Later on my secretary's brother was able to take me into the Presidential Palace Gardens and we drove in just as the President himself, accompanied by Megistu, Chairman of Ethiopia, on a state visit, was driving out.

> We later saw the tomb of Safdarjang, Prime Minister for the Mughal Emperor Muhammed Shah and built between 175-54. It was the last instance of a garden tomb. The sudden vision we had of the splendid edifice framed by the arch of the entrance afforded a breathtaking contrast to the frantic activity of the thoroughfare outside. The peace and tranquillity of this beautiful tomb surrounded by its delightful garden is yet another Indian architectural triumph.

I was to return to Delhi in 1991 and I ever remember it as one of the most astonishing and fascinating places I have ever visited.

By 1990 it became clear that we were receiving, in London, many requests internationally for both training and research fellowships for young trainees in paediatric gastroenterology from many countries. Some of these who brought funding themselves we were able to accommodate in our programme, usually with great mutual benefit. However some more formal approach was required. First an annual international course in paediatric gastroenterology was established which continues today. Second it was clear an award of a qualification was needed. Modelled upon my experience with the Diploma of Tropical Paediatrics in Liverpool, where I had been an external examiner, a year long course for a Diploma of Paediatric Gastroenterology of the Medical College of St Bartholomew's Hospital was instituted. There was a comprehensive teaching course with lectures, seminars and clinical teaching in ward rounds and in the outpatients, and one month's visit to King's College Hospital for teaching in hepatology. The Diploma was awarded after a clinical and theoretical examination. There were 19 candidates over the period 1991 to 2000. Sixteen passed and three failed. In addition to Britain candidates came from eleven other countries.

Among notable fellows was Dr Christine Hauer of Austria who also undertook significant laboratory research with Tom MacDonald. Christine is now a paediatric gastroenterologist in Graz where I had the good fortune to be invited to visit her. Two successful candidates introduced us to parts of the world where we had no previous contact. First there was Mario Vieira in 1992-93 from Curitiba in Brazil. Later he was to establish his own unit there which I had the honour to visit before a conference in Sao Paolo. It was wonderful to see his success in building up paediatric gastroenterology from scratch. Then there was Beatrice Amadi from Zambia in 1995-96 who opened our eyes to the terrible problems of Africa, especially in relation to diarrhoeal disease and AIDS. My colleague Mike Thomson has visited her unit to teach her endoscopy and we have done an important collaborative research study also including Alan Phillips. Mike in 2002 arranged a remarkable fundraising exercise by persuading colleagues to climb the three tallest peaks of Scotland, England and Wales in twenty-four hours to raise money with appropriate sponsorship for Beatrice's department in Lusaka. The Diploma was a wonderful way of making relationships internationally but sadly it lapsed in 2002, for lack of resources.

My many trips to Boston to collaborate with Allan Walker at Boston Children's Hospital and Massachussetts General Hospital must be mentioned. I have also visited his wonderful holiday home in New Hampshire both for holiday with my family and for an editorial meeting for our multi-author book *Pediatric Gastrointestinal Disease* at the Silver Lake. This is a completely unspoilt rural idyll in the White Mountains where one is able to completely escape from the pressures and stress of modern life.

I have only once been back to Kinderspital, Zurich and that was for the retirement of David Shmerling. I have been delighted that I was able to train Christian Braegger who has taken on his mantle. Also another Swiss Raoul Furlano was jointly trained by my unit and Alan Walker's. He is now established as paediatric gastroenterologist in Basel, where I was very honoured to be invited to visit his unit. So I have kept up my Swiss connection begun in 1967.

I must mention my many trips to Singapore, my favourite destination in Asia. The Singaporean Boh-Gee Yap and his wife Pat are amongst my oldest friends and we have enjoyed man occasions in the Raffles Hotel. Both had been trained by me both in Sydney and London and is now a leading general paediatrician in Singapore. It has been wonderful to see paediatric gastroenterology grow and develop there since I first visited Professor Wong Hok Boon in 1969. It is now led by Dr Qak, current president of Asian Pan Pacific Society of Paediatric Gastroenterology and Nutrition (APPSPGAN) and another old friend I have always been interested in Singapore and I have met that remarkable man Lee Kuan Yew, former President of Singapore, at a meeting of The Royal Commonwealth Society in London.

Then I have visited Taiwan on three occasions over thirteen years. I have been delighted to see how Dr Mei-Hwei Chang has led and developed the discipline in Taipei. Taiwan and Singapore are both remarkably dynamic in the development of medical services. The quality of the clinical services now provided in each country in paediatric gastroenterology is the equal of anywhere else I have visited at home or abroad.

Travelling in the far and Middle East I have on occasion come across graves or church memorials of British soldiers dying far from home, for example in Penang, Singapore and Jerusalem. I have then been reminded of Housman's evocative verse:

> It dawns in Asia, tombstones show
> And Shropshire names are read
> And the Nile spills his overflow
> Beside the Severn's dead

A Shropshire Lad I

One of the most memorable trips was to the Gulf and Cyprus in 1990. I stayed in Kuwait not long before the war, totally unaware of any risk. I started in the United Arab Emirates driving from Abu Dhabi to Dubai and then flew to Kuwait and then on to Cyprus. I have been there many times thanks to John Hadjiminas, a former fellow and now a paediatric gastroenterologist in private practice in Nicosia. His father Minas Hadjiminas is a very distinguished paediatrician who has contributed to the prevention of thalassaemia, an inherited disease, a scourge of Cypriots. I also knew a Turkish Cypriot doctor Rif Atun (former HP at Barts) and during one of our trips to Cyprus I and my family crossed over the green line in Nicosia from the Greek to the Turkish side to be greeted by Rif and his family We spent the day travelling around the north of the island, so little changed from the days of British rule. However when we visited the shrine of St Barnabas all orthodox Christians had tragically gone. The crossing itself reminded me of the Mandelbaum Gate. Very few people make this crossing each day. I hope it may soon disappear when Cyprus joins the European Union in the near future.

There also have been wonderful trips to Slovenia with Dusanka Micetic-Turk and Croatia with Sanja Kolacek. Jerne Dolinesk, a young trainee from Slovenia, has regularly been encouraged by Dusanka to attend the Royal Free Annual Course, which she has attended over many years.

I should conclude that I and my family have returned to Sydney many times and travelled in Australia. I and my children and grandchildren arc privileged to have dual Australian and British citizenship. I have seen RAHC move to wonderful new facilities from inner Sydney to West Mead, west of Sydney near Parramatta. The architectural beauties and originalities of the new buildings are in large measure due to the vision of John Yu.

There is not space to mention all my numerous trips, but what a privilege all this travel has all been, and hopefully there has been much practical outcome for the benefit of sick children.

My career, as a paediatric Gastroenterologist, was crowned in June 2010. ESPGHAN presented me with the first distinguished service award of the society in Istanbul. The award was made for a lifetime achievement in paediatric gastroenterology. This was awarded for making a major contribution to the understanding and treatment of paediatric gastrointestinal diseases, for training young paediatric gastroenterologists who are now leaders in the field and for making specific contributions to ESPGHAN as a society. I was also delighted to be associated with the organisation of the CAPGAN silver jubilee meeting in August 2011 at the Institute of Child Health. These meetings demonstrated the continuing role of Britain in the paediatric affairs of Europe and the Commonwealth.

These international associations are of immense importance to me and such organisations are key players in the further development of this paediatric specialty.

CHAPTER FOURTEEN

The Tomlinson Report

Medical life is often one of controversy, whether working in general or hospital practice, but perhaps more so when involved in academic matters. Medical politics is a tough game and often as Byzantine as national politics, because it is usually very hard to know just what is going on in the corridors of power, especially as a young consultant. The controversy concerning the Tomlinson report, fortunately perhaps for me, came in the latter part of my career when I had some, albeit limited, access to the corridors of power.

In this Chapter the controversy concerning the Tomlinson Report's recommendation in 1992 to close St Bartholomew's Hospital and Queen Elizabeth Hospital for Children as part of its policy of hospital mergers and closures in London, will be discussed. As this is an autobiography, this will in large measure be discussed as it impacted upon me, rather than attempting a comprehensive account and detailed history which is for others to do.

On Friday 23 October 1992, I wrote in my journal:

> This is certainly a black Friday! The Tomlinson Report has recommended the complete closure of Barts and its re-location on the London Hospital site and also the transfer of the Queen Elizabeth Hospital for Children to Homerton Hospital. An act of such vandalism and such denial of 869 years of tradition, can hardly be grasped. Surely the government will not act in this way, one might say, but with the facile remarks Mrs Bottomley, the Secretary of State for Health, has made, welcoming the report, it seems all too probable that next January she will act to close Barts and QEHC. This leaves me reeling with 20 years of work in possible jeopardy! I have written to our local MP - faint hope. I shall not vote conservative!

In fact my local conservative MP James Arbuthnot refused my invitation to visit Barts and QEHC. I knew James moderately well, as I was a member of his Dining Club in the House of Commons. He followed the party line. He is very much an establishment figure.

Of course once the government had appointed Professor Tomlinson, an elderly retired academic from Newcastle with considerable administrative experience, to report on the provision of service by the hospitals of London, the rumour mill began to grind. We were surprised to learn that the government apparently wanted to close Barts but astonishingly he himself, did not ever visit the hospital. I duly met him when he did visit QEHC. Tomlinson was socially a pleasant friendly man attended by an even older doctor, a lady general practitioner, who looked after him as he proceeded around the hospital. To his credit he met the consultant staff at the end of his visit. He obviously had been quite impressed by what he had seen at the hospital and even had been surprised as to how busy it was, especially casualty. However he gave nothing away about his likely recommendations, but the mood amongst the consultants was one of head shaking and sadness as he left the hospital.

In fact it was not till 16 February 1993 that Mrs Bottomley announced the government's response to the Tomlinson Report. Yet it was not to be the final word as the government recommended a number of specialty reviews over the following three months, including a review of paediatrics, to decide the best options. However for Barts there were only three options, closure, merger with the London Hospital, or survival as a specialist unit. It was already decided that Queen Elizabeth Hospital for Children was to be detached from GOS governance and handed to Homerton Hospital, which in turn was split from Barts. This wretched splitting and merging was occurring all across London, with terrible consequences for staff morale and profound anxieties for patients. The whole drawn out process was in fact in the end to last more than a year. The paediatricians at the London Hospital immediately launched a bid to have QEHC transferred to them. They were ultimately victorious! I wrote at the time 'These changes in the health service in practice are setting the doctors at each other's throats.' Little did I know how bad it would get!

Clearly though, the paediatric specialty review would be a complete charade, the government had already decided what it wanted to happen, and so it proved to be.

The document outlining the Tomlinson proposals was called 'Making London Better', a ridiculous title for a document, which was to cause so much havoc and to have such unfortunate consequences that persist until this day. The task of preparing a document describing the paediatric gastroenterology service, both academic and service for the review body, now had to be undertaken. It was a heavy task. I called on everyone concerned to help with the facts and figures. A body called the London Implementation Group had been appointed and they were to run the review process.

In March 1993, the stress of events began really to affect me. I wrote 'I really feel very tense, on edge and quite unwell in a vague non-descript way'. I later discovered that many colleagues were similarly affected and some were much worse, requiring psychiatric help. I felt my whole life's work was in danger of being destroyed. How I managed to continue my day-to-day care of patients, supervision of young colleagues etc. I simply don't know. However it all went on and on.

It was in March that I first seriously considered transferring to the Royal Free Hospital. Dr Andy Wakefield had already telephoned me on Christmas Eve 1992 and suggested I consider this. He was an adult gastroenterologist leading a research investigating chronic inflammatory bowel disease at the Royal Free Hospital. I was delighted to receive the invitation, coming at a very low time. It had then lifted my morale and transformed my Christmas. However I did not want to leave Barts and QEHC. The proposed closure of Barts was a terrible and a completely unexpected shock, but at first I could not really believe a Conservative government could close St Bartholomew's Hospital, after all those centuries of excellence. Ever since I had arrived from Australia, right until this moment at the end of 1992, I had maintained my faith in the good judgement of the old establishment, especially the medical establishment. This was about to be shattered. A hospital I saw at the heart of Britishness for centuries, an internationally recognized centre of excellence was about to be closed by a so-called Conservative government of Britain. Surely that could never be!

As described earlier, I came to Britain for one reason alone, to work at Barts. I would simply not have come to Britain to work anywhere else. Certainly I would never have left Sydney to come and work at the Royal London Hospital. If there had not been an opportunity at Barts back in 1972, I would have stayed at RAHC in Sydney. So the situation was very poignant for me and my whole life. As I have indicated earlier Barts Hospital had also become of importance to my wife and family. I had in the early years at Barts/QEHC endured facilities which were had been far inferior to anything in Sydney. Yet by 1993, we had a quite beautifully restored children's ward block at Barts with ideal facilities and a custom built research laboratory staffed by an outstanding team lead by Tom MacDonald. At QEHC we had an outstanding electron microscope unit and team led by Alan Phillips, with good modernized ward facilities, albeit in a hospital requiring re-development. As related in Chapter 12 we had just celebrated the 125th anniversary and ironically we had had great hopes for the future. One thing I decided immediately once I heard the government's plans, was come what may, I was not ever going to transfer my department to the Royal London. My reasons were the poor facilities and my scepticism that the hospital could be re-built by the Public Funding Initiative (PFI) within a decade. On March 29 I wrote 'One of the options I have to consider is going to the Royal Free if Barts closes. This would be a very exciting opportunity'. I did in fact briefly visit the Royal Free for an informal meeting, that Dr Andy Wakefield arranged with the Dean Arie Zuckerman, (whom I had known of old through rota virus) and Cally Palmer of the NHS trust, with others. I had received a very warm welcome, but I had made clear I could not consider transferring to the Royal Free, until the fate of Barts was finally sealed. However it was a huge boost to my morale at such a difficult time to be ' head-hunted' in this way, and very flattering too. However all kinds of rumours were circulating that the government would change its mind and Barts would in the end be saved. The patients had begun a formidable Save Barts campaign with much support and attention, from the *Evening Standard*, London's evening newspaper. Surely this campaign could not fail.

Then in April came the London Implementation Group (LIG) visits for the paediatric review. At Barts this was conducted by Sir David Hull, a distinguished paediatric professor, but it was a terrible ordeal for us all. I felt particularly sorry for Jim Malpas, the professor of oncology who had done so much to secure funds to restore the children's block at Barts with funds from cancer charities. He was particularly upset by Hull's whole attitude and the aggressive style of his questioning of us all. Tom MacDonald was outraged as Hull said he didn't even have time to speak to Tom. Everyone felt our fate was sealed, before we even had made our presentations to him. So it proved to be. I also attended the LIG meeting in the Board Room at GOS where Hull continued his very aggressive style. It was all so terribly depressing. At the end of 1993 I was to write that the year had been the worst in my professional life. Fascinatingly nearly nine years later at York in April 2002 Sir David Hull came up to me and said to me 'Things went well at the Royal Free then?' I replied 'Yes indeed, but even after all these years I would have preferred to have stayed at Barts.' He then went on to say what a terrible time it had been for him too! I was glad and indeed grateful to hear these comments and the trouble he had obviously taken to speak to me. Yet it does not change how I still feel about those awful events of 1993.

In July 1998 his intervention into the controversy following the publication of the *Lancet* paper (see Chapter 15) made a difficult situation more difficult. He wrote an unsolicited letter to the Dean expressing his anxiety that as "the children do not suffer long term bowel disorder, it would seem difficult to justify such invasive studies on clinical grounds". I was disappointed that he did not contact me directly and informally as we each other knew each other. In fact we believed that the children did have a type of chronic or long term bowel inflammation. From my own experience this was proved to my satisfaction by the time I retired in 2000. However his letter led to some confusing correspondence, to which I contributed. The final contact I had with David Hull was as a GMC Prosecution witness in the Hearing, described in Chapter 16.

By January 1994, things began to unravel at Barts, Jane Sallabank, our outstanding ward sister in Lucas Ward, was made redundant and Dr Clive Bartram decided to leave. Although in the event Dr Alison McLean, Prof. Michael Farthing's wife, succeeded him. She was another outstanding radiologist who made a great contribution in my remaining time at Barts.

In February, Andy Wakefield re-activated the Royal Free offer, but I felt I still needed time to reflect. In early March I was with Simon Murch in Paris for a paediatric congress. This provided a good opportunity for me to talk and reflect with him on the Royal Free Hospital offer. By chance we met Roland Levinsky, Dean of the Institute of Child Health, an old colleague of mine at the Opera. He said, 'I hear you are on the move.' This remark both surprised and rather pleased me and curiously spurred me on to accept the Royal Free offer. I later wrote 'If I can get a good offer, I think it is the best thing for me and my department'. On return I had extended discussions with Alan Phillips who throughout this difficult time was a tower of strength. We decided to enter into negotiation with the Royal Free, and Cally Palmer and Martin Else, the then treasurer at Hampstead NHS Trust, visited me at QEHC. Cally also met Tom MacDonald at Barts.

At the end of that month a sad nostalgic event occurred. With the reorganization that the government had already decided upon at Barts by the creation of the Royal Hospitals Trust, our Directorate of Paediatrics, which had linked the hospital with the local community, was dissolved and the Barts department of Child Health came to an end. In future there would be a merged Child Health Directorate involving both Barts and the London. The first director was to be on the site of the London. So I, as last 'physician in charge' arranged a dinner which I called 'Wake for Barts Department of Child Health' in the Consultants' dining room at Barts. I was the last to occupy this position of 'physician in charge, department of diseases of children'. The first had been the very distinguished Sir Archibald Garrod 1904-1910 and so his photograph was on the cover of the menu. Ten consultants were present, the entire consultant staff concerned with children at Barts. Tim Eden who was an outstanding professor of paediatric oncology felt as I did and was to leave soon. It was the beginning of the end of a whole era. The children's beds at Barts were finally closed at the beginning of 2002.

However in May 1994, although we were in negotiation with the Royal Free I felt I had a responsibility to leave no stone unturned in relation to staying if Barts could possibly be saved. It was obvious that QEHC was irredeemably lost on its current site so we explored the option of transferring the bulk of the gastroenterology department (tertiary service) including the electron microscope unit to Barts, retaining gastroenteritis and a secondary service at QEHC and its successor wherever that might be. This scheme was approved by Dr Sarah Benton, the new clinical director of paediatrics, and Dr David Rampton, clinical director of gastroenterology of the new Royal Hospitals Trust, which combined Barts and the London hospitals. It had the backing of Mr T. Battle, director of operations in the Trust, but was shipwrecked by the vehement opposition of Ms Catherine Square, QEHC Hospital Project Manager, and some members of the medical staff at Queens. The proposal was never seriously considered. No option was open to me except to go to the London.

In June 1994, I voted labour for the first and only time in my life at the European election. I wonder how many people have been lost to the conservative party via the decision to close Barts.

In July, the inexorable process leading towards closure pressed on. It was affirmed that the QEHC site was to be closed (this finally happened in 1998) and the hospital's patients and assets were to be split, three-quarters to the Royal London and one quarter to the Homerton Hospital, and GOS would remove all their joint posts etc. Also the Royal Hospitals Trust, which then administered Barts and the London, announced it would close Barts in five years. Sir Derek Boorman, chairman of the Trust, stated that it was too costly not to have all services centred on one site. He stated the Royal London was much better suited to serve the East End and promised new buildings by the turn of the century. All this was discussed at a crisis meeting of Barts Council, the assembly of the consultant staff. The Council expressed its collective dismay at the above decision. There was a move to pass a vote of no confidence in the Board. However in what seemed to me a typical English Public School way, Professor Hudson, Chairman of the Board, would not allow it, as this was just 'a knee jerk reaction', he said! It was remarked, 'What would future historians think of the custodianship of the present consultant staff if this motion was not voted on?' I spoke up and said, 'The very stones would cry out if we did not express our views.' Sadly they did not! I was but a very small voice representing a tiny children's specialty. I as an Australian was struck yet again that senior medical figures in England will almost never challenge the 'establishment'. A comparable situation in Sydney would have been greeted with outrage, publicly expressed. However at the January 1994 meeting of the Council, to their great credit the Barts Council consultants at last did pass a vote of no confidence in the Chief Executive and the Chairman of the Royal Hospitals Trust Board and recommended their resignation. Posterity, I am certain, will applaud, but at the time sadly nothing happened, the government had decided and the Council had become a charade.

Mrs Bottomley also in July re-affirmed her intent to immediately close the casualty department at Barts despite all the protests from city workers etc. and the vigorous Save Barts patients campaign. Obviously the end was approaching. I had met Mrs Bottomley when she had visited QEHC. She was a 'jolly hockey sticks' character with what appeared to me an inflated view of her understanding of the health needs of the children of London. 'That Bottomley Woman' was to become a cry of despair for many of us.

I and my team had now been in detailed private consultations at the Royal Free with Professor Zuckerman and Martin Else who had become the new chief executive officer. On 6 October 1994 I received a letter from Martin Else inviting me and my colleagues to relocate both my academic and clinical services to a new base at the Royal Free. If I accepted then a business case would be submitted to the London Implementation Group to seek their general endorsement and to apply for capital funding. I felt I could no longer continue to play Hamlet with the Royal Free as it was now eighteen months since they had first approached me. I accepted this offer in confidence and awaited developments. I felt elated for the first time for ages. No public announcement was possible because detailed discussions of all the practicalities had to occur.

I went off to the ESPGAN/NASPGN joint meeting in Houston, Texas. I received wonderful hospitality whilst there from Allan Walker and Ian Sanderson and their enthusiastic endorsement with what I had decided, as old friends. I came home on 16 October feeling great, but within days this had completely changed.

I wrote concerning the week ending 23 October 1994, 'This has been a terrible week! Perhaps the worst in my professional life.' The reason was first that on the Monday of my return, Nigel Meadows told me that while I had been away, he had decided not to go to the Royal Free. I respected his sincere decision but it was a great personal blow, as he is an outstanding clinician and I wanted him as part of the team. He had accompanied me on previous visits to the Royal Free and had been a party to all preliminary discussions. He was one of my protégées. I had backed his appointment as Clinical Lecturer. He also told me that 'the long knives were out' for me in some quarters. These exact words were later confirmed to me by Martin Savage. To this day, I don't know who said them of me or just what they meant. Then on Tuesday during William Harvey Day at Barts I was subjected to a harangue from Professor Michael Besser, leader of the Save Barts campaign. Kate Costeloe was very upset at my decision, which apparently was now on 'the grapevine'. I could understand how she felt. I respect her enormously and we remain good friends. On that day I was reeling and I began to wonder if I had made the wrong decision and that Barts would indeed be saved. At lunch-time I went back to our laboratory and Delphine Parrott helped me to calm down and look at things objectively. She was a senior scientist and original mentor of Tom MacDonald who in her retirement had come to our laboratory on a part time basis. Mark Beattie the CICRA fellow at the time and husband of Jane Sallabank gave me welcome moral support. Michael Farthing I met by the fountain that afternoon in the famous square at Barts. He me gave me words of support, which I appreciated and I shall not forget. So after my wobble I decided that clearly the move to the Royal Free was the best option. Although so very sadly, Tom Macdonald had now decided that he also would not be coming with us, as he wanted his own laboratory. He did not like the connection with Andy Wakefield with whom he profoundly disagreed, shades of the future! He had rejected the offer of transferring in my department. The team was breaking up.

Sir Colin Berry, the new warden of the future combined medical school, summoned me to his office at the Royal London shortly after, perhaps alerted by Michael Besser. He made a bid to entice me to stay, namely he agreed for my long-standing application for a senior lecturer post to now go ahead, which I hoped would be filled by Simon Murch. (In fact this did occur the following year). This overture by Berry coincided with the confidential news that the London Implementation Group both approved and would fund our proposed move to the Royal Free. So Alan Phillips, Simon Murch and I went to the Royal Free to see Martin Else. Later we had a celebratory drink for our future at the Royal Free with Andy Wakefield and Roy Pounder. Now all stops were out to plan our new department at the Royal Free. What they had offered us was quite wonderful, a new laboratory and offices were to be built for our requirement and a refurbished ward. Thus my unit on two sites at Barts and QEHC would be now be united on one site, but negotiations to get all the staff members I required took some time and this delayed announcing my transfer. In the event every request I made was granted, quite remarkably. A huge amount of work was involved before I could announce my decision publicly and determine a date for transfer. Detailed negotiation was still required to secure all that we needed both in the hospital and the university. The new department was to be called, to my delight, the University Department of Paediatric Gastroenterology. For me this was a major landmark for the recognition of paediatric gastroenterology and was an event of international significance. I was to be a full Professorial Head taking my place at university committees with the professors of medicine and surgery etc.

How does one cope with stress? For me, my wife was a great comfort and I relied heavily on Alan Phillips and Simon Murch for professional support. Taking my Grandson Joseph into town was a marvellous relief, yet I felt very alone. So I did turn to the church as well. Now serendipitously, January 1995 was the ninetieth anniversary of the foundation of the department of child health. So with the Vicar's support (Rev. Michael Whawell) we arranged a special service of thanksgiving for ninety years in the church of St Bartholomew's the Less, after all we were a religious foundation. Hospital patients took a major part in the service, including a dramatic presentation by some children. It was a marvellous occasion and very well attended. John Dickinson, emeritus professor of medicine, played the organ wonderfully.

Then on 6 March 1995 I went to see Lesley Rees and told her I had accepted the invitation to transfer to the Royal Free School of Medicine within the University of London and I wished to transfer on 1 September. She was pleasant and very understanding, considering the circumstances, which were quite clearly difficult for her. She said I had been made such a remarkable offer that I could not refuse it. Later she was to give me a Barts Hospital tie, which can only be worn by graduates of Barts or by a gift from the Dean. I wore it with pride at my retirement dinner in Barts Great Hall in 2000. By contrast the administrator at QEHC, was very unhappy about my decision. I arranged a meeting at Barts next day inviting everyone, doctors, nurses laboratory staff etc. both in my department and concerned with it, from both sites, so they would be fully informed concerning what I had done and why. I explained to everyone, what I had decided and how difficult it had been for me to make the correct decision.

I wrote on 19 March 'It has been a battering two weeks!' At QEHC the general reaction was hostile, even though the hospital had no future. The unpleasantness of my departure was by no means over, in some ways it had hardly begun. A graffiti in the lift described me as a traitor! To my great shock the administration refused to agree the transfer of a large part of the research funds that I had personally generated over the years from the care of overseas patients. Then to my greater distress my independent clinical rights were taken away. I could only practise in the presence of Nigel Meadows, after 22 years of service to QEHC and to the children of East London. I found this to be quite outrageous and still find it so. My colleagues Chris Wood and Vanessa Wright on the Hospital Executive Team signed the document with no personal apology to me. In 2001 at a dinner I asked Vanessa why she had done it, she replied it was just an administrative matter! The reason of course was that many parents wanted to transfer child patients with me to the Royal Free. At Barts the overwhelming majority of my patients did transfer to the Royal Free and the parents gave me tremendous support. At the same time, they did all they could to try and prevent Barts being closed. The administration of the Royal Hospitals Trust did all they could to try and stop this patient transfer, even to the outrageous extent of opening my mail against my instruction after I left. This was done to prevent new referrals reaching me at the Royal Free. They opened all letters addressed to me at Barts. I shall not mention the names of the administrators opposed to me, as they doubtless felt they were doing their job and are now in post somewhere. None are still where they were in 1995. I shall mention however by complete contrast Sir Anthony Tippet, Chief Executive at GOS/QEHC, who was completely sympathetic and understanding to my move. He wished I had decided to transfer to GOS, which at one stage had been an option. In fact I had unofficial approaches also from St Marks at Northwick Park and from Cambridge. What was so difficult for me was that neither the Royal Free Hampstead NHS Trust nor the Royal Free School of Medicine contacted at any point the Royal Hospitals Trust or Medical School of St Bartholomew's Hospital concerning my transfer, despite my requests to Martin Else and Cally Palmer to do so. All the flack at both Barts and Queens was directed at me and borne by me. Of course I was so privileged to have this freedom of movement to be able to move my unit and the patients I cared for to the place where the best facilities were on offer within the University of London, who incidentally approved our transfer. However it was hard to believe at the time we were all in one health service and one university. All I was doing was trying to secure the best provision of service for my patients and the opportunity for clinical research.

At QEHC, the administration directed a confrontational approach towards me. An aggressive memorandum was sent out. My team and I were subject to a kind of psychological warfare. We were told the whole transfer would fail. We were told that the paediatric service itself at the Royal Free itself was poor and would close etc. etc. Simon Murch who had only just taken up his senior lecturer post was put under great pressure to withdraw from the transfer and stay. Incentives were offered to him. To his great credit, his loyalty prevailed and I remain very grateful to him. I shall now draw a veil over further unpleasantness, which continued in varying degrees until we transferred, more at QEHC than at Barts. In fact there, things became friendlier, no doubt influenced by Lesley Rees's response. Martin Savage very generously hosted a small dinner party at Barts to mark Simon and my transfer. He made a very touching speech, which I shall never forget. At QEHC Alan Phillips arranged a departmental party to farewell me, but after 22 years of service to the hospital and its child patients, the administration did nothing to mark my transfer to the Royal Free. The ultimate demise of that wonderful institution Queen Elizabeth Hospital for Children was to come in September 1998. If I had been given the chance I would have fought for her to the bitter end but it was not to be. The cynical bureaucrats had won.

To this day I remain puzzled what was the real political purpose of the decisions to close Queens and Barts. More precisely, what really was the Conservative government's true purpose to close such distinguished and long-standing institutions.

As for Barts, the hospital was not closed as the conservatives lost the election of 1996 and the incoming labour government preserved the hospital in a reduced state providing specialist units of the highest standards. The medical schools merged in 1995 to become St Bartholomew's and the Royal London School of Medicine and Dentistry within Queen Mary and Westfield College, with the school office located at Whitechapel. The name says it all. How can a medical student be 'patriotic' for such a geographically split school? For myself I have not observed any obvious advantage to flow from this merger, but the list of loss is too long. Suffice it to mention, in relation to quality of life issues, albeit in a minor matter which I observed myself, the long-established and vigorous Barts Gilbert and Sullivan Society, of which I was a vice-president, sadly did not long survive the merger.

Now, the reader may ask why all the fuss that I have outlined above? After all I had the privilege of a superb offer at the Royal Free. Yet I could not be indifferent to the two institutions (with their staff and patients) whom I had frankly, come to love, if the reader will forgive such emotional language. Also 1992 was a year of much pessimism, for the Queen it was her 'annus horribilis', a year when royal marriages disintegrated and with terrible symbolism, Windsor Castle, the heart of the monarchy, was engulfed in flames. Looking back the general pessimism of the time related to these and other events doubtless added to my mood at the time. Was the whole world I believed in falling apart?

Indeed before I received my invitation to transfer, all did seem doom and gloom and premature retirement an attractive option.

CHAPTER FIFTEEN

MMR, Crohn's Disease and Regressive Autism

The controversy concerning measles, mumps and rubella vaccination (MMR) and autism, so well known to readers of the press in the United Kingdom, has its roots in the events described in the last Chapter, as Sir David Hull remarked when I chatted with him in York in 2002. This relates of course to Dr Andy Wakefield's initiation of our invitation to the Royal Free. Although of course Mr Martin Else and Prof. Arie Zuckerman were the main players in the actual overture to me and my department to transfer.

Let me now briefly outline this controversy and how it arose, from my own perspective. Andy Wakefield is an adult gastroenterologist, formerly a surgeon. He has suggested that there are risks associated with MMR. These he now centres particularly upon children with regressive autism but he at first was concerned about a possible role in Crohn's disease. He is a clinical investigator and was appointed senior lecturer and then promoted to reader by the Royal Free School of Medicine. He was a member of the University staff rather than the NHS Trust staff. He was academically accountable to Professor Roy Pounder and ultimately to the Dean. He has not and does not care directly for children, as he is not a paediatrician. His only access to children was indirect, via me and my colleagues in our outpatient clinics in the University Department of Paediatric Gastroenterology at the Royal Free Hospital. He was director of the inflammatory bowel disease study group at the Royal Free, a clinical research unit, investigating chronic inflammatory bowel disease and Crohn's disease.

I had known Andy for many years. I had admired his work, especially his 1989 paper in the *Lancet*. In it, he, Roy Pounder, and colleagues in pathology, had described an inflammation of the blood vessels they called vasculitis as the primary pathological event in Crohn's disease. They had used a very elegant technique to outline the blood supply in those parts of the intestine removed at surgery in patients with both Crohn's disease and ulcerative colitis. They used a red dye to outline the vessels, producing a dramatic picture. I had invited Andy in 1994 to lecture in our annual postgraduate course on paediatric gastroenterology on his latest theory of measles and Crohn's disease. He had associated the increase in incidence in Crohn's disease in children, which was now so obvious to us in paediatric gastroenterology practice, to the measles vaccine. Now this was highly contentious matter, especially as we had heard in 1994 that the government proposed a mass vaccination campaign with measles and rubella vaccine in school age children to counter the perceived risk of a measles epidemic, because of earlier low measles vaccine cover.

After our transfer to the Royal Free, Andy came to see me to discuss the many telephone calls he had received from a number of highly articulate parents who had associated the onset of their child's regressive autism with MMR immunization, and of relevance from our perspective, with major bowel symptoms. He asked whether I would see them myself and whether I and my colleagues would consider a clinical research project? After discussion with my clinical colleagues we decided to meet with Andy to discuss his requests. After these discussions I felt it right that we should do two things. First I should see these children myself and second we should plan a joint clinical research project.

At this point it is important to try and define autism and its important variant regressive autism. This is as difficult to do in a few words as it is in practice for doctors to make the diagnosis. The term autism was first used by an American Dr Kanner in the 1940s to describe a group of children with a remarkable combination of behavioural difficulties. These included poor or absent communication, marked social isolation and an array of unusual behaviours. Since then childhood disorders with similar features have been gathered together under the broader term 'pervasive developmental disorder'. This includes children with autism and so-called autistic spectrum disorder as well as Asperger's syndrome. These latter children do not have the language delay and delay in cognitive development which is such a feature of autism, but do have severe impairment of social interaction and may have repetitive and restricted stereotypical (always the same) behaviour. Diagnosis is difficult and depends on a number of criteria being fulfilled and is often long delayed. Looking back, once the diagnosis has been made, it often looks more straightforward than it did at the time. Those children who develop normally until the first birthday and beyond and then regress with loss of language and cognition are the most poignant cases for parents. These children are diagnosed as regressive autism. As they get older more than half of the children may develop behaviour that is a danger to themselves and others. This gets much more difficult for the parents as the children grow in size and weight. These symptoms include uncontrollable motor activity, persistent aggressive behaviour even assaulting others, marked anxiety and marked sleep disorder. This can be a quite terrible scenario for parents whose lives may be ruined by divorce or reactive depression. Most of these children are boys. This is not the time or place to describe the wide range of things that can be done to help, suffice it to say that for many families the presence of an autistic child can be disastrous for the family itself. It represents one of the greatest challenges to the medical profession there is.

In early 1996 I began to see such children. It was obvious to me that these self selected cases referred to me as a gastroenterologist indeed had bowel problems of varying severity that needed investigation. The parents of the initial children had first made contact with Andy Wakefield but then were referred to me, usually by the child's general practitioner. Thus they were a self-referred group. However as time went on the children were referred directly to me without any involvement of Andy Wakefield. As a result, for just on five years I saw one or two new cases of children with autism and bowel symptoms for most weeks. I did however after several years, in December 1998, ask the NHS Trust administration whether we should continue the work, as it was not properly funded and had just drifted into our work load. The reason I made this request was because these children and their families posed such complex and time consuming problems that they were making inroads into our routine Inflammatory Bowel Disease and Food Allergy Clinics. At first I personally saw all the new cases but as the numbers expanded Simon Murch and sometimes Mike Thomson helped me. From the beginning the junior doctors were involved, as these children were seen as normal NHS patients. The whole thing became a huge team effort. The nursing staff also became deeply involved as these families had so many problems and the dieticians also played an important role as some responded to a milk-free and gluten-free diet. All this happened without planning but in the classical way that things had developed in the NHS throughout my career by clinical need and demand, i.e. it grew like topsy in an ad hoc way. On this occasion, a more formal decision was finally made and the trust affirmed we should continue and promised to seek funding for additional consultant sessions.

When all this began, I did not know much about autism, although serendipitously I had studied a group of children with autism at RAHC, Sydney as I mentioned earlier. I had undertaken a study to determine whether a group of autistic children with bowel problems had coeliac disease. At that time in the late sixties and early seventies, many autistic children had been reported to have bowel problems and anecdotally there had been reports of benefit from a gluten-free diet. This study was published in 1972. My study of seven autistic children with bowel problems had used diagnostic small intestinal biopsy. It had excluded coeliac disease, but in a letter to the *Lancet*, we reported the finding of low levels of alpha-one-antitrypsin in the blood of these children. This low level was later found in other patients to be due to a leak of this protein from the gut. This occurs in disorders where there is a general protein loss, as I had studied years earlier at Prince Alfred. They included patients with inflammatory bowel disorders. Looking back on this work it now seems I was biopsying the wrong part of the gut. I should have biopsied the colon rather than the small intestine, as we were to do twenty-three years later. Since I left Sydney in 1972, I had no further contact with autistic children until 1995.

So I was shocked to see the autistic children with very severely disturbed and often destructive behaviour who came to my outpatient clinic at the Royal Free. Some parents had been given a "hopeless" prognosis in relation to the child's behavioural regression. Tragically this has proved to be all too true for some of these children. It seemed to us that such children may have had a wrong diagnosis of autism. Encouraged by Mike Thomson, we decided to investigate them with lumbar puncture to obtain diagnostic cerebrospinal fluid CSF, as well as EEG's and brain MRI scans to exclude such disease.

Many had quite major bowel symptoms. The first question was, did they have some kind of inflammatory bowel disease? At first our focus was on possible Crohn's disease. Their symptoms were consistent with that possibility. As I began to see the children their clinical features suggested that they have bowel inflammation and so I recommended diagnostic ileo-colonoscopy to exclude chronic inflammatory bowel disease. My endoscopic and pathological colleagues reported that these children did have a curious, morphologically mild, inflammation in their bowel, but it was not classically chronic inflammatory bowel disease. Yet one child was considered at first to have Crohn's disease and to our surprise responded dramatically to enteral nutrition, our standard approach to therapy of new patients with Crohn's disease. This is however a very demanding approach for such children, replacing their normal diet with a liquid diet. Others were given sulphasalazine, an anti-inflammatory drug used in the milder cases of children with Crohn's disease. To my further surprise and pleasure a number of these children had improvement in their behaviour even more than their bowel symptoms. Although this effect did in some cases wear off. It was no miracle cure. The children's improvement plateaued but often relapsed if the medication was stopped.

There was of course the fact that most of these children had regressive autism. Most poignantly of all some parents brought videos which we later played back in the department. These showed happy sequences of smiling children at Christmas or birthday celebrations, but then there were sequences, sometimes only a few weeks later, showing children with vacant faces and obvious slowed development. (This I might add was a new aspect of medical life in the nineties, when parents could come to clinics bearing helpful videos of their children's behaviour.) Some parents had attributed the onset of these behavioural symptoms and also the bowel symptoms to MMR. They showed us videos of the normal child before and the abnormal afterwards. This was very difficult to assess, as regressive autism usually occurs at about the time MMR is given, circa 15 months or so. I consulted colleagues interested in autism and they all felt it was a coincidence. I relayed this to the parents. Most were highly articulate and dismissive of this view. Yet most of the parents were touchingly grateful that at last they had found doctors who would listen to them. Many had been constantly reassured by their general practitioners and consultants, that MMR could not possibly have anything to do with their illness. I was sceptical too, but I felt we simply did not know whether in a highly selected relatively small number of children (in national terms) this could be linked.

From early 1996 Andy Wakefield was keen to develop a research study of this group of children, whose parents had contacted him by telephone. Many parents were pleading for this to be done, some even demanding it. Indeed some years later an angry group of parents ambushed me in a hostile way, because we were not going ahead with more research, albeit of a different nature. The centre piece of the research per se would be to determine whether measles virus, especially the vaccine virus strain, was present in any inflamed tissue which might be found in these children and to investigate a pathogenetic hypothesis. This research could only be contemplated as a by-product of routine investigation. If I considered inflammatory bowel disease was a likely or possible diagnosis, then I would recommend diagnostic ileo-colonoscopy with multiple biopsies. Provided my endoscopic colleagues Simon Murch and Mike Thomson agreed with my recommendation and were themselves prepared to undertake clinically indicated ileo-colonoscopy in these children, then it would be possible for Andy's research to go ahead. After discussions between the three of us we agreed the way forward was to discuss a research project with Andy Wakefield.

In the meantime I began to see children by clinical need. Any research would be a by-product of clinically indicated investigations. I already had ethical approval for two extra research biopsies to be taken in all children who had colonoscopy provided there was parental approval.

So Andy in his laboratory, with immunohistochemistry would seek evidence of measles virus as the first step to develop his research hypothesis. Although later on John O'Leary of Dublin would take over this work using more sophisticated molecular techniques.

In planning such research it was essential that a child psychiatrist be involved to vet the accuracy of any diagnosis of autistic spectrum disorder, so that any laboratory finding was placed within an accurate clinical context. Mark Berelowitz enthusiastically agreed. A team was assembled, an ethical committed application was developed to investigate an hypothesis and was submitted by Andy Wakefield but based upon our clinically indicated diagnostic approach. The Ethical Committee approved the application but in the event the study was not implemented. More modest studies based upon ethically approved research biopsies went ahead.

In view of our anecdotal observation of clinical benefit from sulphasalasine therapy in these children who proved to have bowel inflammation a second study to evaluate the use of a better drug mesalazine (Salofalk), was also planned with the assistance of Dr Herbert Falk of the firm Dr Falk Pharma GmbH in Freiburg Germany. Dr Falk has over the years supported research in chronic inflammatory bowel disease. His firm was developing mesalazine pellets for both adults and children, which would be particularly advantageous for administration to children. A great deal of planning went on. I visited Freiburg with Andy to meet Dr Falk and later Mark Berelowitz also made the trip with him. A randomized, double-blind, placebo controlled clinical trial of the efficacy of this product was planned with behavioural aspects the main end-point. Tragically all this in the end was not to be. Dr Falk was not willing in the end to proceed with the new product in children either in our study or in another completely different study in ulcerative colitis being organized by Prof. Hans Buller in Rotterdam. He wanted first to undertake further studies in adults. This was a great blow. This initiative had been strongly supported by our Dean Arie Zuckermann. It proved impossible to get any other company or any other source to fund this work. This means we have not been able to scientifically prove our use of anti-inflammatory drugs. However I did recommend continuing to use the drug in practice as in my own experience we continued to have good reports of efficacy in many autistic children but not all.

Before this latter initiative Andy Wakefield felt we should discuss our preliminary results in the first 12 children with the Department of Health. He was planning a wider meeting with the health minister Mrs Tessa Jowell and the chief medical officer (CMO) Sir Kenneth Calman to discuss the role of MMR with Crohn's disease. In the absence of Roy Pounder Andy asked me to go with him. I discussed this with the Dean and he recommended that I should not go. He was becoming more and more concerned by the risk of damage to the reputation of the medical school, especially because of inaccurate reporting of unpublished data in the media. Now this was a very difficult issue for me, as I was academically accountable to the Dean and I respected his views very much. However it was not an order, just advice. After much thought I decided to go with Andy to the Richmond House meeting as I felt it important to open a dialogue. At the meeting were the minister and the chief medical officer with David Salisbury and several others. It was quite a friendly meeting. Sir Kenneth Calman and I chatted about our mutual friend Ann Ferguson of Edinburgh but I did clash with David Salisbury, albeit in a friendly way, concerning the evidence on increasing cases of Crohn's disease in children, which he did not accept. There was however an agreement to have a CMO research meeting on the whole topic. We were pleased. But in the event, it was not to be so. In fact a closed meeting run by the Medical Research Council (MRC) was arranged instead.

Going back to our work, the results in our first twelve patients who had had ileo-colonoscopy were of such interest that Andy felt that not just the Department of Health but the medical world, should be alerted to what we had found. The rest of us agreed. I myself was keen to avoid any mention of MMR in this first paper, as at that stage we had no proof of its relevance. I just wanted to describe the bowel changes we had found in children with autism. Thus I saw it as a description of a new clinicopathological syndrome. All we had was anecdote about MMR. Most importantly, all of the paediatricians in the study remained committed to the MMR campaign and are still committed to it. The *Lancet* accepted the paper and it was eventually published in 1998. By then we had studied many more patients than the original twelve with virtually the same clinico-pathological results.

I believe a great mistake then occurred, in relation to this paper, namely the convening of a press briefing to discuss its results at the time of publication. Andy and Prof. Roy Pounder were keen to hold the conference. I refused to attend. I do not believe professional and research matters should normally be discussed in the public media. They should be discussed in scientific and medical media and at the relevant meetings. The press conference was duly held in February 1998. Andy Wakefield, without any evidence, but because of his own fears concerning MMR recommended the single components be given at yearly intervals. Andy had discussed this with the paediatricians in advance and we had told him our opposition. Arie Zuckerman, the Dean (a virologist himself, professor of medical microbiology) disagreed as well. We three paediatricians produced a press release for the day of the Press briefly supporting MMR and we also responded to some other contentious issues that had been raised in the correspondence columns. My worst fears about the media then came true.

All this publicity at the time in February 1998 was extremely unpleasant for us in the University Department of Paediatric Gastroenterology at the Royal Free. We received what can only be called hate mail. One letter we destroyed long ago could only be called a poison pen letter. Furthermore many colleagues at GOS were publicly angry with us. Keith Lindley and Peter Milla rapidly published a letter in the *Lancet*, which described our findings as 'no more than anecdotal. Perhaps the only saving grace for the *Lancet* is the accompanying well balanced commentary', an unkind swipe at both us and the *Lancet*. In fact, most unusually, the editor Dr Richard Horton was in some quarters to be severely, and in my opinion unjustly, criticized for publishing our paper.

In those dark days two people whose opinion I respected very much gave us real comfort. First Dame Sheila Sherlock said to me in the corridor of the Royal Free in relation to the *Lancet* publication, in her brief bluff manner 'Good paper that!'. Then Professor David Baum, President of the Royal College of Paediatrics and Child Health, a little later, when I told him of some of the unpleasant criticism we paediatricians had received from colleagues. He commiserated and said one can only report the facts as one knows them to be true to one's self and give one's own opinion. He felt sure that one day all would be clarified and that our departure from paediatric orthodoxy by speculating about immunization did not put us beyond the pale. We were all made to feel guilty that by questioning MMR in any way we were betraying our calling as paediatricians. It all became very emotive and most unpleasant.

Perhaps for me the worst of all occurred in March 1998, when the Chief Medical Officer sent out a letter to all doctors in the UK plus a number of other NHS Personnel concerning 'MMR, Crohn's disease and autism'. What deeply shocked me was that not only was our speculation concerning MMR denied (as was expected) but also some gastroenterological findings (non-specific colitis) were not mentioned, whereas others were dismissed (ileal lymphoid nodular hyperplasia). In a clever and for me most unpleasant way, this dismissal was based upon quotations from my own writings or those of my team. Coming from textbooks, the references were rather obscure for a general audience, e.g. a quotation from my textbook *Practical Paediatric Gastroenterology* (Walker-Smith, Hamilton and Walker) was taken out of context.

I wrote to Sir Kenneth Calman, as follows, beginning

> I was personally very dismayed by your letter of 27 March 1998, especially after our cordial meeting with the Minister at Richmond House. I was not surprised by your robust defence of MMR vaccination but I was very concerned not only by your attempt to completely discredit our reported association between ileal lymphoid nodular hyperplasia, non-specific colitis and autism but your targeting of me personally on page 5 of your letter. It almost seems as if someone in your department has looked through my publications seeking to discover inconsistencies and so undermine my personal credibility as the senior clinician in the *Lancet* letter.
>
> There are many factual errors….

Then I went on to say

> I have refrained from any public statement to the media since I met with yourself and Dr Wakefield despite repeated harassment to do so. With my two consultant paediatric colleagues in the *Lancet* letter, Murch et al, 'we emphatically endorsed current vaccination policy' yet you have seen fit to target me and attack the whole validity of our gut observations which are quite distinct from the MMR issue.

Only someone in the department of health, very familiar with my writings and my team, could have done this. I felt this was an attempt to discredit me personally. This shocked me, as when I had met both Sir Kenneth and David Salisbury they had shown no adversarial response to me personally, that had been reserved for Andy. Suddenly came this attack. Arie Zuckermann gave me personal support and also thought it quite extraordinary. So I wrote to the editor of the *Lancet* along similar lines. He published a shortened version of my letter.

The CMO eventually replied and denied my interpretation but made no attempt to rebut any of my arguments. There things stayed for the moment.

Then one of those unexpected events occurred. A letter from Professor Alderbal Sabra, Dr Joseph Bellanti and Dr Angel Colon, writing from Washington, was published in the *Lancet*. This letter confirmed our whole concept of ileal lymphoid hyperplasia, which I had just defended. There was a beautiful colour photograph showing enlarged lymphoid nodules in the terminal ileum of a child with attention deficit hyperactive disorder. This was a great public vindication.

We continued to perform diagnostic ileo-colonoscopy in children with regressive autism and bowel symptoms where bowel inflammation was indicated on clinical grounds. If this were demonstrated, then the drug sulphasalazine was prescribed as a suspension in younger children or mesalazine as a capsule in the older children was prescribed, as well as other measures such as relief of constipation when present and dietary manipulation might be appropriate. I believe we were able to help these children, albeit sadly not cure them, the dream of every parent of an autistic child. What a terrible, terrible ordeal many of these parents endure. In many cases, parental life is totally disrupted by these children. We also were able to get their consent in most cases for research biopsies to be taken with ethical approval at the time of diagnostic endoscopy. This was done so John O'Leary's group in Dublin could look for evidence of measles virus. Most parents were keen on this. Some demanded it!

Now it is important to mention the MRC meeting. Simon Murch and I went along as observers to hear Andy's presentation and we made some remarks and answered questions. Andy was uncharacteristically nervous, and the whole atmosphere was like the Star Chamber, totally unlike the usual open scientific meeting. David Candy and Ian Sanderson, fellow paediatric gastroenterologists, had also been invited to attend, but they told me later their judgement on the matters was not sought. Later the committee publicly stated there was no link between bowel disease with autism and MMR vaccination, but did describe Wakefield's work as 'elegant and impressive'.

Eventually another more comprehensive Medical Research Review on Autism was published in 2001 after a number of meetings. I was not invited to attend. However by then I had retired and so 'was out of the loop'. Their report admitted for the first time that autism was increasing, one of Andy's initial claims. However it stated 'epidemiological evidence does not support the proposed link of MMR to autistic spectrum disorders'. I am sure this is true, but that is not really the issue. The issue is that there appears to be a small highly selected group of children where there is a risk, which would not be picked up by epidemiological studies.

Now to mention in more detail the new dimension that had come to our work by collaboration with Professor John O'Leary at Trinity College Dublin, a well-known virologist. Using a very sophisticated molecular biology technique he in fact began to find evidence of measles genome in tissue from our children with autism who had been endoscopically biopsied. I myself heard his principal young investigator Dr Uhlmann present this work at a meeting of the Pathology Society of Great Britain in London. A particular difficulty for me I must mention now, is the lack of my own personal expertise and knowledge concerning the specialized molecular techniques that John O'Leary uses in his laboratory Tac Man PCR is a term I shall not attempt to explain but I am given to understand this is a state of the art technique used to demonstrate small numbers of viral particles within tissue, which he uses in his laboratory.

Since the work has been published, criticism of a technical nature has been made. Such a situation poses a difficulty for a clinician where one does not have personal technical expertise, one has to make a human judgement based upon the quality of the person doing the work and his reputation. For me I have complete faith in the integrity of his findings and the quality of the work coming from John O'Leary's laboratory. However his findings are merely a beginning. Scientific rigour demands these must be confirmed independently in another laboratory.

O'Leary's work was completed and ready for publication in March 2000 but was only published after an agonizingly long wait in the journal *Molecular Pathology*, in 2002, long after I had retired. The finding of measles genome in tissue from our children with autism in this publication does not prove anything, but mean there was for the first time hard evidence concerning measles virus in children with autism who have bowel inflammation. There was now a case to answer concerning the possible role of measles in the gut inflammation of children with regressive autism. Yet there was no evidence whatever to link the measles virus or MMR directly to autism itself.

In early 2002 with this evidence, although I had retired over a year before, I felt as senior clinician in the 1998 paper I should make a statement. I did this in a letter which was not only published in the *Lancet* on 23 February, but Richard Horton, the editor, wrote an editorial concerning it. He concluded 'A clear research agenda into the causes, developmental abnormalities, and treatments of the autism-spectrum disorders is needed.' What I said in part was as follows:

> Am I too naïve to ask all people of goodwill on both sides of this debate to speedily agree on an independent research agenda that will finally resolve this matter? Such an agenda must involve non-epidemiological research focusing on the bowels of these children. It is self evident that this whole question is going on far too long and is causing so much heart-ache in parents.

After publication of the letter, I was astonished by the invitations for me to appear on TV and to speak on radio, all of which I resolutely refused. I have always wanted to avoid any fuelling of further worries concerning MMR for the perplexed parents of children trying to decide what is best for their own normal infants, as they are blown hither and thither by contrary reports in the media.

Since 2002 I have not attempted to keep abreast of the scientific controversy concerning whether measles virus does have any role in autism. I am in 2012 unaware of John O'Leary's current opinion. However the general consensus in 2012, as enunciated by Mr. Justice Mitting, is that the measles hypothesis in autism proposed by Andy Wakefield has not been confirmed.

This account largely first written in 2002 has been autobiographical. What I have written is obviously not a comprehensive account of this incredibly complex controversy but my own albeit incomplete story. It has been and remains a deeply disturbing chain of events. It has been for me the most difficult problem to deal with in my entire career. It has caused me and others much pain. Much more pain was to come in 2004 and beyond when the GMC became involved.

At the time of publication of this Chapter in the first edition in 2002, I remarked that the 'truth' was not known and that litigation was pending in 2003. This I deplored as I did and I do not believe adversarial litigation will help the children concerned. It has certainly hindered disinterested research and I believe has delayed it. In fact legal aid was withdrawn from that class action. In 2004 an investigative journalist made allegations against Andy Wakefield and me with Simon Murch. These are discussed in the next Chapter.

My greatest hope for the future remains that research will identify therapies which will ultimately be able to alleviate and hopefully cure this deeply distressing disorder of children with regressive autism and bowel inflammation and more importantly that its pathogenesis will be fully understood so that this disorder can be prevented.

CHAPTER SIXTEEN

The Trial

In February 2004, I received a telephone call at my home, from the Editor of the *Lancet*, Dr Richard Horton. Little did I realize that for the next eight years I would be pre-occupied with the matter, which he then raised with me.

A journalist had made allegations to him, against Andy Wakefield, myself and Simon Murch. These focused in large measure, upon the *Lancet* article published in 1998 referred to, in the last Chapter. The paper concerned the clinico-pathological findings in 12 children within the autism spectrum who had bowel problems and were shown to have evidence of non-specific colitis. But some of the allegations were more extensive. The Editor invited me to a meeting to discuss these allegations in his office, attended by the three doctors. At the meeting he recommended that an urgent investigation of these allegations should be undertaken, by the Royal Free School of Medicine, as we were three academics. This meeting was duly convened the very next day at the Royal Free Hospital, by the Vice-Dean, Professor Humphry Hodgson. It was attended by Simon Murch, Mike Thomson and myself, as well as by the Vice-Dean, accompanied by the Editor of the *Lancet*. This meeting to investigate the allegations, was held in the Centre for Paediatric Gastroenterology. A detailed response to the allegations was subsequently published in the *Lancet*.

COMPLAINT

Someone must have been telling tales about Josef K, without doing anything wrong [1]

Before the meeting I was invited alone to the office of the Vice-Dean. At this time, I had been completely retired from clinical medicine for over four years. This office had been very familiar to me in times past. There I had met the former Dean many times. It was a plain office, typical of academics. There

[1] By permission of Oxford University Press, Inc

was little ornamentation. It was an ordinary place. When the Vice-Dean told me that the journalist was considering reporting me to the General Medical Council, it became an extraordinary place.

I was already aware of the allegations made from the meeting with the Editor, the previous day. So I knew that these were no more than half truths and full of misunderstandings and misinterpretations of medical matters.

So it was the Vice Dean, who first alerted me to the fact that a complaint to the General Medical Council (GMC) was likely to be made against me by the journalist who had made the allegations to the Editor.

> *think of yourself, think of your relations, of our good name* [2]

I remained apprehensive for three months with the words of the Vice-Dean reverberating in my head. Then an official of the GMC wrote to inform me that a journalist had made a complaint against me. My heart sank. I thought of my wife, my children, my grandchildren and my friends. Tom Stapleton, my former professor in Sydney, now in his old age said to me "What would your father say?" Although dad had died thirty years before, I did wonder what he would think. A sense of outrage and injustice surged over me. My reputation, my very honour, indeed all that I stood for, was being questioned.

Little did I realize that many, many, anxious weeks, months and years were now to be devoured by what was ultimately known as the Hearing. I would have to endure this sense of outrage for so many years to come.

THE WAIT

> *But cannot find the least thing I am guilty of with which I could be charged* [3]

I knew I had done nothing wrong. Yet six long months were to pass before another Official of the GMC wrote to me informing me that charges were being prepared against me. I later learned that charges were also being prepared against the other two doctors.

Through the good offices of the Medical Protection Society I secured the legal services of a dynamic team of solicitors and barristers.

> *I cannot inform you that you have been charged with anything or, rather I do not know whether you have been or not.* [4]

Then I had to wait and wait. Although I knew that I was not guilty of any

---

[2] By permission of Oxford University Press, Inc

[3] *ibid.*

[4] *ibid.*

wrongdoing yet this made the wait no easier. Through my lawyers I became aware of repeated postponements and inexplicable delays concerning the announcement of charges against me by the GMC. It was at this time that colleagues began to draw my attention to "The Trial" by Franz Kafka. As time went on this analogy seemed ever clearer to me as I read the book once more.

Extraordinarily, two years were to elapse from the time I was informed that charges would be formulated against me until I received the "Draft Charges" against me from the GMC. The charges chiefly concerned my clinical care of 12 children. Yet no parent had made a complaint to the GMC. The correspondence from the GMC revealed that the only person who had made a complaint against me was the original journalist.

A feeling of shame [5]

Over thirty charges were made against me. Some charges were most unpleasant as they included astonishing charges of dishonesty. I knew that at no stage had I been dishonest, but I felt it was deeply shameful to be in the position in which I now found myself.

The chief issue appeared to concern whether the 12 children had been investigated for clinical need or for research planned by Andy Wakefield. In fact I had investigated all these children to find out what was wrong with them, gastroenterologically and in many of the children, because of the severity of their regressive autism also to investigate them, in order to exclude metabolic brain disease or other brain pathology incorrectly presenting as autism. This investigative approach, which was quite routine in paediatric practice, required two invasive procedures ileo-colonoscopy and lumbar puncture. Consultant paediatric gastroenterologists performed colonoscopies routinely every Monday morning at the Royal Free Hospital. Lumbar puncture was a relatively simple procedure, as performed by the junior middle grade paediatric staff.

I learnt my comprehensive diagnostic approach for clinical illness for patients who are referred to a tertiary clinic, at the Hammersmith Hospital under the direction of Professor Christopher Booth as described in Chapter 6. This approach fostered the direct application of science to the investigation and treatment of patients. When I transferred from adult medicine to paediatrics it was my dictum that children deserved to be as extensively and thoroughly investigated as were adult patients, provided that the investigations were ethical and safe and that the child was sedated etc. to minimize any stress.

---

[5] By permission of Oxford University Press, Inc

The purpose of accurate diagnosis is to ensure that appropriate and effective therapy be given to the sick child. The detailed background to this approach in paediatric gastroenterology is discussed in Chapter 11.

Some charges against me seemed trivial. These included matters of documentation and provenance, as well as my personal style of letter writing, which often mentioned innovative/research ideas in routine letters to general practitioners. It seemed to me, that "someone" with the allegations in front of him or her, had trawled through the children's clinical notes looking for any item no matter how trivial which might lead to charges. It was clear I was to be given no benefit of any doubt and that my reputation and experience counted for nothing at all. This proved to be correct, right to the last statement of the Hearing!

THE DELAY

But in general we don't proceed with trials we're not certain to win [6]

I naively anticipated that after such a long time that the GMC would announce a date for a Public Hearing, quite swiftly. This was not to be. Five months were to crawl by until I finally received a notice of the Hearing date as well as the final charges against me. This was three years and five months after the journalist's original complaint. Neither the GMC nor their lawyers offered any explanation or apology to me for this astonishing delay. By now I had discovered that the GMC and their lawyers were effectively one and the same. They were both concerned with prosecuting me rather than finding the truth. At the beginning I was naïve, almost unworldly in some ways. I had thought that the GMC would conduct an enquiry to determine the truth! This proved not to be the case. Although later on, during the Hearing from time to time, the prosecution would mention inter alia the enquiry aspect of the Hearing. It was never made clear to me by the GMC what the prosecution meant by this term.

I could only assume that all these delays reflected my belief that the prosecution/GMC were absolutely determined to convict me.

THE HEARING STARTS

On the one hand, he was told, it was in everyone's interest to bring the trial to a swift conclusion, on the other hand the hearings had to go into every aspect thoroughly…[7]

The Hearing finally began in July 2007. The GMC /prosecution indicated to

[6] By permission of Oxford University Press, Inc

[7] *ibid*

my lawyers that it was anticipated that the Hearing, involving all three doctors, would probably last three months. After six weeks the prosecution announced that this would not be possible. The prosecution planned the next session for an incredible five months later. No explanation was given for this inexplicable delay. I was simply astonished and shocked by the cynical way the Hearing was being managed. In fact this second session was followed by six further sessions. Eventually these sessions totalled eight in number. The Hearing itself concluded in May 2010. This was approaching three years from its start. There were a total of 202 Hearing days. The GMC never communicated to me any reason for or explanation concerning, these repeated and escalating delays. My heart was filled with despair. Would the Hearing ever end? Would I die first? I was 73 years by the time the Hearing ended.

THE HEARING CHAMBER

He had assumed he would recognize the building from a distance [8]

I discovered that the Hearing was to be held on the third floor of an austere modern building. This glass fronted building stood on a busy street. Few of the many people who passed the building each day, would have any idea of the existence of the tribunal which was being held within.

was not calculated to instil much respect in people [9]

"The Chamber" used for the Hearing proved to be a large long room, which could be divided into two, by means of a screen. It was devoid of any of the grandeur, which one might associate with the term "chamber". There were no stars in its ceiling but those who had suffered in the Star Chamber of Stuart times would recognize the atmosphere as the prosecution got underway. Indeed I came, in time, to feel that it took on the persona of the Star Chamber of old.

On the right hand side were large glass windows, looking out onto another anonymous glass fronted office block. The remaining three walls were bare of any ornamentation. Very significantly, there were no symbols of justice upon its walls. There was no crown. There were no symbols of any kind of legitimate authority. It was not a room designed to dispense justice.

Along this long right side were several tables where the members of the adjudicating Panel, the legal assessor and the GMC officials would sit. On the long left side were the tables for the legal teams for the three doctors,

---

8 By permission of Oxford University Press, Inc

9 *ibid*

where two barristers, one or two solicitors for each and the doctor himself would sit. On each side behind the tables and the chairs, were masses of legal files, stacked high. During the Hearing these would grow higher and higher, even to the point of collapse. A similar stack was present at the short far end of the room, behind the tables, where the GMC/prosecution lawyers sat, three barristers and two solicitors. At the short end of the room adjacent to the principal entrance in the left wall, a small table was placed where the defendants and the witnesses would sit. This was some distance from the prosecutor at the other end. So microphones were an essential feature of the Hearing. The long distance and the transmitted voice of the prosecutor was later to give me a sense of the unreality of the whole proceedings. The prosecutor was a remote figure apparently speaking on the radio! To achieve privacy in conversation between defendants and their lawyers etc. one had to speak sotte voce or even in whispers. Yet I found as I sat in the defendant's chair that sometimes due to peculiar acoustics I could overhear distant confidential conversations.

Thy don't show much consideration for the public [10]

Behind the chair for defendants and witnesses was an area cordoned off for a "gallery", for both the public and the press. In fact it often proved to be quite difficult for the words of the Hearing to be clearly heard in the "gallery" even with microphones.

I found this "chamber" to be a deeply deceptive room. I regarded the absence of traditional symbols of justice to be highly significant. There were no visual assurances that justice would be done in this room. It seemed to me that the purpose of this room was to deceive the defendants into thinking that this was a room where normal "business" meetings would be held. The implication was that the Hearing was a normal business meeting. This was far, far from the reality, as all the lawyers and Panellists knew from long experience. I saw it as a dishonest room where a defendant might be lulled into a false sense of normality. Thereby entrapment by the prosecution might occur. The chairs and the tables had stainless steel fittings. These came to symbolize instruments of torture in my mind. Indeed by the end of cross-examination I came to regard the room as a "Torture Chamber".

THE HEARING PROCEEDS

Once the legal teams and the defendants were seated on the left and the

[10] By permission of Oxford University Press, Inc

prosecution lawyers at the far end of the room, the proceedings began by the Panellists processing in, at a slow pace, from a door just to the left of the prosecution desk. There were five panellists. Three were doctors. Two were lay people. Three were women. Two were men. The chairman was a general practitioner, most appropriately. He would understand from personal experience how sick children came to be referred to a specialist department in a teaching hospital like the Royal Free Hospital. However no panellist had had any particular experience with children. None of them were paediatricians. None were gastroenterologists. None were university academics. Clearly the GMC considered the composition of the panel to be politically correct. My heart sank when I knew the composition. I considered that I was not being judged by my peers. No member of the panel had any relevant expertise in the areas to be covered by the Hearing. I thought it would be hard work for my lawyers and for me as well, to explain to the panel the immense complexity of the topics to be discussed. So it proved to be.

The panellists were not a jury. They were five people chosen by the GMC. I was told that the lay members had had previous experience on such GMC panels, as indeed had the medical members. Their role was first to decide whether any of the charges were found to be "proved" by them. Then, if the charges were found to be "proved", they would decide whether this represented serious professional misconduct and finally if that were the case, they would decide the appropriate sanction.

The legal assessor processed in with the panel. He was a distinguished Queen's counsel. He sat on the left of the chairman who in turn sat in the middle, on the right side of the room. My lawyers had alerted me to the fact that there was no judge in the proceedings. The legal assessor was there to advise the Panel solely on any relevant legal matters. He was not a judge equivalent.

It has to be a black jacket [11]

I noted an interesting contrast between the lawyers (defence and prosecution) and the doctors on the one hand and on the other the Panel. The former were dressed almost universally in dark suits, my own was almost black. Some of the young lawyers wore very sharp pin-stripe suits, dark in colour. All this created a very sombre and serious atmosphere. I liked this as I felt it was appropriate to the reality and indeed the gravity of my situation. By contrast the Panel dressed in clothes of a somewhat lighter hue and less formal style.

---

[11] By permission of Oxford University Press, Inc

A distinguished Queen's Counsel led the prosecution/GMC legal team. This Lady Prosecutor practised law within a very adversarial system. During her cross-examination of me, I came to think of her as the Lady Inquisitor. Her style was often hectoring, and inquisitional, in manner. She began the Hearing with a long prosecution polemic but the defendants' counsels had no opportunity to make a statement at that time. She then went on to call many, many witnesses of fact, for the prosecution and two expert witnesses Professor Ian Booth of Birmingham (paediatric gastroenterologist) and Sir Michael Rutter (child psychiatrist) as well. I considered it was inappropriate to have a child psychiatrist adjudicating on whether or not a lumbar puncture was indicated. I had never heard of a psychiatrist, being concerned with lumbar puncture indications. One of the many other witnesses was Sir David Hull (See Chapter 14). The evidence of witnesses consumed the first session.

I was sad to discover that some former colleagues were witnesses of fact for the prosecution. Yet I was pleased to find that they made no criticisms of me. Remarkably one witness of fact for the prosecution who was a mother of one of the children involved, revealed to me after she had given evidence, that she thought that she was going to give evidence for me, until just before the Hearing.

The second session, months later consisted of the evidence in chief and cross-examination of Andy Wakefield.

Eventually after a year I at last came to give my own, evidence in chief, in the third session of the Hearing. I had an outstanding Queen's Counsel acting for me, ably supported by a dynamic young Junior Counsel.

This was followed by my cross-examination by the Lady Prosecutor which proved to be the must difficult and unpleasant event of my professional life. It was a terrible ordeal. She was very hard hitting in her prosecution. One afternoon, a few days after she had begun her attack, I told the chairman that I felt exhausted. This caused an immediate flurry of activity within the chamber. At the chairman's initiative and with the powerful support of my own Counsel, the session was then concluded, for that day. This was a great relief for me. That night I wondered whether I should continue. However the great sense of injustice I felt concerning the way the GMC/prosecution was treating me, lead me to decide to fight on. My wife was a great support concerning the rightness of this decision. She had been a great support to me during my cross-examination. I was also grateful to my daughter, son and loyal friends who regularly attended the Hearing. Such loyalty will never be forgotten. Otherwise I had a great sense of isolation. Whilst I was giving evidence, I was forbidden to have any contact at all with my own legal team whilst I was giving evidence. I had developed a great sense of respect, for my legal team and even friendship after four years. I felt a real sense of loss when I was no longer able to speak to them. There was a great sense of elation, comparable to seeing old friends again when at last the end of my evidence, came.

The Prosecutor during my cross-examination, often used a very harsh tone. She shocked me profoundly on one occasion when she suggested that I had treated the 12 children like "guinea pigs". I told her that I found this allegation to be upsetting. In reality I felt like raging at such an appalling allegation. Yet I calmly but vigorously denied the charge with what I hoped, was with appropriate dignity. I wondered whether the Prosecutor really wished to link me to the Nazi doctors tried in Nuremberg and with the like of Dr Mengele of Auschwitz. It shocked me to the core.

She had made much of the Press Briefing convened by the Dean held at the Royal Free Hospital prior to the publication of the *Lancet* paper in 1998, in her cross examination of Andy Wakefield. At the Briefing he had introduced the issue of separate immunizations, rather than MMR, a matter not discussed in the *Lancet* paper. This should never have been mentioned at the Press Briefing. It was clear from the evidence of the video of the Press Briefing, shown to the panel, that I was not present. I had stayed at home as I did not approve of press involvement, in such medical matters. I made this point in my evidence.Yet the prosecutor gave me no credit for this. I also made clear in my evidence to her, that Andy Wakefield was not academically accountable to me, as he was a member of the Department of Medicine. As such he was accountable to Professor Roy Pounder. The Panel could see how high profile Professor Pounder was in these matters, from his forceful statements as recorded in the video of the Briefing, which the Panel were shown. However he did not appear at the Hearing.

> *Charges are not brought lightly, and when the court does bring charges it is firmly convinced of the guilt of the accused and can only be persuaded to change its mind with difficulty* [12]

My Counsel had introduced a great deal of documentary evidence from my own personal files. This material was not available to the prosecution before the Hearing. Items such as an original letter, hitherto unknown to the Hearing, which preceded a reply letter, known to the Hearing were immensely important for the clarification of facts. Or so I believed. Yet the Prosecutor in large measure ignored this large body of evidence except on a few occasions,

---

[12] By permission of Oxford University Press, Inc

when she interpreted it to be beneficial to the prosecution. I came to believe that the prosecution had been absolutely convinced of my guilt before they had even met me or heard my evidence, based upon the documentary evidence and witness statements they had had ab initio. Nothing that I could say in evidence, nor anything I could produce in documentary evidence would change this perception. I formed the impression that the GMC had instructed their Counsel to prosecute as hard as possible.

Throughout the cross-examination, the prosecutor largely ignored my curriculum vitae as well as my reputation as a clinician and my national and international reputation. This of course was later to be a feature of the panel's determinations. It was as though my reputation etc. did not exist. One example concerned my ability to order lumbar punctures. She scorned the fact that paediatric gastroenterologists were ordering/doing lumbar punctures. This ignored the fact that I had a role in general paediatrics at Barts from 1973 until my transfer to the Royal Free in 1995. Much time was lost in her prosecuting this idea and my QC defending my position. Likewise it was clear that Ian Booth largely ignored my reputation. This was very strange, as I had known him since he was a junior doctor at Queen Elizabeth Hospital for Children. We had been co-authors of a paper on colonoscopy with Christopher Williams in 1982. Furthermore he had clashed with me in the past concerning the need for small intestinal biopsies and tissue diagnosis in some situations. His critical comments on my clinical assessment of the children suggested to me that he was treating me as a novice. The prosecutor leaned heavily on his emphasis on my initial assessment of some children. He and she appeared to suggest that when I changed my mind after new clinico-pathological information this was somehow wrong.

During my cross-examination I became very tired of being asked to comment on letters written by Andy Wakefield and others, as well as documents I had not seen before. I felt that I was being asked to speculate concerning the meaning of these letters. I sometimes felt as though I was trapped inside some of these letters.

In the end, I gave evidence for 27 working days (nearly six chronological weeks). It tested my stamina at the age of 71 years. My lawyers told me that this was for a longer period than any other doctor in the history of the GMC. I do not understand why the prosecution in particular, should have considered the charges against me to be of such a serious nature as to justify the great length of my cross-examination. It therefore was natural for me to conclude my evidence by saying "It has been a marathon". It was hardly surprising that the chairman readily endorsed this comment by saying "It really has".

I was later told by a friend that a colleague had remarked that despite my years I had appeared "sharper" during the cross-examination, than at the time of my retirement. For the first and probably the only time since the Hearing began, I laughed. Clearly cross-examination was good for the "little grey cells".

THE EVIDENCE AND FINAL SUBMISSIONS CONCLUDE

Two expert witnesses, Dr Victor Miller (paediatric Gastroenterologist) and Dr Neil Thomas (paediatric neurologist) and one witness of fact, Dr Christopher Williams (endoscopist) strongly supported my position in most ways. Interestingly I personally knew Ian Booth (GMC expert) better than I did Victor Miller, as Ian Booth had been secretary to BSPGHAN, when I was president. I also had sat on other committees with him

The evidence of the expert witnesses, was followed, by the evidence in chief, and cross-examination, of Simon Murch. He was able to confirm my clinical assessment of the children. He agreed with me, that all the colonoscopies performed in the Lancet children, were indeed clinically indicated. Thus my evidence, on this subject, was backed up by Victor Miller and Simon Murch. For the prosecution, only the evidence of Ian Booth, was against my evidence.

The final submissions were made in turn by the Counsel for the GMC/ prosecution and then the Counsels for the three doctors in the sixth, seventh and eighth sessions of the Hearing. Finally the Legal Assessor gave his brief legal advice and the Panel went into a private session described as "in camera". The panel continued their deliberations for six months albeit with an interval of 1½ months when they did not meet.

ENDLESS DELAYS

There is no session today [13]

Repeated and endless delays were perhaps the most characteristic feature of the way the Hearing was managed. Some non-sitting, whole or half days were arranged in advance, but others just inexplicably emerged. There were sometimes huge gaps between sessions. Sometimes nearly half a session was taken up with non-sitting days. The panel appeared to have all the time in the world. There was no sense of urgency whatever. They finished early on Friday afternoons and found early starts to be next to impossible.

---

[13] *ibid*

While his trial was inexorably pursuing its course, while the court officials were sitting over the trial documents up there in the loft? Did it not look like a torture, approved by the court [14]

The planned and unplanned recurrent delays induced in me a deep sense of despair. I asked myself whether this ordeal would ever end and indeed at times whether I would survive it. It was a form of slow torture. The GMC, the prosecution and the panel appeared quite indifferent to any possible effect that the delays might have upon me. The only person to ever show concern was the Legal Assessor who referred to the delay on two occasions, but to no measurable effect.

So I went to the lawyer and complained. He gave me long explanations, but firmly refused to do anything [15]

I vigorously complained to my lawyers about the delay. They considered that a formal protest would not help my case. Although, they did publicly refer in a gentlemanly manner to the great length of the Hearing. It was without effect.

THE CENTRAL MYSTERY

It's the organization that's guilty [16]

The central issue for me over all the years from the time of the first complaint had been made to the GMC by the journalist, was the following. Who or what was behind the decision ab initio to take his complaint against me so very, very seriously? Other related questions remained unanswered, for example Why was I pursued in such a zealous way by the GMC/prosecution? Was there a department or organisation behind these decisions? I could not understand why I had been forced to give evidence, especially in cross-examination, for such a long time. I asked myself were the charges against me so heinous that they demanded so great a time and such intense cross-examination? Once again I pondered the central mystery of the Hearing for me. Was there another influence behind the GMC, an invisible Deus ex machina?

I never had an answer to these questions.

PANEL DECIDES

[14] By permission of Oxford University Press, Inc

[15] *ibid*

[16] *ibid*

you feel like throwing everything up, taking to your bed, and ignoring everything [17]

After a further six months delay, the panel at last announced "their determinations of fact" i.e. their decisions concerning which "facts" the panel regarded as "proved". I was relieved that, the appalling charges of dishonesty were found not proved. However the panel had decided that I had been doing research rather than clinical care in the twelve children. I knew this not to be true. I concluded that I had been in fact trapped in my own letters as well as those of Andy Wakefield. These letters, which I had written so many years before had been re-interpreted by others, (the prosecution and their witnesses). Yet this interpretation of the prosecution had been accepted by the panel, rather than my own. My evidence was given a year after the Hearing began, after the prosecution and after a number of prosecution witnesses had given their interpretation of my letters. My evidence that the colonoscopies, which I had recommended were all clinically indicated, was ignored. So the panel had found things to be "proved" which I knew not to be true.

Once again despair engulfed me, coupled now with humiliation. The "overpowering sloth of sadness" as described by Isherwood overcame me. I felt like staying in bed forever as each day dawned.

YET MORE DELAY

The panel adjourned once more. Two long months were to elapse before the Hearing resumed for the next stage. I had hoped and prayed that a medical outcry might develop after the panel's determinations of fact were made public. I hoped that informed medical opinion would see through these determinations to the underlying reality, namely that the so-called facts, were weakly based. Furthermore that they were in large measure disproportionate to the charges made. I also had hoped there would be comment as well, concerning the extraordinary length of the Hearing. Some of my colleagues did act quietly and confidentially. No outcry developed.

NEXT STAGE

The Prosecutor began by insisting with some vehemence that I was guilty of serious professional misconduct. Furthermore she harshly recommended the sanction of "erasure" to the panel. She stated that I was a threat to Public Health and to children. Yet I was 73 years old and had been completely retired from clinical practice for almost ten years. She advocated, that this, was the correct approach in view of the panel's finding, that I had performed research

[17] By permission of Oxford University Press, Inc

rather than clinical care in the 12 children, some 15-16 years earlier. I knew this not to be true. I was in despair yet again. I had letters of support from the parents of the children. None had complained. They had been full of praise for my care of their children. I knew I had always acted in the best interests of the 12 children.

My Counsel told the panel that if they chose "erasure" as the sanction against me, that this would destroy me. I felt a coldness, around my heart when he said these words. I feared he might be right.

FRIENDS AND COLLEAGUES

well liked and respected [18]

The final session of the Hearing was an opportunity for my Counsel to present evidence of mitigation in my favour. I had many friends and colleagues to support me. Over 100 testimonials were presented to the panel, all written in full knowledge of the panel's determinations of fact. Two medical knights (Sir Christopher Booth, doyen of British gastroenterology), Sir Nicholas Wright (warden of Barts London Medical School), a senior colleague from Boston USA Professor Allan Walker and one of my former trainees Dr Robert Heuschkel from Cambridge were character witnesses for me. All spoke powerfully on my behalf.

The testimonials and testimonies produced mixed emotions in me. Some mentioned very private matters, which embarrassed me, when read out in public. But my dominant emotion was immense gratitude. I also had the feeling that the testimonials sounded rather like my obituaries. Yet I felt it was a rare privilege to know how well my friends regarded me. This was a unique privilege. I was deeply touched by what was written and said. However I was left wondering whether the panel comprehended or cared as I looked at their faces. One panellist's eyes roved around the room while my Counsel spoke, another's eyes tended to shut intermittently. In the end the testimonials were all to no avail.

I had also appreciated very much those who had attended the Hearing Sessions to support me. My wife, daughter, son and grandson attended. However a number of colleagues Neil McIntyre, Alan Phillips, Ian Sanderson, John Dodge, Rob Heuschkel, David Galton, Evan Stone and Robert Douglas attended the Hearing. I shall not forget.

THE MARK OF CAIN

---

[18] By permission of Oxford University Press Inc

The panel indeed had not cared. The testimonials and testimonies were discounted, including my lifetime award in paediatric gastroenterology by ESPGHAN. The panel demanded the maximum sanction possible, as they did for Andy Wakefield. This was the harshest sanction possible. However Simon Murch was shown great mercy by the panel and he got off scot-free. I applauded this merciful decision. Andy Wakefield also received the maximum sanction of erasure.

A sense of utter devastation swept across me. I had been shown no mercy whatever. I had wasted the six years of my life fighting these unjust charges. My honour, the very core of my being, had been assailed and assaulted. I felt I now had the mark of Cain on my forehead. Furthermore upon reading carefully the Panel's determinations it was unclear to me in most instances, why the Panel had reached their decisions and upon what precise evidence.

TO APPEAL OR NOT TO APPEAL?

The only thing I can do now is to retain a calm clarity of mind right to the end.[19]

My lawyers told me that there was one last chance to redeem the situation. This was to make a legal challenge to the High Court. Yet they told me they first had to determine how likely was success, before embarking upon this strategy. The lawyers and I had detailed meetings and conversations. They told me that there was a significant chance for success. They assembled a number of powerful grounds for appeal against the panel's determinations. After a calm review of these grounds I thought it right to appeal. An Appeal to the High Court was duly lodged, supported by the Medical Protection Society.

WAITING AGAIN

My innocence doesn't simplify matters at all[20]

I felt passionately that my honour had been impugned by the whole process in the years, leading up to the Hearing and the years of the Hearing itself. I was shocked that my reputation for personal probity and professional ability at home and abroad had counted for nothing with the GMC/Prosecution, the prosecution expert in gastroenterology and finally with the Panel itself. I was so disappointed. All I could now do was to wait yet again. During this time several friends gave me very real support, including Alan Phillips, Bill Dinning, Evan Stone, Robert Douglas, Jim Malpas, David Galton, Neil McIntyre and

[19] By permission of Oxford University Press Inc

[20] *ibid*

Deirdre Kelly as well as Baroness Gardner. I shall never forget this support at a dark time.

POWERLESSNESS

No one, he said, could influence the setting of times for the hearings [21]

Eighteen months passed without any listing for the date of my Appeal to the High Court. My barrister had estimated the need for a 10 working days i.e. a two week appeal. My lawyers relayed to me that court officials informed them that such an appeal length was unusually long.

As a result obtaining a judge to conduct the appeal posed practical problems. This long silence became increasingly intolerable but my lawyers told me that any formal complaint could be counter-productive.

KAFKA NO MORE

My Appeal was finally heard by the High Court in the Royal Courts of Justice, Mr. Justice Mitting presiding. Accompanied by my wife and daughter we entered the Royal Courts of Justice in the Strand with my solicitor. We had first to negotiate the tough airport–like security. Then we passed into the beautiful gothic Great Hall with its smooth polished mosaic floor. Portraits of judges and historic scenes decorate this vast hall with its cathedral like proportions. We walked up an elegant stair case, then along a cloister–like corridor on the first floor, to the Court Room. It was not very large but had a very high ceiling. The judge's bench was high above everyone else. The barristers sat in the front on either side, mine on the left and the GMC on the right, with respective solicitors behind them. Then behind, were double pew-like rows of seats for the public gallery, where we sat. I was to say nothing during the Appeal. My appeal was listed Walker-Smith versus GMC. At the age of 75 years I had become a rebel.

We all rose for the gowned judge. The be-wigged and gowned QC's could then begin their respective arguments. I thought that here at last, was a place where justice would be delivered. The court-room was a place for fairness, not a kangaroo court. After 4½ days instead of the planned 10 days the judge reserved his judgement and the public session concluded. The GMC had appreciably softened their attitude toward me. Their lawyers acknowledged that I believed subjectively, that I was doing clinical care, but stated that my correspondence etc. showed that I was doing research. My counsel denied this. The GMC also admitted, that some errors had been made by the GMC Panel. Over a thousand people sent me support on Facebook. This gave me

---

[21] By permission of Oxford University Press Inc

quite a boost. As well, some parents of children with autism and one patient from the *Lancet* paper, attended in the gallery. Local friends Sue and Richard van Maanen, Allan Hitching, Arthur Tilley, Paul Harcourt and Graham Sawyer all boosted my morale as well at this difficult time.

LET RIGHT BE DONE

Right was done at last, after eight years, when Mr. Justice Mitting made his judgement on 7 March 2012. He stated that the GMC panel's "overall conclusion that Professor Walker-Smith was guilty of serious professional misconduct was flawed, in two respects inadequate and superficial reasoning and, in a number of instances, a wrong conclusion." He concluded that the panel's "determination cannot stand. I therefore quash it". "The end result is that the finding of serious professional misconduct and the sanction of erasure are both quashed". He also said that it would be a misfortune if what happened to me ever happened again to anyone else.

When I heard the decision, I said to myself Hallelujah! Justice is done at last. Wonderfully British justice had not failed me, after eight long years. I do hope that no one will ever have to face such a drawn-out ordeal again.

This quotation was referred to by Clare Dyer (British Medical Journal 2012, 344.3) when reporting a new Medical Practitioners Tribunal Service launched by GMC on 11 June 2012 to be heard by a judge. She stated it was the biggest change of medical regulation in UK in 150 years.

RIGHT HAD BEEN DONE

The quotations in Italics are taken from "The Trial" by Franz Kafka using the translation by Mike Mitchell published in the Oxford World's Classics 2009. Permission to publish from Oxford University Press Inc has been granted.

I am grateful to Don Hill who first drew my attention to the parallels between my Hearing and Kafka's trial and to David Galton who made the same observation. He published "Kafka revisited". Quarterly Journal of Medicine 2010 103 541-542. The full text of the judgement of Mr. Justice Mitting is found on the Internet http://www.bailii.org/ew/cases/EWHC/Admin/2012/503.html.

CHAPTER SEVENTEEN

Time for the Family: Aspects of the Personal Life

THE MOST IMPORTANT event in my adult life was my marriage to Elizabeth Cantley Blaikie on 29 August 1969 in St Giles Church of England in Greenwich, Sydney. She had come to Australia from Scotland in 1966 by sea, as a British migrant, for the incredible sum of £12 under the Australian government's immigration programme at that time. Her support over the years has been priceless. Our greatest blessing has been the birth of our three children Louise, Laura and James. This has been followed by the marriage of Louise to Paul Letchford with the further blessing of our six Grandchildren Joseph, William, Morgan, Chloe, Lily and Stephanie. James, after graduating with a degree in politics from the University of Bristol, began an exciting career in advertising and communication in London. He is now at the leading London agency Abbott Mead Vickers BBDO. He and Suki have given us the blessing of our seventh Grandchild Edith.

I don't propose to expand here upon my family life other than to say my medical life has required sacrifices, especially from my wife, but my children too. I have had a very busy consultant position ever since I was married which has made huge demands upon my time. In addition when I have been at home I have often been preoccupied with work-related issues and very often I have been on call for one of the hospitals. At first this responsibility was all the time except when I was away, but reduced to one in three nights and weekends from 1995 after our transfer to the Royal Free. So I have not given to my wife and children the time I would have liked and they deserved. It is quite different for my grandchildren for now I do have time.

I also have had the great privilege of having many dear friends, some of whom (mostly medical) I have mentioned but others I have not. They are now in several countries. Apart from my medical friends I have often neglected them too. Some of them have sustained and supported me in ways which have been incalculable. For this I am so very grateful.

I am all too conscious that the reader may find what follows rather banal and conventional but I do want to describe here, quite briefly, some aspects of my personal interests and activities. If these were not mentioned, this autobiography would not give a balanced account of my life. Although there is real risk of recording here what others may regard as matters of trivia.

Poetry has played an important part in my life, in a small but precious way. Just a few poets have meant much to me. Perhaps the most important has been A.E. Housman.

I cannot remember exactly when I first came upon '*The Shropshire Lad*' and the poems of A.E. Housman. Yet it must have been some time whilst I was at University, for during the 1950s I purchased a LP record of James Mason reading '*A Shropshire Lad*' and other poems. I still have this record and there can be no doubt that this record kindled in me a real love of Housman's melancholic yet curiously comforting poems. Several of his lyrical poems such as 'Loveliest of trees, the cherry now' and 'When smoke stood up from Ludlow' have on occasion really uplifted my spirits.

I was so thrilled when I first saw Shropshire itself and visited beautiful Ludlow and saw many places named in his poems. I realize that in reality his Shropshire is a poetic place, a land of lost content, i.e. a place of imagination rather than a precise geographical area. However its beauty and his evocative words describing so many places added to my appreciation of the poems. So some years ago I joined the Housman Society. I have only been able to attend a few of their meetings, including the annual commemoration in Ludlow on two occasions. Most notably my wife and I went to the dedication of a stained glass window in Westminster Abbey, attended by Alan Bennett and also Enoch Powell. We had quite a long chat to that irascible old man, who had been a Professor of Greek at Sydney University in the past. More recently I visited Trinity College in Cambridge where Housman spent his latter years as Kennedy Professor of Latin from 1911 to his death in 1936, the year I was born. We saw some of his original manuscripts in the Wren Library. I was particularly interested to see his bible with pencil strokes beside particular verses, especially in the Old Testament. He purported to be an atheist but it was also interesting to read in a letter to Kate Symons dated 29 September 1930 that he told her he was preparing to meet his God. He even wrote a hymn 'For My Funeral Service' whose content is at least theist if not overtly Christian. For me its last verse is one of the most powerful he ever wrote, addressing God.

We now to peace and darkness
And earth and thee restore

Thy creature that thou madest
And wilt cast forth no more.

More Poems XLVII

What he truly believed must be forever unknown. His poems and life still have the power to fascinate me. I saw Tom Stoppard's play *The Invention of Love* in 1997 with my Daughter Laura at the National Theatre, arranged by the Housman Society. It is a very clever play using the free form of memory to describe aspects of his life.

Another poet who has mean much to me is Rudyard Kipling, whom Housman very much admired. I suspect many many Anzac Days and Remembrance Days have given me my particular affection for his words in the Recessional:

Judge of the nations, spare us yet
Lest we forget, lest we forget!

However I have to confess that his poem 'If' is without doubt my favourite poem. He gave a remarkably discerning summary of Sydney in his Song of the Cities.

SYDNEY

Greeting! My birth-stain have I turned to good
Forcing strong wills perverse to steadfastness
The first flush of the Tropics in my blood,
And at my feet Success!

I have recited at our departmental annual Christmas shows, some poems by the nineteenth century Australian poet, Banjo Paterson, author of 'Waltzing Matilda', beloved of nostalgic Australians when abroad. My especial party piece has been 'A Bush Christening'.

Stephen Spender is a poet whom I have come to much appreciate who himself much admired Housman. His brief poem 'To My Daughter' I have found especially powerful and I quoted it at my Daughter Louise's wedding in 1991.

Bright clasp of her whole hand around my finger
My daughter, as we walk together now.
All my life I'll feel a ring invisibly
Circle this bone with shining when she is grown
Far from today as her eyes are far already

I had the great good fortune to meet the aged white-haired poet in 1985 when he attended a book launch of his final book *Collected Poems 1928-1985*. I myself wrote a brief poem about this in 2007.

THE POET

Meeting you was brief and short.
Yet as you looked at me,
Did you discern a soul
Touched by your youthful words and deeds
So long ago?
White-haired and tall you stood.
One whose inner life you shared with all.
Never we were to meet again
And yet your momentary look,
Still remains with me today.

During my professional life I have been able to read all too little but I have particularly enjoyed reading history and historical novels. I have now accumulated quite a large library of books begun when I was a child and brought with us when we moved to London. I still retain a book which I labelled as No.2 in my library when I was about eight years old. It is *Little Treasure Island, Her Story and Her Glory* by Arthur Mee, published not long after the 1914-18 War ended. It is a book of extraordinary British patriotism, Empire-wide patriotism, embarrassing to the modern reader who may ask the question, could he have been serious? He described the Union Jack in these terms:

> It is red with the blood of heroes, it is blue with the blueness of the sea, it is white as the stainless soul of Justice. It is the flag of the free, the very breath of life to you and me.

Yet these expressions of the most heartfelt compassionate patriotism must be seen as a symptom of recovery, indeed of resurrection after the appalling horrors of the First World War, concerning which he stated in the same book. 'Man in these five years has fallen from the height of power to grovel in holes like the beasts of the field'.

Arthur Mee's Children's Encyclopaedia had a huge influence upon my childhood perception of the world. Its optimism, its lyrical descriptions of works of art, things of beauty etc. and above all its hundreds of pictures over which I would pore for hours on end, had a profound effect on my life time interests and tastes in art and literature as well as other things. When I first saw the ancient Graeco-Roman theatre at Taormina, it looked curiously familiar. I discovered why recently while browsing through Mee's Encyclopaedia, before writing this Chapter. I came across a photograph long familiar from childhood which I had quite forgotten, illustrating the theatre at Taormina. This Encyclopaedia has influenced me more, I believe, than any other book or indeed books I read in childhood. In fact it was a small library of ten books in a special bookcase which my parents gave me as a very special gift. When I look today at the much thumbed volumes I realize after all these years how special was this gift.

Light novels used to attract me a great deal and I especially enjoyed the works of John Buchan such as *John Macnab* and D.K. Broster's *The Flight of the Heron*, recalling the family links with Scotland. The latter novel with its memories of the rebellion of Bonnie Prince Charlie in 1745 fed a major interest in the deeds of the Prince, which I continue today. I have visited the Palazzo Muti in Rome where he was born and eventually returned to die.

Indeed I have visited Rome five times and with my love of antiquity I have found the city to be of one of endless fascination. H.V. Morton's *A Traveller in Rome* I have found an invaluable guide and his writing evocative, for example concerning the Palazzo Muti he wrote:

> For seventy years this building was the headquarters of 'The King over the Water', and now in its shabby condition it could not be a more appropriate memorial to the sad fortunes of the exiled Stuarts. No Englishman can surely pass it without a thought of the lives fretted away there, of the futile plots and schemes, and spies who gleefully reported every event that occurred in those old rooms where typists now thump their machines and cooks prepare dishes that smell so strongly on ground floor.

The historic novels of Mary Renault I came to enjoy very much indeed especially *The Last of the Wine* and the *Alexander Trilogy*. All this connected with my deep love for Greece and the ancient world kindled first by Darcy Grigg as a schoolboy at Shore and Mee's Encyclopaedia. In more recent times I have dipped into more serious historical works and modern biography. I have always been intrigued by the French Revolution and especially the fate of Queen Marie Antoinette. It is an old interest as book no.10 in my childhood library which still graces my library is *Marie Antoinette* by Alice Birkhead, a school prize received by my mother in 1914. So I avidly read any new books on the subject, such as Antonia Fraser's recent book also called *Marie Antoinette*.

I have an endless fascination with the history of monarchy. I have much enjoyed Gordon Brook-Shepherd's books on the Austro-Hungarian Monarchy, especially *The Last Hapsburg*. Not surprisingly I have become a member for some years of the Constitutional Monarchy Association. Through it I have been pleased to make new friends who hold similar views to my own.

London provides many fine opportunities to indulge historic interests. My favourite is the British Museum. It is a quite wonderful place. It celebrates the achievements of the human spirit for three thousand years and more. I relish the Graeco-Roman sculptures, especially the Elgin Marbles, the bust of Alexander the Great and the remnants of the Mausoleum. The central court with its marvellous glass dome constructed to honour the millennium have transformed the whole environment. I have often entertained friends and colleagues in the Court Restaurant. It is a particular delight looking down on the inner court.

I have had little time to attend concerts apart from an annual concert in the Royal Albert Hall of Christmas music to which I have taken my children over many years and more recently my grandchildren. I do enjoy relaxing listening to classical music and Classic FM is my favourite radio station. I began to learn the piano as a small boy, with my grandmother (nana) as my teacher, but she was a great disciplinarian and I was not well hand-to-eye co-ordinated, so it was not a success. This I regret, as both mum and dad played the piano well. My time as a choirboy set me on the road of appreciating English choral music and later on I came to particularly enjoy Handel's works, especially Zadok the Priest. Handel's Largo had been the favourite piano piece nana used to play. His Water Music has become an especial favourite. Although very conventionally I am afraid, Mozart is the composer I most enjoy. As this autobiography has been written, many have been his works I have listened to on CD. I particularly enjoy his concertos for flute, harp and clarinet. Then Vivaldi's works, especially the much-hackneyed Four Seasons I find a delight. Elgar's Cello Concerto and predictably his Pomp and Circumstance are firm favourites. However it is Allegri's Miserere that gives me the most intense emotion of all. The only living composer who gives me comparable intensity of emotion to Allegri is John Tavener.

I am an inveterate collector, at first of stamps, and then of commemorative pottery, (especially Royal Events) and more recently of antiquities. In pride of place is a Roman glass flask and an ancient terra cotta, retirement gifts from my colleagues at the Royal Free. Quite where to put them all is becoming a problem of space, as I grow older and go on collecting.

I have dabbled with watercolour as a very amateur painting over some years now. Liz and I have had pleasant summer art holidays at Inniemore on the Isle of Mull taught by Sue Murdoch, an inspirational teacher. I have learnt to do thumbnail sketches in my little sketch book, which I use as souvenirs on visits abroad. All I feel able to do is to give some feeling of place. I have joined the Medical Art Society and usually exhibit some very amateurish pictures in their exhibition each year as well as the annual art exhibition of the Royal College of Physicians.

As to collecting paintings I have inherited a few from the family, notably a beautiful watercolour portrait of a young lady dated 1883 from the Australian painter Julian Ashton and a fine Australian landscape from Lister Lister. We have been friends with two modern artists first there is Karolina Larusdottir the Icelandic painter and we have several of her paintings. Then there is Sandra Pepys, daughter of Professor Jack Pepys mentioned earlier. We have a number of her paintings, including wonderful oil paintings of Jerusalem viewed at dawn from the Mount of Olives and another of the 'Cypress Trees of Bolgheri' in Italy.

Photography has been an interest since I was given a Zeiss Contina on my fifteenth birthday, at first with colour slides and latterly with colour prints. I graduated to a compact camera and now a digital camera but I myself have never really graduated to much more than taking snaps, especially of the family in recent years.

Pets, especially dogs, have meant a lot to me and my family. I mentioned in early Chapters my childhood pets. After marriage we had a delightful cocker spaniel Ruari Boy but he had to endure months of quarantine when we moved to London from Sydney. He never really recovered from this and became very disturbed. We finally had to give him away. We were later given a small mongrel black dog Flossie. Not long after, Liz was captivated by a golden retriever puppy which she could not resist. We named him Louis and for the next 12 years he became a central figure in our family. He died in 1999. We now have a very active border terrier Hamish.

An immense tragedy befell our family in 2004 when our dear daughter Laura aged 29 years died in Sydney. Words cannot adequately deal with such a loss. However her death triggered in me the urge to write poetry, which I have never had before. I published a short book of poems, called *Poems of Love and Death.*

LOSS

Choosing to go, you I cannot summon back,
Yet I store the hours we spent together
Walking the shore in Bondi's winter,

Till erasing that fell day, I almost believe
I shall see you home again once more.
Sometimes I glimpse you amidst the throng
Or fashion loving gallery crowd.
So sad it is that we shall walk no more
But I yearn for that eternal day,
On another shore, when together shall we be.

A further tragedy occurred in 2005, when my nephew Stephen died aged 33 years. The two Cousins Laura and Stephen had died just a year apart. I attended their funerals in East Lindfield, Sydney.

FUNERAL DAYS

Once more a house of grief,
Wet and cold,
In Lindfield again,
Once more a funeral for youth and beauty.

33 years was all he had,
But our Lord had no more.
For me His life alone,
Keeps the flame of hope alive.

Are the cousins together now,
On another shore?
My hope can only be,
That this is so.

Both lives were rich in love,
Given and received.
Much love flowed out,
On their funeral days.

However great happiness has occurred since the first edition with birth of two further Grand-daughters Lily and Stephanie. In addition our Son James has married Suki and their first baby Edith was born in April 2012.

CHAPTER EIGHTEEN

Reflections on Anglo-Australia, the Empire and the Monarchy

ANGLO-AUSTRALIA is not a name to be found on any map, now or in the past. Yet that is the country in which I grew up. Sadly it has passed away and I mourn its passing.

Yet there are still powerful resonances of Anglo-Australia in the Australia of the first decade of the twenty-first century. Three spring to mind, first the fact that Australia remains a constitutional monarchy with Elizabeth II, Queen of Australia, second the fact that the Union Jack still flies proudly in the first quarter of the Australian flag, third and more personal to me, the fact that my old school Shore, officially known as Sydney Church of England Grammar School, retains this name at the wish of both the school and its old boys. There are affectionate memories of the Church of England in Australia with its traditions of tolerance, kindness and a beautiful liturgy, which the more trendy and up-to-date Anglican Church of Australia with its increasing diversity may not always inspire.

In Britain the resonances are less obvious but nonetheless powerful. Three spring to mind first the size of the 'Aussie Diaspora' living permanently in Britain and instanced by the vigorous and active London branches of Shore Old Boys Union, the UK branch of Alumni of University of Sydney and the Britain-Australia Society, there are also the considerable contributions individual Australians have made to life in Britain, in this book two people have been mentioned, Charlotte Anderson who was the first woman to be a Professor of Paediatrics in the UK and Lord Robert May, a past President of the Royal Society, second, the presence of Australian troops (as one of the four former old Dominions) at the Queen Mother's Funeral, third, the invitation to Professor Kim Oates, Chief Executive Officer of the Royal Alexandra Hospital in Children in West Mead Sydney, to attend her funeral. The Queen Mother had been Patron of the hospital for many years and had shown great interest in it, inviting chief executive officers to tea at Clarence House over many years. However it has to be admitted that nowadays, young Australians are usually better informed about the old links with Britain than are British youngsters concerning old links with Australia. The Britain Australia Society, of which I am a member, does its best to maintain these links but its membership is increasingly aged and it is making a determined effort to attract young people.

Whilst the term Anglo-Australia was not used in my youth, it is a term that historians and commentators have used to describe the reality of Australia after federation up to the nineteen sixties. In fact at the end of the nineteenth century a book of Australian Ballads used the phrase 'The Greater Britain Under The Southern Cross'. So Britannic Australia or British Australia would seem to be more accurate terms, especially as Scottish and Irish influences were just as powerful as were English ones. This was certainly true of my family where my father was entirely of Scottish stock. However historians speak of Anglo-Australia. The value of this notion of Anglo-Australia is that it indicates the intimate bilateral relationship, based upon kinship between the peoples of Australia at that time, and those of the British Isles or the old country, as it was often affectionately then known, in Australia. In my young days, those who came from the old country we called English, Scottish, Welsh or Irish. We would never have described such people as British because we Australians were British too as were New Zealanders, Canadians etc.

We did not however, at that time, appear to have the same close relationship with these latter people who in fact, were often kinsfolk too, and like us, were all parts of the British Empire. So also were Indians, Africans etc. but these were not our own kinsfolk. It was the bilateral family relationship with the old country, that was so important rather than the imperial connection per se. It was the relationship with the land from whence we had sprung that counted. Even as late as 1968, when I told my mother of my engagement to a British girl, she said, 'You mean Scottish, we are British too.' Although three of her grandparents were Australian born, my mum throughout my childhood referred to England as home, although she had never been there and was only to visit England once, in her late sixties. She was no less an Australian because of her affection for the land from whence her forbears had come. Dual loyalty was the norm in her day. It is easy for journalists in the *Evening Standard* and the *Guardian* to mock such sentiments. In their day such sentiments were enough to inspire a generation of young men, young Australians, to fight and die on the other side of the world for the Empire they saw as much their own as it was any Scot or Welshman's. Such sentiments were still alive in my childhood, witness the young Australians from the RAAF who fought in the Battle of Britain in 1940.

1947 was the year when I first became aware of the British Empire in a serious way at the age of 11 years. Although from my earliest memories we had celebrated Empire Day as our annual fireworks day and I can vaguely remember talk of 'The Empire' and phrases like 'that is the kind of spirit which built the Empire' were quite common. In 1947 I clearly recall actually being taught at school about the history and geography of the British Empire in a formal way at Shore, when I was in Form IIB. There in history lessons, we learnt about the colonization of North America, the conquest of India, the British settlement in the South Pacific and the colonization of Australia. There in geography lessons we learnt about the 'all red routes to London'. The British Empire was then at its greatest extent, at the time of its eleventh hour. At that time the British Empire was always indicated by the colour red on maps. So the All Red Route meant that one could make a journey from Australia to London both east and west without leaving British territory. The western route travelled by sea from Perth to Trincomalee in Ceylon, then to Aden and on via the Suez Canal, calling if one wished at the Holy Land, i.e. the British Mandated Territory of Palestine. Then through the Mediterranean via Cyprus, Malta and Gibraltar and on to London at Tilbury Dock. Alternatively the eastern route by sea took the traveller via Fiji to Vancouver in the Dominion of Canada, where there was a change to train via the Canadian Pacific Railway which took the traveller across Canada and then by sea to the colony of Newfoundland. The journey thence continued across the North Atlantic to Tilbury.

1947 proved to be the year when the Empire began its rapid decline. The retreat from Empire was to be almost complete 50 years later in 1997 when Hong Kong was handed over to China. In 1947, I can remember the excitement of H.C.W Prince as he told us of the current events of that year, when the Indian Empire was to be disbanded. India was to become independent and to be split into Hindustan and Pakistan on a basis of religion. Ceylon was to become independent within, and Burma was to be independent outside the Commonwealth. Of course the name Hindustan was not used and the name India continued but shorn of much of its territory. Later on one boy O'Dowd who joined our class showed the practical consequences of the British withdrawal to us. He and his family had left India following independence and he regaled us with tales of the Raj. We of course saw ourselves as Australians, who had quite a different relationship to Britain than the Indians had ever had. We were their kinsfolk, and after all New South Wales had been self governing since the 1860s. Mr Prince taught us how all the territories in India,

Africa etc. which had not been largely settled by British people were being prepared for self-government and ultimately independence. The aim was to give these countries independence in peace and prosperity with democracy.

There was at that time nothing, implicit or explicit, to suggest that Australia as a fully self-governing nation would want in any way to weaken its own real but loose imperial link with Britain. This was the time of 'the silken bonds of Empire which shall never he unloosed'. For us the Union Jack was our flag. I wrote as a schoolboy essay in 1948 'The Union Jack stands for British power and freedom all over the world. Our flag stands for the memory of three great men (St George, St Andrew and St Patrick), and is a symbol of freedom, justice and peace.' In my diary of January 26 1954, I recorded that at home we had flown the Australian flag for the very first time on Australia Day for that year. We always had a flagpole at home and flew the Union Jack on special days, we had never flown the Australian flag before, clearly times were changing.

In fact most British colonies were given their independence between 1947 and 1960. A trickle of others, including Rhodesia/Zimbabwe in 1980, were given independence later, culminating in Hong Kong being handed over to China in 1997. Interestingly this date was exactly 500 years from 1497, when John Cabot arrived in Newfoundland to claim England's first colony and exactly 50 years after India's independence.

My own direct experience of colonial life has been rather limited. This was a brief call at the port of Aden in 1962, which I mentioned earlier, two family holidays in Gibraltar and three short trips to Hong Kong before it was handed over to China. The last of these included a Commonwealth Conference on Diarrhoea and Malnutrition there in 1994. As described earlier, I also had a trip to the then Rhodesia in 1966-67 during the period of Unilateral Declaration of Independence (UDI) which cannot count of course as colonial rule. I have also visited many Commonwealth countries, including Canada, New Zealand, India, Pakistan, Cyprus, South Africa, Malaysia, Brunei and Singapore. In addition I have visited former British territories, namely Ireland, Jordan, Israel, Kuwait, United Arab Emirates (Trucial States in Imperial times) and Egypt who did not join the Commonwealth. In all these countries I have looked for echoes of British Rule. Perhaps the most constant is the pillar-box. I have photographed such pillar-boxed from Kuwait to Penang. It it interesting that this symbol of mass communication is one of the most visible of the physical relics of the British presence.

However the relationship between all these places and Australia was and is totally different to the bilateral relationship between Britain and Australia.

So returning then to my theme of Anglo-Australia, I personally don't believe that this retreat from Empire was inevitable, especially as far as the former Dominions were concerned. I am interested in the idea that modern Britain herself, from the time of Prime Minister Harold Macmillan onwards became a very reluctant imperial power, contrary to much international, especially American, opinion, which regarded Britain divesting herself of Empire in a grudging manner. Macmillan spelled this out to Sir Roy Welensky of the Federation of Rhodesia and Nyasaland, when he told him that the British had lost the will to govern. Indeed citizens of the United Kingdom often tended to become 'ashamed of the Empire' in some curious way from 1960s onwards, as if they had been brainwashed. This in some intellectual circles has been followed by an apparent shame of any expression of nationhood. I sometimes wonder today whether some English people have lost all sense of patriotism. In May 2002 it was reported that the University of Warwick banned students flying the English flag before or after the world cup! This was not Northern Ireland, this was England. I appreciate that the National Front with all their bigotry and racism have tried to hijack the English flag. However the world cup combined with the Golden Jubilee and then the Commonwealth Games in Manchester have appeared to liberate people's natural patriotism and London has become bedecked with the English flag as well as the union jack. The English flag has been reclaimed by the English people in 2002.

A good example of the British government's continuing desire to end the Empire completely, come what may, is provided in recent times, by the British government's efforts to shed Gibraltar. This is despite the overwhelmingly democratically expressed wishes of her people to remain British and the fact that Britain had fought in the Falkland Islands to drive out the Argentinians because the Islanders also wished to remain British. It was even reported in March 2002 that the Gibraltar government was offered a 'sweetener' in the shape of £35 million of European Funds as an inducement to the colony to integrate with Spain. Naturally this offer was refused. Approximately 15,000 people demonstrated their resistance to Prime Minister Blair's proposal to sign an agreement with Spain. Chief Minister Peter Caruana called this a 'betrayal'. I agree with this. Of course Spain's behaviour is totally hypocritical as it refuses to even discuss giving up its comparable Moroccan enclaves Ceuta and Mellila.

In my view it is quite improper for an Imperial Power who is also a democracy to abandon a colony, the majority of whose inhabitants wish to remain within the Empire. For me the watchwords of the British Empire are summarized in the motto of London House, 'Empire and Liberty'. The British

Empire could never have survived in its latter days without consent, witness the example of the American Colonies once consent was withdrawn. To pick up an Empire and then dump it when convenient is a totally unacceptable behaviour for a democracy. An imperial power morally should not abandon the democratically expressed wills of its imperial subjects even if they become a financial liability. John Humphreys on Radio 4 posed the question why does the British government want to give up Gibraltar? The answer provided by Michael Ancram was summarized in one word - Europe. The Blair government wanted to have Spanish support in furtherance of its agenda of greater integration with Europe. I would pose the question. Why did the Macmillan government seek to weaken the Imperial ties with Australia, etc? The answer again was Europe.

I have a particular affection for Gibraltar, apart from happy holidays there, as my great-great Grandmother Mary-Ann Trindall née Adams was born there. Her father John Adams was in the British Army serving in the Royal Military Artificers in the Peninsular war against Napoleon, at the time. He later emigrated to Australia with his wife and children, after discharge from the army in England.

I do believe that Britain's retreat from both the Indian Empire (the Raj) and the colonial empire was inevitable but the retreat from the British Commonwealth (the old Commonwealth) in the case of the Dominions was not. I see it as a kind of betrayal by the British Government of Britain's own people who had gone out voluntarily or involuntarily to settle her Empire. At no point were the people of the Dominions asked via a referendum whether they wished to weaken or end the imperial connections, not imperial rule. Such direct rule had gone long before, in the case of NSW nearly a hundred years earlier, no one advocated direct rule from Whitehall.

One who resisted this trend by the British government to divest herself of the Dominions, was an Australian Prime Minister. During my childhood, university life, and early life as a young doctor from 1949-1966, Sir Robert Menzies (Knight of the Thistle and Lord Warden of the Cinque Ports) was Australia's Prime Minister. He famously said he was British to the boot heels. Our Australian Passports during his time had on their cover 'British Passport' and we were (mostly) proud to call ourselves British subjects in a British country. When I enrolled at the University of Sydney I described my citizenship as British. As late as 1967 travelling in the west country of England with mum and dad we always filled in our citizenship as British in hotel registers. Towards the end of our trip I discovered that the hoteliers were often discreetly crossing this out and writing in 'Australian'. In fact, English people at that time were often somewhat incredulous and even irritated that Australians should describe themselves as British. I know of a paediatric colleague from Perth, Western Australia, who was accused almost of fraud, because he wrote his citizenship as British, when he had clearly been born and grown up in Australia. Many English friends were curiously outraged that Menzies still appointed British Governors-General for Australia. The last such was Lord de Lisle. However to be fair there were others who rejoiced in the old Anglo-Australian links and remained proud of the Empire. In fact those English and Scottish families who did still have family ties with Australia were those most likely to appreciate our shared imperial links. In Scotland I was struck by the warmth of the family feeling towards Australia in many places. Scotland had of course taken a disproportionately large share in terms of people voluntarily emigrating to the Empire and to Australia and Canada in particular.

For me I was proud to be British (Australian too!) and I was a warm supporter of Menzies and his anglophile views. When I arrived in England in 1962 I was quite shocked to find how strong was the anti-imperial view among many doctors. My consultant chief Chris Booth at Hammersmith Hospital was in fact a republican. To this day we chide each other with our respective republican and monarchist positions. My English colleagues sometimes mocked or alternatively teased me concerning my royalist views and the associated concept of Australian loyalty to the old country. Clearly in a typically superior way, many English intellectuals felt Britain had moved on from such an outdated view. I felt that some of them regarded me as a quaint colonial to express such views as seen from their snobbish metropolitan perspective. One doctor friend, David Harvey, could even become angry when I expressed such loyalist opinions.

So by the 1960s not only Prime Minister Macmillan but also many British people had lost the sense of interconnection with Australia and other parts of the Empire and appeared eager for these links to go. Why this change occurred in Britain so rapidly at that time, I have not yet been able to discover, either then or now. Perhaps it may relate to a desire to be free to enter Europe without any complications, or was there a kind of national depression related to poor economic performance and above all the terrible suffering during World War II? It would be a good topic for historical research.

The real blow for Anglo-Australia had come in the Commonwealth Immigration Act 1962 when Britain began to demand work permits for Australians coming to Britain. Most importantly it abolished the right of entry and residence to the United Kingdom for Australians, which they had possessed since the country's foundation. I believe if the British people had been asked to agree this decision it would have been overwhelmingly denied. I have never myself quite recovered from the shock and sense of outrage that Australians were required to enter the land of their ancestors and of their sovereign lady through immigration in a non-British category, in contrast to republican Irish and former German enemies from the EEC who did not. Inevitably Australia responded in a tit for tat manner, restricting the entry of citizens of the United Kingdom to Australia by visas etc. Nothing has ever done more damage to the bilateral closeness between Britain and Australia than these outrageous restrictions of travel and working between these kindred nations. As a direct result of this and more than any other event, by 2001 John Howard Prime Minister of Australia, on a visit to Britain with former Australian Prime Ministers to commemorate Australian Federation in 1901, was forced to state the reality, that Australia was no longer a British nation.

In fact I met John Howard during that visit on an historic occasion organized by the Alumni of the University of Sydney of the UK, in the Great Hall of St Bartholomew's Hospital, hosted by that remarkable woman, the then chancellor of the University of Sydney Dame Leonie Kramer, and organized by Baroness Gardner. She is the redoubtable former Australian dentist who was chair of the Royal Free Hampstead NHS Trust when I moved to the Royal Free in 1995. Former Prime Ministers Sir John Gorton and Bob Hawk were also present. When the latter arrived he was very excited and delighted to report to all and sundry, that 'the pommie Prime Minister had confused the Americans and Australians'! Clearly this had made his day. Indeed most unfortunately the British Prime Minister Tony Blair had made a slip of the tongue in the House of Commons. When he meant to be praising Australians, he had said Americans. This of course delighted the anti-British lobby in Australia. Interestingly in another context, Tony Blair was criticized in the cynical British press some time later for giving a eulogy for Australia on that occasion. Sadly I, and probably most people in the UK, were not aware at the time that Blair had said this, as the British media had not even bothered to mention it. It was also a great privilege to meet Sir John Gorton, who sadly died in May 2002. He became Prime Minister in astonishing and unique circumstances. His predecessor Harold Holt disappeared in the surf off Melbourne in December 1967. No body was ever found and speculation has continued ever since as to what happened. Was he taken by a shark? Gorton was an old boy of Shore and a staunch monarchist.

Later in that week I was privileged to attend another reception for Australia Week at Australia House where the former Prime Ministers of Australia were also present. On that occasion I was able to speak to Gough Whitlam who was obviously not in good health but was mentally very alert. We discussed the first performance of *Jesus Christ Superstar* at the Capitol Theatre in Sydney in the early seventies where I had seen him first. I found it remarkable and encouraging that two such powerful critics of Britain and the Australian Monarchy as Whitlam and Hawk should yet feel it important enough to visit Britain to celebrate the Act of the British Parliament in 1900 which had created the Australian Federation on 1 January 1901. The only former British Prime Minister to attend the Australia House reception was Baroness Thatcher. I had quite a long chat with her. I was most impressed but I have always been an admirer. To me she was a conviction politician whose own view of the public good was more important to her than personal popularity. She told me how much she admired Australia. She is a Vice-President of the Britain-Australia Society. However her main theme was her concern about the European Union and she gave me a virtual lecture on the continuing threat posed by a re-united Germany. She concluded our conversation by saying 'Beware Germany'. This left me a bit perplexed at the time, but was explained when her book *Statecraft* appeared in April 2002. This suggested Britain should withdraw from the European Union. Yet this view has an interesting connection in this Chapter, inasmuch as the decision of Britain to apply for membership of EEC dramatically changed Australia's attitude to Britain. So although I have somewhat strayed from my theme of Britain's prime responsibility for the weakening of links with Australia I am now returning to it.

Australia and the *British Embrace* by Stuart Ward (2001) provides hard evidence to sustain this view and I wish to quote from him:

> When it came to dismantling the old familiar ties to the Mother Country, Australia was pulled along reluctantly in the wake of changing British policies and priorities. In the case of Britain's EEC membership application, it is significant that revision of sentimental attachments and the more optimistic appraisal of Australia's national future began to emerge after it had became painfully self-evident that the British Government was determined to pursue national interests and a national destiny that could no longer be reconciled with the traditional conception of an organic Anglo-Australian community.

He suggests that the United Kingdom's EEC membership application in 1961-63 caused a sea change in Australian perspective on its future relation with Britain and the meaning of its own nationhood.

To this day I feel angry and bitter that the British Government never seriously entertained a Commonwealth of kinsfolk (a free trade association), i.e. UK, Canada, Australia and New Zealand as an alternative to the European Union. To this day the twelve thousand mile journey to Australia seems a far lesser journey than that twenty miles to France when one considers language, common traditions, way of life and commitment to parliamentary democracy as well as shared history and shared wars.

Many British readers may be surprised by the loyalist views that I have expressed and still hold, because I am proudly Australian, born and bred. Why have I continued to hold the views of my adolescence throughout adult life? Why did I not change to a republican and Australian nationalist position, as most people living in Britain today would have expected me to do? To be honest I simply do not know the answers. The influence of my parents, especially my mother, no doubt played a part, the views expressed by masters at Shore at the time such as Darcy Grigg and the headmaster L.C. Robson, played a part no doubt, the warmth of the welcome I have experienced on my first visit to Britain by the Borthwicks and so many others, my love of Britain's fascinating past, the happiness and excitement that royal occasions engender in me and perhaps my continuing membership of the Church of England have all played a part. Have I ever felt that I am out of step with events? Yes, one such occasion I recorded on 30/9/93 when I wrote while visiting Liverpool as external examiner for the Diploma in Tropical Paediatrics as follows:

> Liverpool brings me strong feelings of retreat from Empire and reminds me of a feeling that I often have of swimming against the tide of history!!!

I wish here to say only a few words concerning the modern Commonwealth of Nations. The 'New Commonwealth' as it is now often called, is clearly quite distinct from the former Empire, having reached the present position via a transition through the British Commonwealth. The pivotal moment, of course, was the decision in 1949 for the newly created Republic of India to remain within the Commonwealth with King George VI as a symbolic Head of the Commonwealth, in a personal role. This led to a number of newly created republics and later independent monarchies such as Malaysia, Tonga and Lesotho remaining within the Commonwealth. For a time the concept of a Crown Commonwealth united by a shared monarch was considered but the broader concept of the Commonwealth prevailed. At the time of the Queen's Jubilee there still were still 15 sovereign nations apart from the United Kingdom, described as Her Majesty's realms that have Queen Elizabeth II as their monarch. These are Antigua and Barbuda, Commonwealth of Australia, Commonwealth of the Bahamas, Barbados, Belize, Canada, Cook Islands, Grenada, Jamaica, New Zealand, Independent State of Papua New

Guinea, Federation of Saint Christopher and Nevis, Saint Lucia, St Vincent and the Grenadines and Tuvalu. The governors general of these countries were entertained at a dinner party at Buckingham Palace in April 2002 for the Golden Jubilee. However there is no separate international organization for this group of nations. They are all part of the Commonwealth, which now has a majority of republics.

In this autobiography it is not appropriate to give a history of how the Commonwealth evolved, just to record my own experience of it. I have been privileged as President of the Commonwealth Association of Paediatric Gastroenterology and Nutrition (CAPGAN) from 1994-2001 to see something of the modern Commonwealth in action. It is in fact one of the most remarkable multi-cultural, multi-racial organizations in the world and a remarkable channel for engaging its developed members such as UK, Canada, Australia and New Zealand with developing country members in Asia, Africa, the South Pacific and the Caribbean. From a medical perspective, it affords a remarkable way of sharing knowledge, technology and research in a bi-directional way. Professor Ralph Henrickse, a South African settled in Liverpool, remarked in 2002 that Britain is too widely connected in medical affairs ever to be isolationist. Commonwealth medical organizations are a channel to prevent this happening.

On behalf of CAPGAN, I have attended regular meetings at Marlborough House, the international headquarters of the Commonwealth, with both the Commonwealth Secretariat itself hosting meetings of Commonwealth Non-governmental Organizations (NGOs) and one particular action group, PARA 55. This group takes its name from the Durban Declaration of the 1999 Commonwealth Heads of Government Meeting (CHOGM) concerning the terrible threat posed by AIDS to the Commonwealth in particular and the world in general. Paragraph 55 states:

> Heads of Government expressed grave concern over the devastating social and economic impact of HIV/AIDS, particularly in sub-Saharan Africa. They agreed this constituted a global emergency, and pledged personally to lead the fight against HIV/AIDS within their countries and internationally.

PARA 55 was the initiative of a remarkable woman Marianne Haselgrave of the Commonwealth Medical Association. On behalf of PARA 55, she invited me and Peter Sullivan on behalf of CAPGAN to work with CAMHADD to organize and host a Commonwealth working group at Marlborough House on mother-to-children transmission of HIV infection, in December 2001. Tragically there is an increased risk of AIDS mothers with active disease passing on the HIV virus to their breastfeeding infants. Exclusive breastfeeding, i.e. breastfeeding without any other intake, including water, may however appreciably reduce the risk, but we recommended that more work needs to be done and indeed funded. However we did endorse the use of anti-retroviral drugs such as nevirapine. Even one dose to the mother significantly reduces mother to child transmission, but tragically Thabo Mbeki's government in South Africa refused to make the drug available at public health clinics and hospitals the policy has changed under the government. This has changed under the present government. Delegates came not only from UK but South Africa, Kenya, Zimbabwe, Botswana and Uganda. Indeed the Uganda High Commissioner Dr Kiraye opened the meeting and took an active part in it. This was very much the modern Commonwealth in action.

Such practical activities are the feature of the modern multi-racial Commonwealth. Although the Commonwealth Secretariat is still based in London in Marlborough House since 1965, thanks to the Queen's generous loan of that royal palace. This building was commissioned in 1709 for the Duke of Marlborough after his great victory at Blenheim. Later it became a Royal Palace and was the home of Queen Mary, widow of George V, from 1936 till 1953. PARA 55 often meets in the former state dining room where there is a large painting of the Four Generations showing the future Edward VIII in a skirted sailor's suit presenting a bouquet of flowers to his great-grandmother Queen Victoria, accompanied by his father, future George V and grandfather, future Edward VII. The wearing of skirts by boys in the Royal family till the age of eight years was the practice at the time. The name breeching was given when they began to wear trousers. Poignantly Edward VIII was to dine in this room in 1936 before he went upstairs to break the news to his mother that he was to abdicate. I have found it uplifting to meet in such an historic environment.

Britain herself, however, is no longer the leader of the Commonwealth. She, in fact, is quite often in a minority position on various matters. Sadly in Britain today, there appears to be remarkably little interest in the Commonwealth and its affairs, especially from the media, except at times of Jubilee, Commonwealth Games and crisis. Such a crisis occurred in March 2002 on the occasion when the Commonwealth Troika of John Howard of Australia, Thabo Mbeki of South Africa and Olusegun Obasanjo of Nigeria recommended the suspension of Zimbabwe from the Commonwealth for one year. This decision was very fortunate for the survival of the Commonwealth as a credible body, the Commonwealth having previously suspended Fiji and Pakistan for lack of democracy. In relation to the theme of this Chapter, as I read the British media at the time of this decision, there seemed to be some reluctance to give credit to John Howard for his role in achieving this unexpected outcome, apart from a conservative party spokesman. Clearly the intelligentsia in the media still have a patronizing attitude towards Australia. From Australia's perspective, it is however both a great credit to her prime minister and also a demonstration of the importance of the Commonwealth for Australia, giving her an important role in the wider world, this time in the affairs of Africa.

However Africa poses an enormous problem for the Commonwealth and for the world at large. Political corruption and above all mismanagement has been a feature of post-colonial Africa. Many countries have been independent for 40 years and it is incredible that many incompetent governments still 'blame' the colonial powers. In fact Britain provided better public health and general health infrastructure for many countries in Africa which were administered by Britain in the colonial era. Zimbabwe's government has virtually ruined the country. When I was there in 1966, it was a net grain exporter and at one stage it had a strategic grain reserve of one million tons. Now it receives, in 2002, United Nations Food Aid. More intolerably, from the world perspective, Zimbabwe was elected in 2002, despite its suspension from the Commonwealth, to the UN Commission on Human Rights and even more astonishingly Robert Mugabe attended the UN General Assembly Special Session on Children in New York despite the country's record on AIDS in children. What terrible cynicism is this? At least the Commonwealth has courageously taken a stand on Mugabe even if the United Nations has not.

The Commonwealth Games in Manchester in July 2002 were a great success for the Commonwealth tradition of the friendly games. They showed how much the Commonwealth can mean in sport, witness the huge size of the Australian team, however the opening ceremony was too parochial, a street party for Mancunians with the Commonwealth teams as guests combined with token imperial echoes symbolized by the Grenadier guards. The Head of the Commonwealth herself seemed to find it difficult to juggle these strange juxtapositions. Fortunately though there was in the closing ceremony a wonderful celebration of the multiracial, multi-cultural heritage of the Commonwealth which Manchester was able to lead from its own multi-faith community. The profile of the Commonwealth was given a great boost by the Manchester games. The friendly spirit of the games was well shown by the reception for the slowest runner of the Marathon from the tiny territory of Norfolk Island.

In Australia herself, apart from the Commonwealth Games where Australia excelled, the media too are not so interested in the Commonwealth. Both they and the average Australian often appear confused by the term Commonwealth itself. This relates in part to the fact that since federation the Australian nation has called herself the Commonwealth of Australia and also confusion with the old British Commonwealth. The fact that the Commonwealth is quite unrelated to the issue of constitutional monarchy in Australia, has not been appreciated in some circles.

So sometimes the term is seen as referring to the old bilateral relationship between Australia and Britain whereas, as I have made clear, the new multi-cultural and multi-racial Commonwealth is totally different. As an example, in this new Commonwealth, when the Queen dies, it is not automatic that her successor as sovereign will be the new Head. This would be a Commonwealth decision and not a hereditary matter.

Turning now to the Monarchy itself, it is clear that Queen Elizabeth II herself has mightily contributed to the smooth transition from Empire to Commonwealth. A peaceful transition has occurred in the majority of the nations of the former Empire. What is remarkable is how well she indicates her personal sympathy and understanding, on the one hand for people like my mother who loved England as home before having ever visited the country and on the other hand, for people who are commonwealth citizens of many races, unrelated to kinsfolk from the British Isles. In a reception at Buckingham Palace which she gave in March 2002 to celebrate her 50 years as Head of the Commonwealth, I saw for myself how she is really interested in and cares for people of all racial backgrounds and cultures. This dedication to her task, which she clearly expressed at the time of her coronation, has been in my view one of the most underrated factors in the remarkably smooth transition from Empire to Commonwealth, (in most cases albeit not all, vide Zimbabwe). She has rather surprisingly, considering her own background and imperial origins, become a multiracial symbol. This is an astonishing achievement and a stabilizing factor in an unstable world. She brings a little oasis of sincerity, kindness and dignity to a world often characterized by cynicism, cruelty and triviality. She also has, as the *Daily Telegraph* remarked on June 2, 2002, an instinctive ability in Kipling's words 'to meet with Triumph and disaster/And treat those two impostors just the same' (from his poem '*If*').

From my earliest memories I can remember talk of the King. In fact the only artefact I still have from the wartime years is a framed picture, which was in my bedroom as long as I can remember. It shows an illuminated poem 'At the gate of the year' by the American poet, M. Louise Haskins (1875-1957),

'Quoted by His Majesty the King in an Empire Broadcast'. The year was 1939. It still hangs in my study.

> I said to the man who stood at the gate of the year,
> Give me a light that I may tread safely into the unknown,
> And he replied - Go out into the Darkness and put your hand into the hand of God.
> That shall be to you better than a light and safer than a known way.

I was so pleased to see that this poem became a feature of the Queen Mother's funeral service in April 2002 and to learn that she had the poem engraved on bronze plaques at the entrance to the King George VI Memorial Chapel in St George's Windsor.

However for me, I first really became aware of the importance and indeed excitement of the monarchy at the time of the Royal Wedding of the then Princess Elizabeth to Prince Philip in 1948. We as a family sat up very late to hear the Royal Wedding live on the wireless. This was the first of four such wireless occasions in my childhood. The second was the funeral of King George VI, the third the Coronation of Queen Elizabeth II and the last a non-royal event, Churchill's funeral.

It was perhaps the death of King George VI on 6 February 1952, more than anything else, which made me aware of how much the Royal family meant to my own family.

I vividly remember my mum quietly weeping as she did the washing up, after hearing on the wireless that our king had passed away in his sleep at Sandringham. She said that she felt as if we had lost a member of our own family. There followed in Australia a remarkable period of national mourning lead by the Prime Minister Sir Robert Menzies. The whole family listened to the wireless in the early hours of the morning to hear the funeral service live from England. Later we saw black and white newsreel film in the cinema. I clearly remember the sad image of the three mourning queens, Elizabeth II, Queen Elizabeth the Queen Mother and Queen Mary.

At Shore, the Head Master L.C. Robson marked the occasion by an address in the school chapel at a special service. His words were recorded in *The Shore Weekly Record.* In part as follows:

> Today we have met in circumstances of peculiar sadness, to give expression to our sorrow at the death of His Majesty King George VI. The death of a sovereign is always a circumstance of great solemnity to the nation. It is especially so in this case, as it was also when his illustrious father, King George V died sixteen years ago. Each in his turn was called upon to assume this exalted and responsible

office when perhaps he would have preferred a quieter life. Each overcame his own temperament and was moved by the highest sense of duty to meet the enormous demands of kingship. Each was called upon to meet the stupendous mental and physical demands of a long and dangerous war. Each without doubt sacrificed his health to his duty.

Though during the war most of us were far from danger, we all have heard stories of the devotion of Their Majesties to duty in London and elsewhere, even at times when their place of residence might have been and probably was a target of high priority to the enemy.

The school cadets wore black armbands for three months.

By contrast there followed the happy events of the Coronation in June 1953. Not only did we listen on the wireless and later see the colour film, but we had a family party at 68 Shirley Rd of the wider family. My Uncle Roy Trindall made an amateur film of the family celebrations for posterity. This showed how we had decorated our home with photographs, bunting and flags.

Next year came the greatest royal event I have ever experienced, the Royal Visit to Australia. Remarkably this was the first visit by the reigning monarch to Australia. King George VI had planned to travel to Australia and New Zealand after his memorable tour of South Africa and Rhodesia but his illness (lung cancer) defeated him. The anticipation before the event was great. In my diary for 27/1/1954 I wrote 'How wonderful to think the Queen will be in Sydney next week' I also described 'the magnificent decorations' for the visit 'The GPO is terrific. David Jones has a wonderful Union Jack on one side.' David Jones is a large department store.

On 5/2/1954 I wrote

Today we saw Her Majesty Queen Elizabeth II. What an amazing enjoyment. We got up at 5.30 a.m. and all four of us (i.e. dad, mum, Judith and me) caught the quarter to seven train which was packed and we got into dad's rooms at about half past seven. Even at this early hour an expectant throng, some in Macquarie St, having spent the night there, lined the route. Uncle Roy and Auntie Dot joined us and he took a film. However there was plenty to watch all the time and when the Queen came we had a magnificent view of her and HRH. She looked radiant and both of them looked up at us. After lunching there we went to Government House where we joined a merry crowd who were singing 'We want the Queen' and patriotic songs. Later to our amazement we heard the Queen had gone to Parliament and we managed to get two feet away from the Royal

> Car on its return. In the evening we saw the fireworks from Wollstonecraft Railway Bridge.

So for our family it was a very exciting day. The view we had from dad's rooms at 'Locarno' high above Macquarie St (the Harley St of Sydney) was wonderful. The mood of general happiness and celebration continued throughout the Queen's visit to Sydney. She attracted the largest crowds ever recorded before in Sydney, wherever she went. It was reported in the newspapers on 5 February that one million people in Sydney saw the Queen and Duke. They even attended a Royal Surf Carnival at Bondi Beach. We actually glimpsed the Queen again on several occasions. My sister went with her school to see her at a school event in the Royal Show Ground. I went and saw her drive through ranks of children assembled in St Leonard's Park. Finally mum, Judith and I walked to the middle of the Harbour Bridge and saw the Royal Yacht *Gothic* as she slowly sailed down the harbour to the heads. 'A magnificent end to a historic event'.

Some years were to pass before the next great Royal event celebrated this time by my own family of Liz and two daughters Louise and Laura, now in England in Woodford Green at the time of the Queen's Silver Jubilee in 1977. I took my daughter Louise to St Paul's Cathedral to see the Queen arrive in her golden Coronation Coach, a marvellous sight. Louise aged 8 years sat on my shoulders for several hours! The great family event however was a street party in Tudor Close. Louise and Laura (aged 18 months) had a great time with friends new and old. It was a very happy and neighbourly time. At Queen Elizabeth Hospital for Children, the great jubilee event occurred during the Queen's tour of east London. She stopped outside the hospital in Hackney Road and alighted to be greeted by hospital staff and patients. Our loud cheers rang out across Hackney Road. It was a great moment. The hospital was held high in the Queen's affections as it was there that she made her first speech in public as Princess Elizabeth in 1944 at the Annual Court of Governors as President of the hospital. Her father King George VI was a great supporter of the hospital and continued to send regular gifts there especially at Christmas. He had visited it several times with his wife after whom the hospital was named.

We were on holiday in Norfolk, at the time of the next great Royal event, the Royal Wedding of Prince Charles and Lady Diana Spencer on 29 July 1981. My QEHC consultant colleague Dr Bernard Laurence asked us to join him and his family to watch the wedding on his television. Our two families which now included James (aged 3 years) watched in a party atmosphere.

In 1982 I had interesting indirect contact with the Queen Mother. I had been invited as visiting professor back to the Royal Alexandra Hospital for Children. As part of my lecture programme I was asked to give a talk on Queen Alexandra, as the hospital had been named after her in 1904 and until her death in 1924 she had remained as hospital patron. She was then succeeded by the then Duchess of York, later to be Queen and finally Queen Mother. Queen Elizabeth the Queen Mother remained patron of the hospital from 1924 till her death in 2002 and regularly welcomed hospital superintendents such as John Yu to Clarence House when they were in London. From 1904 till 2002 there have only been two patrons. I sent a draft of my paper to the Queen Mother and I was delighted to get a letter from her secretary Martin Gilliat who stated that 'It gave Her Majesty very real pleasure to read the draft of your lecture on Queen Alexandra, the first Patron of the Hospital, and The Queen Mother found it to be of absorbing interest.' I was delighted by these comments, as were my colleagues and friends in Sydney.

In August 1995, I watched in the Mall the great procession to honour the VJ (Victory over Japan) fiftieth anniversary. It was wonderful to see so many marching from all the countries that had ever been under the crown both commonwealth and non-commonwealth. What a remarkable list of nations, it was a kind of valedictory of the Empire. I saw Prince Phillip who paused just in front of me and he was loudly cheered only a little more than Tony Blair, not yet Prime Minister. The greatest moment came for me when the Lancaster bomber flew over the Mall during the silence releasing poppy petals which spread remarkably over the length of the Mall. I still have one in my journal. Finally I attended sunset ceremonies outside Buckingham Palace with the lowering of the Commonwealth flags, which surrounded Queen Victoria's memorial. I remembered the fireworks in Sydney harbour I had seen fifty years before.

I have also been privileged to meet members of the Royal Family over the years. I met both Prince Philip and Princess Anne on visits they made to RAHC. Some years later I was to meet her again in her role of Chancellor of the University of London first at Barts and lastly at the Royal Free in 2000. I met Prince Charles at Great Ormond St Hospital. I was wearing the scarlet MD gown of the University of Sydney. Sensibly he asked me if I was wearing an Oxford gown. When he heard that I was from Sydney, he remarked 'But you are not staying here permanently?' He was amazed when I said I was. He went on to tell me that he had spent some of the happiest days of his life in Australia at Timbertop. I met Queen Elizabeth the Queen Mother at Queen Elizabeth Hospital for Children for its 125th anniversary celebrations. On that day she insisted upon walking right along the length of the ground floor of the hospital so all could see her. She noticed a Burmese doctor in the crowd and quite spontaneously and unprimed, she said to him 'So nice to see you from Burma'. The doctor's resulting joy and happiness were absolute. This was the last of several visits she had made to the hospital, the first having been in 1931 as Duchess of York to dedicate the Princess Elizabeth Ward. I was presented to the Queen at the Society of Apothecaries during her visit in 2001 and had a short chat with her about children's gastroenterology problems.

This was all crowned for me by the reception in Buckingham Palace to celebrate the Queen's fifty years as Head of the Commonwealth in March 2002 when my wife and I met again the Queen, Prince Charles and Prince Edward for the first time. The subsequent death and funeral of the Queen Mother lead to a great outpouring of national grief in April 2002. The sheer press of people waiting to see the Queen Mother's body lying in state confounded many of those commentators who anticipated a nonevent. Even more remarkably on the day of the funeral itself, nearly one million people lined the route. I myself saw the earlier funeral procession in Horse Guards Parade with my Grandson Joseph. I was so pleased to see representatives of the armed forces of Canada, Australia, New Zealand and South Africa in the procession. The Queen Mother had been the patron of the Royal Australian Army Medical Corps. Another echo of Empire was the Kohi-noor diamond of India gleaming in the sun as her crown surmounted the coffin. This was most appropriate as after all she was the last Empress of India. Indeed at the funeral itself in Westminster Abbey the insignia of the Imperial Order of the Crown of India was carried before the coffin, with her other orders. In Horse Guards Parade, the moment the coffin borne by the King's Troop the Royal Horse Artillery passed by, a wave of total silence washed across the crowd, a wave of almost palpable sadness and loss. It was wonderful to see Prince William, tall erect and king-like in his bearing, the future hope of the House of Windsor and our Monarchy. I queued for five and half hours the following day to see the lying in state in Westminster Hall. This was a quite unforgettable occasion. As we entered Westminster Hall, the previously chatty crowd became completely silent. We saw in front of us the brilliantly illuminated personal standard of Queen Elizabeth, the Queen Mother covering the coffin and surmounted by her crown. It was placed upon a purple catafalque standing on a pink-carpeted platform. At each corner of the platform stood four statue-like yeomen of the guard in their brilliant scarlet and red Tudor garb. Then all around was the remarkable ambience of the solemn dark almost brooding majesty of the ancient Westminster Hall. The building was commenced by

William II Rufus with the great hammer beam roof dating from the time of Richard II. This was the place where Guy Fawkes and King Charles I, Queen Caroline and Warren Hastings had stood trial. This was where King George V and King George VI and Churchill had lain in state. All the glory and traditions of this ancient monarchy, nation and former empire were encapsulated in this unforgettable vision. Such a vision of beauty, for many, symbolized what ordinary people love most about our monarchy. The funeral service itself, traditional and majestic, went on to symbolize all that is finest in monarchical and ecclesiastical traditions.

Remarkably, ab initio the BBC were out of kilter with the national mood. The BBC was all too ready to use the day of the Queen Mother's death and thereafter to voice criticism of the monarchy. An example was provided by Jenny Bond who remarked concerning the Royal Family, 'A family not noted for its unity'. This was a scornful remark, mean-spirited and cruel to make concerning a mourning family.

For me the mean-spirited criticism of Royalty by the BBC had reached its zenith at the time of Princess Diana's death when within 24 hours they were showing film of unfortunate details from her life. They seemed to have forgotten the ancient admonition 'Speak no ill of the dead' which by convention for centuries has applied to the days and weeks immediately after a person has died. Britain used to be known around the world for good taste. This is sadly not true now for large parts of the British media. The *Daily Telegraph* however captured the mood of the nation with its cartoon of a long queue 'The Monarchy is working', after all a million people had lined the road of the final procession. After the event the *Evening Standard* raised the issue of the Murdoch press's attitude to the Monarchy 'We're not calling for the abolition of the monarchy. We're just calling for a grown-up debate.' Many in Britain and Australia feel that the Murdoch press's true intent is to bring down the monarchy first in Australia and then in the United Kingdom.

I was in Australia at the time of referendum concerning the future of the Australian monarchy. The newspapers including the Murdoch press appeared to be almost entirely for the republic, as were the media, in general. The Prime Minister John Howard and the government were for the monarchy but nearly all the arguments in the public arena were for a republic. In the event with Australia's system of compulsory voting, the monarchy won 55% to 45% for the republic. The republicans, being bad losers, stated this was due to the wrong question being asked. In this regard it is interesting that the Australian Capital Territory, which includes Canberra, was the only capital city to have a republican majority. I can imagine the political fat cats thinking of all the perks that would come their way if a republic came in. By contrast it was astonishing how high the vote for the monarchy was in some parts of rural NSW. Bill Clinton, his highest vote never achieved more than 36% of the American population to vote for him. Whatever the future may hold for the Australian Monarchy and whether or not there was indeed some tactical voting, this democratic vote, in my view, was a truly remarkable endorsement of the democratic constitutional order that Australia enjoys as a constitutional monarchy. It made me really proud that the people of Australia could make such a mature choice, free of political correctness and despite the media's strong recommendations. Even more importantly Australia has given the monarchy a whole new dimension of democratic legitimacy throughout I believe, all her fifteen realms. Plans to changing to republican status in some of these have been shelved following the Australian referendum.

The Queen's golden jubilee visit to Australia in 2002 to attend the Commonwealth Heads of Government Meeting (CHOGM) was attended by enthusiastic crowds. By chance I was again in Australia. 25,000 people lined the route to farewell her from Brisbane. The response of the people on the street consolidated their democratic vote rather than the cynical press with their own agenda of self interest.

So, throughout my life I have been a stalwart supporter of the monarchy both in Australia and Britain. I feel it both symbolizes the best in our shared past and is a bastion of democracy. Furthermore I believe its spiritual dimension symbolized by the anointing of the monarch during the coronation ceremony is of immense importance. In addition the Queen and other members of the Royal Family have given me and my family much happiness over the years.

In growing up in Australia, I looked to a larger patriotism than to the nation of my birth alone, to a much wider patriotism symbolized by the unifying role of the Crown throughout the world-wide British Community. My life has seen Britain first retreat from Empire, and now a retreat from the United Kingdom has begun with the beginnings of fragmentation into her component nations. The ultimate goal of the European Union appears to be the partition of England herself into regions. Where will the great retreat from Empire end? Will it ultimately end with the disintegration and disappearance of Britain herself within an amorphous United States of Europe?

On 29 April 2011 Prince William married Catherine Middleton in a deeply moving and beautiful ceremony in Westminster Abbey. It was a day of unalloyed celebration and happiness, which spread across the capital and indeed across the world. Cynics were silenced at least for a short time. There was a surge in the popularity of the monarchy in Australia. In one report, such support was surging, to 55% with only 35% for a republic. Like so many others, my family celebrated with a party at our daughter's home with our grandchildren. It was a day when the old certainties of my childhood returned.

Then in December 2011 the Queen had a particularly warm welcome in Australia when she attended the Commonwealth Heads of Government meeting in Perth. However a yet more memorable occasion occurred in London in June 2012 when the Queen's Diamond Jubilee was celebrated by a river pageant. My family & I joined the enthusiastic crowds. In June 2012 the monarchy stands tall.

CHAPTER NINETEEN

Ecclesiastical Reflections

THE MONARCHY and the church have been linked in my thoughts from the time of the Queen's wedding but clearly the church has been a much more important influence in my life than the monarchy. This goes back to my earliest memories with evening prayers, before going to sleep each night, led by my mother. She also told my sister and me stories of Jesus's life and the Bible etc. More importantly were her strong Christian and strict moral convictions coupled with her personal example of love, care and compassion. My mother, sister and I used to worship regularly at St Giles Church, Greenwich, a suburb of Sydney, adjacent to Wollstonecraft. As related earlier I also attended daily chapel services each week day at Shore. I was for a time a Sunday school teacher at St Giles. My wife and I were married there in 1969 and our first child Louise Juliet was christened in St Giles.

At school one of my friends, Phil Stewart, a vicar's son, used almost to pursue me, trying to convert me to his evangelical views. He encouraged me to go to a Mission at St Matthew's Church, Manly where I heard a great preacher Dr Howard Guiness. Later at University I was to attend the University church of St Barnabas where Dr Guiness was the minister. He was later to be a missioner at the University itself. His thinking did have a powerful influence upon me. However I did go to him with one concern, namely, I had never had the evangelical experience of being born again. On the occasion I asked him shortly before a talk, he told me he could not answer this as he was preparing to speak. He did however pass me on to another missioner who explained this was not really essential and I did join the University Evangelical Union.

The Anglo-Australian link is obviously very clear in relation to the Church of England, both in the United Kingdom and in Australia. This is reflected in the identical variations in churchmanship, which occur in each country. The interactions are now bilateral. Non-Anglicans and especially non-Christians may not appreciate fully that the Church of England and the Anglican Communion in general, is a broad church, embracing a very broad range of Christian opinion. On the one hand there are convinced Protestants with a Calvinistic view, on the other hand Anglo-catholics who are so close to Rome in some cases, that almost the only difference from Rome is that they do not acknowledge the Pope as head of the church. In between are the so-called liberals. These in England, in recent years, have been in the ascendancy amongst the clergy if not the laity. They can even embrace those who are not far from agnosticism.

Sydney has traditionally always been at the extreme protestant end of this spectrum. This is not in general true of the church elsewhere in Australia. In North Queensland Anglo-catholics are in the ascendancy.

The protestant evangelical wing of the church is very obvious at St Andrew's Cathedral, Sydney. I wish now to pause and say more of this cathedral which I have mentioned earlier, as it has played an important part in my life and has doubtless influenced my opinions. In fact my father rather remarkably remembered being taken there in 1905, aged five years, by his mother for a service to mark the centenary of the battle of Trafalgar and he recalled the great organ playing *The Death of Nelson.*

I have attended service there many times over the years as I described earlier. Perhaps the most spectacular occasion concerns the enthronement of Dr Hugh Gough as Archbishop of Sydney. He was a most impressive man and a convinced evangelical. Like all his predecessors he was an Englishman, demonstrating again the close links between the two countries. He had been Bishop of Barking but he was the last of the English line. It also became a family tradition to attend the cathedral on Good Friday for the long three-hour service recalling Jesus's words from the cross from 12 midday until three o'clock.

In March 2002 on a visit to Sydney, I returned with my sister Judith to the cathedral to find that it had been re-ordered with the chancel having been changed from one end of the cathedral to the other. This had led to the cathedral as a whole being completely renovated and restored. The present day St Andrew's Cathedral seems to have had much of its mystery swept away. The church's doors are wide open to the world and the sun streams in. This is indeed splendid to beckon the non-believer into the church. However the cathedral now has a curious feeling of emptiness or hollowness, with little or reduced feeling of a sacred place. I had a similar feeling in the Gross Munster in Zurich where at the reformation Zwingli had swept aside all ornamentation apart from the stones themselves. The old St Andrew's Cathedral I remember so well, was a place with a much more religious or mysterious feeling. There is a diminished sense of transcendent beauty, which for me, is central to a sacred place. An example of where it exists very much for me is York Minster. This emotional response on my part is a bit curious, as my own theological sympathies are more with the evangelicals than the Anglo-catholics. However the concept of the church as a sacred indeed holy place, rather than a mere preaching house which could be anywhere, is something I have learned to appreciate. This has developed as I have travelled the world, over the past forty years, being exposed to various Christian traditions, Roman Catholic, Orthodox etc. as well being related to my Anglo-catholic exposure in recent years at St Barnabas Woodford Green.

In London, similar evangelical opinions to those of the Sydney diocese are held. For example in All Souls Church, Langham Place, the clergy have in general abandoned the wearing of robes, as well as the clerical collar. Incredibly in my view, at the York Synod of 2002, a general abandonment of robes was discussed but a decision was postponed till 2003. To me this is symbolic of dumbing down, sweeping away all mystery and the sense of specialness in church services and for me another step towards sweeping away the very Anglican persona itself.

Although in England the liberal ascendancy has often held sway and Anglo-catholics are high in profile if not numbers, evangelicals are of increasing influence as exampled by the Holy Trinity Brompton (HTB) phenomenon. All Souls Church, that most evangelical of churches, was for me a safe haven in my early days in London from 1962-1964. I was deeply influenced by the teachings and evident ardent faith of Rev. John Stott, perhaps the most remarkable Christian I have ever met. I had heard him preach before, as an Evangelical Union Missioner to the University of Sydney and indeed in St Andrew's Cathedral. During those two years in London I attended All Souls (as often as my medical life would allow). I remember sharing this with my close friend at London House, the historian David Wollman. Also my sister Judith whilst she was in London worshipped there with her friends.

When we settled in England in 1973, we moved to Wanstead and attended Christchurch parish church with Rev. Paul Bowen as rector. The Book of Common Prayer was thankfully used for services but the church was Anglo-catholic in its practice. Our family valued his ministry very much and our daughter Laura was christened in Christchurch with great pomp one evensong. Liz and I became lifelong friends with Paul and his doctor wife Elizabeth, who moved in retirement to Canterbury. When we moved to Woodford, what a contrast All Saints parish church provided. It was a return to the evangelicals. Although at that time the Book of Common Prayer was still used there was no wearing of colourful mass vestments, no incense and a very protestant atmosphere. Rev. Michael Cole was the vicar. This church has strong historic links with the diocese of Sydney, as Bishop Goodwin-Hudson coadjutor Bishop of Sydney had been vicar of All Saints.

Our Son James was christened in the church of St Bartholomew's the Less in 1978 rather than All Saints as we as a family did not fit in well with the church and Barts had become so much part of family life. Although our three children did attend Sunday school at All Saints, over the years church practice steadily moved away from the Book of Common Prayer and the 'clappy happy style' came in. Neither I nor my children could abide this. So my wife, especially, became involved with St Barnabas Church, Woodford Green where Canon Alan Cross is vicar, by contrast another Anglo-catholic who does not recognize women priests. I myself do not fit easily into this tradition.

Thus I have worshipped over my life at both ends of the Anglican spectrum. Over the years I have moved from a convinced evangelical position (albeit liberal rather than conservative in theology) to one which is broader but still protestant yet more liberal than I was. By contrast my wife has moved from a Church of Scotland position to the catholic wing of the Anglican Church at St Barnabas Church Woodford Green.

Clearly I have obviously been influenced in my religious views by the dramatic changes which have occurred in society as a whole since my youth, and more importantly by the changing views of my own family and dear friends, both in Australia and in Britain. These remarkable changes in the way we live today have indeed been a feature of life in the English-speaking world as a whole.

All these differences of worship practice I mentioned above, which I have experienced, are not directly related to this change. Over my lifetime, I have seen the wider influence of the church decline dramatically in both Australia and England, but especially in England. This makes me sad. To be an Anglican churchgoer in England at the beginning of twenty-first century is quite unusual. The decline of the church's influence in public affairs is all too obvious. Christianity itself is under constant attack yet as W.F. Deedes, that remarkable columnist in the *Daily Telegraph*, remarked, you can insult Christianity to your heart's content but if you write or speak in 2002 about the religion of Muslims or Jews to cause them offence, you may well be in trouble.

I have had the great privilege of hearing and sometimes meeting Archbishops of Canterbury over many years, Geoffrey Fisher, Michael Ramsay, Robert Runcie, George Carey & Rowan Williams. Carey is the only one with whom I have met to talk with, for any length of time. He is clearly a convinced Christian of great sincerity and personal bravery, as his trips to the Holy Land in the midst of bloody strife have shown. However unlike Michael Ramsay he did not come across as a great charismatic and intellectual figure. By contrast I can remember Archbishop Ramsay holding in rapt attention a packed audience of university people, students and teachers alike, in the Great Hall of the University of Sydney in 1959. In complete contrast I was surprised to hear Archbishop Runcie make a mocking joke about Prime Minister Thatcher at a University of London function, in the presence of the Chancellor, Princess Anne. This was not good form in my book.

At present the Archbishop, Rowan Williams, is a great theologian. For the future my own hopes centre upon Bishop Richard Chartres, Bishop of London whom I have met twice. I was struck by his evident spirituality and pastoral care at the funeral of a good friend Betty Busby, sister of my old friend John Yu. Bishop Chartres had been a wonderful pastor to Betty for twenty years in her remarkable fight against cancer, which she described so well in her memorable book *The Rice is Boiled. My Life, My Cancer* by Chen Yu (Betty Busby).

So clearly, great changes have occurred in recent years in the Church of England itself and the Anglican Communion as a whole. They both urgently need charismatic Christian leadership of a high order in these changing, yet challenging times. I believe the church is ready to reverse her old decline and to go forward as she is doing in many parts of Africa and elsewhere in the developing world. I remain an optimist.

A great issue for the church and society as a whole, both in Britain and in Australia, is the need to re-draw the lines, limiting total freedom of action. How we live today in the second decade of the twenty-first century is clearly so different, even from ten years ago, let alone the world of my birth in 1936. Old codes of conduct have been torn up. Much of this is good but in my view we still do need some codes, new limits to the anarchy of total freedom. Humans do, I believe, yearn for some guidelines or limits even when not always personally adhered to. Paradoxically perhaps, in my experience this is especially true in youth, although often not admitted. Surely the need for some limits to absolute freedom of action is in the hallmark of civilization.

For me in recent years, it is in matters of morality and in the application of the faith that changes have occurred in my own views. There is however no change in my fundamental belief in the resurrection of Jesus Christ and life after death. Many welcome changes have occurred in the realm of morality. The very strict even rigid morality, with all the associated sanctions, which was a particular feature of Sydney evangelicals and indeed much of society in my younger days, for myself, I have replaced with a more compassionate and broader view of the complexity of the human situation and of what God may require of us. This is in accord, I believe, with the compassionate and loving nature of Jesus Himself expressed in His own Incarnation.

Human nature is very frail, as we all know. St Paul says in Romans 7.15

> For what I would, that do I not, but what I hate that do I.

People are by nature individuals. Both their life circumstances and the society in which they live may pull them in different directions from the strict moralities as enunciated by an authoritarian church in the past and indeed still today by Pope Benedict XVI. Yet I believe that no person, anywhere in the world, is outside the care and concern of a loving, all seeing God.

In this autobiography, I have elected, beyond an account of my own childhood, not to invade the privacy of my own family and friends. In this regard, I link my own precise religious views and precise views concerning morality, with the issue of personal privacy. So I shall draw a veil now on my own exact views, without elaborating further in this difficult area.

All I wish to say by way of conclusion is that I believe I am a Christian, albeit not a very good example of one. I believe that death may be followed by resurrection. Indeed I see the new dawn that each day brings, after 'the perils and dangers of the night' as an imagery of death and resurrection. As we boys sang the hymn to the Trinity 'early in the morning' in the sun-filled Mowbray House Chapel so long ago, we unwittingly were celebrating the 'golden deluge of the dawn' which John Bayley describes (In *Housman's Poems*) as 'the bliss to be alive' and baptized'. The ancients of course well knew the symbolism of the healing and life giving power of the, sun. On the Isle of Delos, the shrine of Apollo the Greek God of sunlight is flooded anew each morning with the dazzling brilliance of the sun. A never to be forgotten moment in those Greek Isles, is the sun rising from the dark blue Aegean Sea. This new dawn that every day brings is a powerful symbol of everlasting hope for all mankind, of all faiths and of none. But for me I hold to the Anglican tradition of Christianity, appreciating particularly the forms, ceremonies and especially the words and music of the church, as I experienced them so long ago in Shore Chapel.

In the end, all I believe we can do, is to put our trust and hope in the loving mercies of God, as shown to us in the gift of his son Our Lord Jesus Christ and experienced by us through the power of the Holy Spirit.

I have begun a course for Master of Arts in Christianity and the Arts at King's College the Strand, London. The theme relates to the idea of beauty in western theology and also involves teaching at the National Gallery concerning art as a theological medium. I have enjoyed this immensely. I am studying mostly with people much younger than myself, which is very stimulating intellectually. We have a charismatic teacher Professor Ben Quash. Perhaps my experience of Correggio in Parma (See page 189) played a part in my decision to undertake the course. However the encouragement of my friends Bill Dinning & David Galton were of key importance.

CHAPTER TWENTY

Medico-Historical Postscript

SINCE RETIREMENT in September 2000, I have been actively engaged with the history of medicine until 2009. There have been two aspects, first the Wellcome Trust Centre for the History of Medicine and second the Faculty of the History of Medicine of the Society of Apothecaries of London. In the former I was granted the privilege of occupying a desk in a room I shared with my old mentor Sir Christopher Booth, a distinguished medical historian. In the latter organization I was the course director for the Diploma of History of Medicine annual course, taught every alternate Saturday in the Wellcome Building in Euston Road, London.

As outlined in earlier chapters, my interest in the History of Medicine goes back to my medical student days. Unfortunately immediately after graduation, I was not able to find much time for medical history until I began my interest in the history of coeliac disease in the early seventies with the collaboration of Dr Bryan Dowd, a paediatrician and classical Greek scholar in Sydney, culminating in a paper we wrote in the *British Medical Journal.* This was entitled 'Samuel Gee, Aretaeus and the Coeliac Affection'. It was published in 1974 to honour the 850th anniversary of the Royal Hospital of St Bartholomew after my arrival at Barts, where Dr Samuel Gee had published his original observations in 1888. In 1988, to mark the centenary of this publication in the St Bartholomew's Hospital Reports, with Dr Parveen Kumar who cared for my coeliac patients when they became adults, we hosted an international meeting on coeliac disease in both children and adults. The meeting had a small historic component which I enjoyed organizing.

Then in 1993 I took the only sabbatical of my career, to work under the supervision of Dr Tilli Tansey and Prof. Chris Lawrence for three months at the Wellcome. I had obtained a scholarship which funded Dr Ramand Kamam, my successor at RAHC, to do my work at Barts and Queens for three months. I studied Diarrhoeal Mortality in Infancy in the Edwardian Period. I was interested in this topic because there were remarkable similarities between the situation in England in the early 1900s and the present situation in relation to infantile diarrhoeal disease in much of the developing world today. I became very interested in Sir George Newman (1870-1948) during his period as Medical Officer of Health in Finsbury, a deprived inner urban borough of London. I later published a paper in *Medical History* in 1998 entitled 'Sir George Newman, infant diarrhoeal mortality and the paradox of urbanism'. I really enjoyed my three months as a scholar, free from the burden of clinical responsibility for the first time in 33 years! I also enjoyed the intellectual life within the Wellcome, especially talking to the professional historians such as Bill Bynum and Roy Porter who were enormously encouraging. I also enjoyed the beautiful library of the History of Medicine in the Wellcome Building. It is a place of serenity, peace and beauty, a place to savour and enjoy, a safe harbour from the bombardments of modern life. Above all it is a place to read, to relax, to study and above all to reflect. Indeed it was this time to reflect which I valued most. In the rest of my life there had been and was to be so little time to reflect. I was continually being driven by events - clinical events and medical political events with almost no time for independent reflection, except perhaps when I was with colleagues travelling to meetings abroad, when we did have time to chew the cud.

Ever since that period in 1993, I have been an active member of the Twentieth Century History Group, an important section of the Wellcome Trust Centre concerned with recent history led by Tilli Tansey. She is a young dynamic woman who was trained as a physiologist but has found life as an historian to be more challenging. I have enormously valued her critical but constructive comments concerning my historical endeavours. I did in fact force myself to make time out of my routine work to be an active member and attend some of the activities of the group. My most memorable involvement with this group was to be after my retirement in June 2002, when I had the privilege of being chairman of the Witness Seminar on Cystic Fibrosis. These seminars are occasions when active participants are invited to attend and speak in front of a small audience about their own experiences as witnesses to the subject being discussed, trying to answer the questions.

What was it like at the time? Why did things happen the way they did? Everything said is recorded, typed up and the printed record reviewed by speakers, chairman etc. for accuracy of record and then is published. It provides a remarkable record of living history.

After my retirement, I went into the Wellcome Trust Centre about three times a week to continue research into the History of Medicine, especially related to George Newman and to gastroenterology, both paediatric and adult.

I also participated in the general activities of the centre.

I found it most exciting to find a substantial archive of letters written by George Newman from the age of seven years till seventy years (1877-1947). Apparently Quakers such as the Newmans like to keep family correspondence throughout their lives. The letters were written chiefly to his favourite maiden aunt but also to his mother, sister and occasionally to his father, with a few in his latter days to his wife when he travelling abroad. These letters give a wonderful window into the life of one man growing from boyhood to maturity and then on to old age. Winston Churchill has remarked 'History with its flickering lamp, stumbles along the past, trying to reconstruct its scenes, to revive its echoes and kindle with pale gleams the passions of former days.' My own elation was great when I stumbled upon Newman's correspondence in the Wellcome Library for the History and Understanding of Medicine. It illuminated for me in a quite wonderful way the man whose professional doings I had been studying. Now I could study the man, behind the remarkable medical officer of health, and read for example his boyhood enthusiasm when he wrote from Bootham School of his decision to study medicine to his aunt in 1886.

> I now begin to see what vast advantages my lot is to slave living in a glorious English rural home, learning at the finest Quaker school in the country; I have the great choice of life being free to take almost what I asked of this world's trades and professions. I have selected God helping me, the greatest, grandest and most useful profession of the times and may I succeed. What a constant of blessings through my happy life'.

This led me to study his childhood and to visit his old school, Bootham, in York. There, the archivist Mrs Margaret Ainscough was able to assemble a remarkable amount of information concerning George Newman the boy, even with photographs and an original essay he had written in 1886 on famines in India.

My historical involvement with the Society of Apothecaries and teaching was quite different. This I began before retirement at the Royal Free Hospital in 1998 following my appointment as Society of Apothecaries Lecturer in the History of Medicine, when I established a special teaching module for medical history with Prof. Neil McIntyre for medical undergraduates. This module was for a month and was a period when we hoped to inspire students in the history of medicine.

A key aspect of this module were weekly outside visits. These included the Wellcome Library and The Wellcome History of Medicine Galleries in the Science Museum. These contain a truly remarkable collection of the artefacts of medicine through the centuries of interest both to doctors and to laymen. Sue Weir, a dynamic trained nurse and now a very lively professional guide who led us to the Chelsea Physic Garden (founded by Society of Apothecaries in 1673), the John Hunter Collection in the Royal College of Surgeons and the nineteenth century operating theatre of the old St Thomas's Hospital, which has survived astonishingly intact, as well as St Bartholomew's Hospital and the old Royal Free Hospital in Gray's Inn Road. I myself led a trip to the British Museum to focus on the Graeco-Roman world. Sue and I were very pleased by the enthusiastic response of the students to these visits but also a little surprised be their lack of knowledge of the history of London and indeed the main outlines of British history. Several had studied history at school but all they seemed to remember were in depth studies of Hitler and Stalin and the second world war. They seemed to know almost nothing about the British Empire and what they did know seemed to be tinged with curious embarrassment about the period. For me I liked the direct contact with students for a reasonably long period of time. This was so lacking in my routine paediatric teaching of students at the Royal Free, where I only saw the same students on one or two occasions. This module was successfully taught for four years with very positive formal feed-back from the students. My perception that the historic dimension can enrich one's vocation in medicine was strengthened by this experience of the Royal Free in the History of Medicine module. The Royal Free students who elected to do this module had immense intellectual vigour and zest for life and the module gave them a time for reflection.

However after retirement I was appointed course director for the Diploma course in History of Medicine for medical post-graduates (doctors both in-practice and retired) and medical under-graduates as well as a few other interested people. I took over a very successful course directed by Robin Price over eleven very successful years. At first I had the assistance of Kim Edmunds of the Apothecaries who was the key to the good organization of the course. Both professional historians and amateur historians (doctors) are involved in giving talks on alternate Saturday mornings, across the whole wide range of medical history from antiquity to recent times. There is then an option to write a dissertation and to sit an examination in order to obtain the diploma itself but this not compulsory.

At this point a brief description of the Worshipful Society of Apothecaries will be given as it is an example of living history. It is both a Livery Company of the city of London, with a royal charter granted by King James I in 1617, and also a member of the only non-university licensing body in Britain, the

United Examining Board.

The original Apothecaries Hall was burnt down in the great fire of London but the present Hall dates from 1668 to 1672. The Hall is a magnificent chamber hung with the portraits of kings and the former masters of the Apothecaries. Apothecaries were those who dispensed medicines and they clashed with the physicians who prescribed medicines in the eighteenth century. Eventually the Apothecaries were granted the right to both subscribe and dispense and can be seen now as the ancestors of modern general practitioners.

I became a Yeoman of the Apothecaries in 1973 and in due course in 1983 a Liveryman, which entitled me to be admitted to the Freedom of the City of London in a brief ceremony and so to vote for the Lord Mayor of London. I also became an examiner in medicine in the Society of Apothecaries from 1978-1983, the first paediatrician to become an examiner. I used to bring child patients from Barts to be examined as part of the final examination by candidates for the Licence in Medicine and Surgery of the Society of Apothecaries (LMSSA) in the ancient Hall of the Apothecaries itself. The children and their parents enjoyed the occasion and they were given a small financial recompense. It was strange though, to conduct a modern examination amidst such ancient but beautiful surroundings. From time to time over many years I have attended memorable dinners in the Hall itself The Faculty of History of Medicine, is a distinct entity within the Society itself to foster the History of Medicine.

London provides many and varied opportunities for the medical historian. I liked the intellectual life of the Wellcome Trust Centre for the History of Medicine of America. I also enjoyed the on-going interaction with Chris Booth, Tilli Tansey and Gordon Cook and others. I joined the council of the Osler Club. This is a medico-historical club which honours the memory of Sir William Osler, a great Canadian physician who had a distinguished career in Canada, USA and who finally was Regius Professor of Medicine in Oxford. He was a great clinician and was author of a major medical text which ran to many editions but also had a great interest in the history and philosophy of medicine and a great source of inspiration to many. The club meets regularly for presentations related to the history of medicine. I have made four presentations to it over the years, on the History of the Queen Elizabeth Hospital for Children, Sir George Newman, Quaker pioneer of Child Health, Smallpox, Queen Mary II and Walter Harris and History of Paediatrics also belong to another club which has medico-historical interests and that is the Harveian Society which honours the memory of William Harvey, the first to recognize the true role of the heart in the circulation of the blood. Finally

I was on the council of the newly formed British Society of the History of Paediatrics and Child Health.

For doctors I believe there is a great educational value for the history of medicine. It alerts us to what has gone on before. It can both inspire and challenge the medical student and practising doctor. I believe knowledge and study of the history of medicine could provide some inspiration 'so that ideals do not die and hopes perish', to use the words of Alcuin of York (735-804) in today's National Health Service. Could it even be that such knowledge might be one factor raising morale in today's medical profession?

For me an historic perspective is of immense value when looking to the future. As the Queen said in her Christmas broadcast in 1999. 'We can make sense of the future if we understand the lesson of the past'. Modern technology provides a great way of revealing, for example, my great interest in the hitherto inaccessible small intestine only became possible by technological advance, so I do believe with St Augustine 'the new is in the old concealed, the old is in the new revealed'. Historical study of such technological advance is now a major area of study.

I retired from the Wellcome Centre for History of Medicine in the summer of 2008 and as Course Director for the Diploma in History of Medicine in the summer of 2009, after nine years. So this was a second retirement for me, this time from the History of Medicine. I was sad to give up these activities. However I continue as an active member of the Osler Club and the Harveian Society. I was president of the Osler Club from 2007-2009 and the Harveian Society in 2009. It was notable that I had such strong support of members from both during my long GMC ordeal. During my cross-examination by the lady prosecutor I wore the medallion of the President of the Osler Club under my shirt. Aequanimitas was a quality much admired by Sir William Osler. It was this stoic quality that I tried to emulate during my ordeal.

Index

Aden 57, 58, 246, 247
AIDS 100, 102, 192, 254-56
Alexandra, Princess 149
Alfred, Duke of Edinburgh 46
Allerton family 31
Allman, Mr & Mrs 17, 19
Amadi, Beatrice 177, 192
Anderson, Charlotte 89, 90, 96, 112, 116, 119, 120, 160, 163, 244
Anderson, K.D. 24
Anderson Stuart, Sir Thomas, 36-38, 44
Andrews, Ethel (Auntie Ethel) 3, 5, 9, 14, 15, 74
Anne, Princess 261, 270
Antwerp 61
Aquitania 10
Aramaic 59-61
Araya, Magdalena 116, 123, 126, 150
Arbuthnot, James 195
Asperger's Syndrome 208
Atun, Rif 193
Auricchio, Salvatore 97, 103, 184, 188
Auschwitz 227
autism 70, 115, 178, 206-19, 221, 235
Backhouse, Rev. Nigel á Beckett 17
Balgowlah, Sydney 3-5
Banchini, Giacomo 187, 188
Barnes, Colin & Marian 71, 104, 137
Barrett, Martin 77, 125
Bartram, Clive 146-199
Barts (St Bartholomew's Hospital) 51-71, 74, 77, 94, 96, 106, 116, 119-26, 128-41, 144, 146-55, 158, 159, 161, 165, 167-70, 174-81, 185-87, 189, 191, 193, 195-05, 232, 261, 169, 273, 276, 177
Bates, Maggie 154
Batty, de Witt Bishop 12
Baum, Prof. David 214
Bavin, L. 7, 16
Beattie, Mark 200
Bellanti, Joseph 215
Benedict xvi, 271
Benton, Sarah 200
Berelowitz, Mark 212
Berry, Sir Colin 202
Besser, Michael 202
Betjeman, Sir John 121, 122
Bhan, Raj 190
Bird, Antony 20
Bird, Dick 143
Bishop, Ruth 114, 142
Blackburn, Ruthven 41, 156
Blackburn, Sir Charles Bickerton 36, 41
Blair, Tony 248, 249, 251, 261
Blomfield, Jeanette 115, 116
Bodley Scott, Sir Ronald 74
Boorman, Sir Derek 200
Booth, Sir Christopher xi, 68-72, 82, 102, 121, 150, 221, 232, 250, 273, 277
Booth, Ian 226, 228, 229
Borthwick, Brian & Ethel 5, 74, 88

Borthwick, Florence (Auntie Flo) 5
Borthwick, Jean 74
Borthwick, Tom (Uncle Tom) 5
Boston 96, 97, 109, 151, 152, 187, 192, 232
Bottomley, Virginia 195, 196, 201
Bourquin, Donnie & Annette 104
Bowen, Rev. Paul 138, 268
Boyce, Malcolm 129
Bradhurst, Peter 27
Brain, Michael 70, 71
Braegger, Christian 148, 192
Branski, David 185
Brierley, Bill 23, 24
British Paediatric Association (BPA) 125, 132, 156, 157, 160, 161
British Society of Paediatric Gastroenterology, Hepatology & Nutrition (BSPGHAN) 122, 160-62, 229
Brock, Lord 77
Brompton Hospital 74, 76-78, 139
Brooks, W.W. 74
Brown, Roderick 140, 168
Bruce, Terry 144
Buchan, John 240
Burgess, John 53, 78, 80, 81, 88
Burrel, Jimmy 25
Busby, Betty & Colin 71, 270
Buswell, Joan 31, 127
Buswell, Lell (Auntie Lell) 29-31, 54, 97, 127
Buswell, Richard 9, 17, 23, 31
Bye, Billy 44, 72
Calman, Sir Kenneth 213, 215
Cambridge 30, 36, 68, 107, 133, 151, 182, 187, 204, 232, 237
Cameron, Don 88
Campbell, Colin 146
Candy, David 216
Carey, Archbishop George 69
Carter, Christine 178
Castellanata, S. 187
Chang, Me-Hwei 193
Charles, Prince of Wales 260-62
Chartres, Bishop Richard 270
Chong, Sonny 148-50
Churchill, Randolph 77
Churchill, Winston 10, 263, 275
Clark, Eve 111
Clark, Jackie 154
coeliac disease 67, 71, 94, 105, 114, 115, 120, 123, 133, 140, 141, 145, 148, 152, 155, 157, 158, 168, 184, 209, 210, 273
Commonwealth Association of Paediatric Gastroenterology & Nutrition (CAPGAN) 101, 173, 189, 194, 254
Connolly, Kevin 75, 77
Cook, Gordon 277
Correggio 272
Costeloe, Kate 50, 139, 167, 174, 202
Cotterill, Andrew 135
Couture, François 68
Cox, Patrick 121, 122, 125, 129, 139, 167
Cremer, Brian 88
Crohn, Burrill 86
Crohn's disease 77, 85-87, 104, 109, 144, 146, 147, 155, 169, 174, 176, 178, 180, 207-18
Crohn's in Childhood Research Appeal (CICRA) 135, 140, 146, 140-52, 168, 175, 178, 182, 202
Crosby capsule 67, 70, 94, 105, 175 176
Cross, Canon Alan 269
Curtin, John 10

Cyprus 193, 194, 246, 247
Dacie, John 68
Davidson, George 112
Davis, John 68, 102
Dawson, Sir Anthony xi, 119, 124, 125, 129, 130, 133, 134, 137, 141, 144, 146, 149, 168
Dey, Lindsay 158
Diana, Princess of Wales 260
Dick, Bob 53, 54, 88
Dickens, Charles xiv, 28
Dickinson, John 203
Dillon, Michael 152
Dinning, Bill 233, 272
Dodge, John 232
Dods, Sir Lorimer 43, 52, 92, 93, 110
Dolinesk, Jerne 194
Domizio, Paolo 148
Dorman, David 113
Douglas, John 149
Douglas, Robert 232
Douglas-Hume, Sir Alec 129
Dourmashkin, Robert 149, 150
Dowd, Bryan 92, 93, 273
Dudgeon, Prof. Alistair 145
Dunlop, Sir Derreck 73
Eden, Tim 199
Edinburgh 35, 38, 46, 51, 65, 71-73, 78, 80, 81, 84, 85, 111, 112, 150, 168, 213
Edmunds, Kim 276
Egypt 50, 58, 59, 247
Eldershaw, Pat 28
Elizabeth II 43, 171, 244, 253, 257-59
Elizabeth, Queen Mother 36, 43, 172, 244, 258, 264, 265
Elliott, Elizabeth 169
Ellis, Dick & Liz 137
Else, Martin 177, 199, 201, 202, 204, 207
England, Debbie 178
ESPGAN (European Society of Paediatric Gastroenterology & Nutrition, later ESPGHAN) 78, 103, 144, 165, 183-86, 203
European Society of Paediatric Gastroenterology 112, 114, 160, 184
European Society of Paediatric Gastroenterology Hepatology and Nutrition (ESPGHAN) 144, 159, 177, 184, 185, 194, 233
Evans, Philip 125
Falk, Herbert 212
Farthing, Michael 114, 169, 202
Feizi, Ten 71, 74
Fell, John 175
Ferguson, Ann 150, 213
Ferriera, Roque 169
Fisher, Archbishop Geoffrey 11, 269
Fletcher, Charles 68, 75
Ford, Sir Edward 44
Forster, 'Bish' 24, 25
Fox, Alexander 171
Fox, Dick 88
France, Norman 141
Freier, Serem 78, 185
Fulton, John 92
Furlano, Raoul 192
Gallipoli 20, 29, 59
Galton, David 71, 232, 233, 235, 272
Gardner, Baroness 234, 251
Garrod, Sir Archibald 158, 199
Gaze, Harold 107
Gee, Samuel 158, 273
George V 2, 9, 25, 46
George VI 2, 20, 171, 253, 258-60, 263
Gibraltar 61, 246-49

Glasgow 3, 32, 64, 73, 80, 81
GMC (General Medical Council) 199, 218, 220-26, 228-30, 233, 234, 235, 278
Gorton, Sir John 251
C Gough, Archbishop Hugh 267
Goulston, Stan 83
Goulston, Kerry 35, 89
Graham, Billy 44
Great Ormond St Hospital 125, 132, 158, 161, 261
Greece 15, 26, 28, 65, 78, 152, 240
Grigg, Darcy 20, 25-28, 60, 240, 253
Guandalini, Stefano 184, 187
Guy, Bishop & Mrs 78, 108
Guiness, Howard 266
Hadjiminas, John 193
Hadorn, Beat 112, 115, 116, 118
Hamburg 61
Hamilton, Dick 108, 164
Hamilton-Fairley, Prof. Gordon 137
Hammersmith Hospital 53, 66, 68-72, 74-77, 83, 89, 94, 102, 104, 107, 112, 151, 221, 250
Harcourt, Paul 235
Harper, Margaret 158
Harries, John 141, 161, 165, 185
Harris, Owen 88
Harris, Richard 42
Harrison, Dorothy 84, 88, 90, 95
Harrison, John 164
Harrison, Mary 135, 145
Harveian Society 277, 278
Harvey, David 69, 107, 250
Harvey, William 36, 277
Haselgrave, Marianne 254
Haskins, Louise 258
Hauer, Christine 192
Henry, Duke of Gloucester 13
Heuschkel, Rob 148, 151, 152, 175, 182, 232
Hill, Don 235
Hitching, Allan 235
Hodgson, Humphry 219
Holy Land 78, 80, 108, 246, 270
Horton, Richard 214, 217, 219
Housman, A.E. 193, 237, 238, 271
Howard, John 251, 255, 256, 263
Hudson, Prof. 200
Hughes, William Morris 12
Hull, Sir David 124, 198, 199, 207, 226
Hunter, Bob 78
Hunter, Dafydd 136
Hutchins, Paul 135, 151, 173
Hyer, Warren 151
India 143, 183, 189-91, 246, 247, 253, 262, 273
Interlaken 105, 112, 114, 116, 120, 145, 184, 189
IRA bombs xiv, 136
Isle of Mull 65, 81, 242
Italy 19, 61, 187, 188, 242
Jackson, Michael 173
Jackson, Tony 140, 168
James, Geraint 68
Jenkins, Peter 26
Jowell, Tessa 213
Kafka, Franz 221, 235
Kamath, Ramanand 116, 150
Katz, Prof. Julian 92, 121
Kelly, Deidre 159, 162, 234
Kelsy-Fry, Ian 134, 135
Kennedy, John, assassination of 76
Kenrick, Ken 114
Kilby, Anne 144
King George V battleship 9
King George V Memorial Hospital, Sydney 47

King's College, London 27
Kipling, Rudyard 24, 191, 238, 257
Krasilnikoff, Peter 107
Larusdottir, Karolina 242
Laurence, Bernard 140, 168, 260
Lawrence, Prof. Chris 273
Lebenthal, Emi 165, 185
Lee, Margaret 149
Leighton, Lord 15
Letchford, Joseph, William, Morgen, Chloe, Lily and Stephanie (author's grandchildren) 203, 236, 243, 262
Letchford, Paul 138, 236
Libby, Gerald 144
Lightwood, Prof. 100
Lionetti, Paolo 187
Lindley, Keith 214
Lipson, Lisa 66, 150
Liverpool 55, 62, 191, 253
London House 66, 68, 69, 72, 75, 81, 108, 248, 268
Lutyens, Edwin 191
MacDonald, John & Geoff 93
Macdonald, Tom 150, 155, 168, 174, 179, 185, 192, 197-99, 202
Mackay, Helen 158, 159
Mackellar, Dorothea 25
Malpas, Prof. Jim 122, 134, 198, 233
Mangiwa, Jan 116
Manly, Sydney 3, 4, 10, 14, 266
Manuel, Peter 145, 150
Masefield, John 29
McIntyre Neil 232, 233, 275
McLean, Alison 199
McNeish, Sandy 160, 161, 185, 189
Meadows, Nigel 139, 201, 204
Mearns, Margaret 140
Mee, Arthur 239, 240
Meath-Baker, Judith 78, 108
Medical Art Society 242
Melbourne 41, 43, 46, 85, 89, 90, 94, 96, 97, 114, 116, 119, 120, 142, 144, 160, 251
Menzies, Sir Robert 59, 181, 249, 258
Meszaros, Andor, 19, 47
Meynkohn, Heino 104
Middleton, Arch 113, 126, 144
Middleton, Bob 86
Middleton, Kate 264
Milla, Peter 161, 166, 214
Miller, Victor 161, 229
Mistilis, Steve 83, 85, 88
Mitchell, John 135
Mittal, Santosh 189
Mitting, Mr Justice 218, 234, 235
MMR vaccine 207-18, 227
Mollin, David 68, 70
Montgomery, Viscount 10
Morgenthaler, Willi 111
Morrow, Sir William 41, 47, 48, 69, 83, 90
Morson, Basil 86, 87
Mortimer, Graham 92, 93, 110
Morton HV 188, 240
Mowatt, Ashley & Kathleen 137
Mowatt, Alex 151, 161, 165
Mowbray House School 7, 11, 12, 16, 32, 271
Mowll, Archbishop Howard 4, 30, 31
Murdoch, Sue 242, 263
Murch, Simon 139, 148, 164, 167, 174, 176, 177, 179, 181, 199, 202-04, 209, 211, 213, 216, 218, 219, 229, 233
Nazer, Hisham 145, 150
Neale, Graham 70
Newman, Sir George 274, 275, 277
Nicholls, Michael 35
Nicholson, Sir Charles 36

Nicholson, Gordon 88
Nussle, Daniel 107
Oates, Kim 244
O'Leary, John 212, 216-18
Osler Club 277, 278
Osler, Sir William 13, 277, 278
Packard, Bob 83
Palmer, Cally 198, 199, 204
Pappworth, Maurice 71, 72
PARA 55, 254, 255
Parma 187, 188, 272
Parrott, Delphine 202
Partin, John 109
Pascoe, Toby 28
Paterson, A.B., ('Banjo') 25, 238
Peak, Howard 11, 49, 66, 127
Peak, Judith (née Walker Smith, author's sister) 9, 10, 12, 14, 15, 31, 33, 62, 64, 66, 75, 127, 259, 260, 267, 268
Peak, Stephen 243
Pepys, Jack 76, 242
Pepys, Sandra 79, 242
Phelan, Peter 85
Philip, Prince, Duke of Edinburgh 110, 258, 261
Philips, Ellen & Mary 170, 171
Phillips, Alan 135, 141-43, 145, 155, 165, 170, 172, 173, 176, 180, 182, 185, 192, 197, 199, 202, 203, 205, 232, 233
Pilcher, Bishop Venn 21
Pink, Ilfra 71, 77
Pocock, Wendy 68, 69, 71, 97
Porteous, Norma 119
Portman, Bernard 115
Pounder, Prof. Roy 202, 207, 213, 227
Powell, Enoch 237
Prader, Prof. Andrea xi, 90, 96, 97, 103, 105-07, 121
Price, Liz 145
Price, Robin 276
Prince, H.C.W. 24, 246
Prince Alfred Hospital Royal Sydney 2, 12, 13, 23, 40, 41, 43, 46, 47, 53, 66, 69, 72, 78, 83, 84, 86, 87, 89, 90, 93-96, 127, 147, 181, 210
Proctor, Thea 49
Qak, Dr 193
Quakers 275
Quash, Ben 272
Queen Elizabeth Hospital for Children, London 86, 107, 113, 119, 122, 129, 131-33, 136, 161, 171, 172, 195, 196, 205, 228, 260, 261, 277
Rahere 121, 153
Rampton, David 200
Ramsay, Archbishop Michael 44, 269, 270
Read, David 71, 78
Rees, Lesley 133, 134, 203
Renault, Mary 240
Reye, Douglas 95, 112
Rice, Steve 145
Richardson, Colonel John 20
Richardson, Captain Rupert 20
Robson, L.C. 17, 23, 253, 258
Rome 15, 26, 78, 82, 153, 188, 240, 267
Rossi, Prof. Ettore 107, 165
Rossiter, Mary 140, 144
Rowe, Peter 116, 118, 119, 142
Royal Alexandra Hospital for Children, Sydney 14, 43, 51, 71, 89, 91, 96, 109, 244, 261
Royal College of Physicians, Edinburgh 71-73, 80, 84, 85

Royal College of Physicians, London 66, 71, 72, 76, 158, 185, 242
Royal Free Hospital, London 88, 102, 125, 138, 139, 143, 151, 167, 180, 182, 197, 199, 207, 219, 221, 225, 227, 275, 276
Royal London Hospital 197
Rundle, Bob 41, 42
Sabra, Aderbal 215
St Andrew's Cathedral, Sydney 10, 12, 163, 267, 268
St Andrew's Church, Zurich 105
St Barnabas Church, Woodford Green 269
St Giles Church, Greenwich, Sydney 21, 236, 266
St Mary's RC Cathedral, Sydney 33, 60
St Thomas's Hospital 46, 48, 88, 102, 276
Salim, A.F.M. 170
Salisbury, David 213, 215
Sallabank, Jane 199, 202
San Francisco 108, 109
Sanderson, Ian 140, 150-52, 162, 165, 180, 201, 216, 232
Savage, Martin 140, 169, 177, 202, 205
Sawyer, Graham 235
Scadding, Prof. J.G., 74, 75, 139
Shmerling, David 96, 103-05, 107, 112, 114, 184, 192
Schmitz, Jacques 184
Schwachmann, Harry 96, 97, 152
Scotland 2, 3, 64, 65, 78, 80, 137, 192, 236, 240, 250, 269
Scott, Ron 31, 35
Scowen, Prof. Eric 124
Setchell, Garth 25, 31, 35
Shahrier, Mamoun 170
Shand, William 169
Shaw Savill Line 54, 57, 60
Shepherd, Ross 136, 143
Sherlock, Prof. Sheila 102, 162, 214
Shiner, Margot 143
Shooter, Prof. Reggie 134
Shore School, Sydney 4, 12, 13, 16-18, 21-32, 35, 47
Silverman, Fred 109, 163
Simpson, E. Barclay 75, 108, 122
Singapore 8, 39, 88, 89, 180, 183, 190, 192, 193, 247
Sinnett, Peter 41, 42
Skene, Ian 61, 62
Skyring, Alan 78, 83, 112
Slim, Viscount 30
Society of Apothecaries 262, 273, 275-77
Soeparto, Pitono 116, 145, 150
Soothill, Prof. John 132
South Africa 68, 97-102, 247, 254, 255, 259, 262
Southwell, Phil 38, 41
Soutter, George 66, 81, 97, 99, 100, 117
Spence, Sir James 92
Spencer, Jo 168
Spender, Stephen 238
Stamp, Terence 101
Stapleton, Prof. Tom 52, 89, 91, 92, 95-97, 107, 110-12, 116-19, 123, 125, 126, 220
Stevens, Sam 26
Stewart, Jimmy 67, 70
Stewart, Phil 31, 266
Stone, Evan 232, 233
Stott, Rev. John 268
Strandvik, Birgitte 184, 185

Suez Canal 58, 59, 246
Sullivan, Peter 186, 189, 254
Taiwan 183, 193
Tanner, Stuart 115, 162
Tansey, Tilli 273, 274, 277
Taylor, John Herman 77
Thatcher, Margaret 252, 270
Thom, Peter 35
Thomas, Neil 229
Thompson, Gilbert 70
Thompson, Phil 38, 41, 42, 126, 127
Thomson, Edgar 47
Thomson, Mike 139, 175-178, 181, 192, 209-11, 219
Tiley, Clem 28
Tilley, Arthur 235
Tindall, Don 41, 42
Tink, Arnold 94
Tippet, Sir Anthony 204
Tizard, Prof. Peter 68, 102
Todd, Ian 144, 169
Todd Report
Torrente, Camilla 182
Torrente, Franco 182, 187
Tomlinson Report 124, 133, 144, 170, 171, 174, 195-06
Trindall, Richard (author's grandfather) 16, 35
Trindall, Rosina (nana) 4, 9, 10, 31, 32, 241
Trindall, Dot (Auntie Dot) 32, 259
Trindall, Roy (Uncle Roy) 16, 29, 36, 259
Turner, Brian 116, 118
Turner-Warwick, Dame Margaret 76, 158
Turtle, John 38, 41, 42, 44, 88
University of Sydney 27, 34-45, 47, 91, 93, 112, 170, 244, 249, 251, 261
268, 270
Unsworth, Joe 152
Utrecht 94, 96
Van Maanen, Sue and Richard 235
Victoria, Queen xiv, 36, 255
Vieira, Mario 192
Visakorpi, Jarmo 96, 114, 184
Von Hagens, Gunther 39
Wagner, Alexander von 15
Wakefield, Andy 197, 199, 202, 207, 209, 211-13, 215, 218, 219-21, 226-28, 231, 233
Walker, Allan 151, 152, 158, 164, 165, 186, 192, 201, 232, 235
Walker-Smith, Alexandra Buckingham (author's mother) 2-4, 6-12, 15-17, 27, 28, 30, 31, 33, 37, 46, 51, 54, 59, 73, 83, 84, 97, 108-10, 112, 240, 241, 245, 249, 253, 257-60, 266
Walker-Smith, Angus Buchanan (author's father) 1-7, 10, 12-15, 21-23, 26, 27, 29, 30-33, 36, 39, 42, 46-48, 51, 54, 55, 57, 59, 63, 64, 73, 83, 92, 97, 108, 109, 112, 117, 125-27, 163, 181, 220, 241, 245, 249, 259, 267
Walker-Smith, Elizabeth (gran) 3, 4, 14, 15, 65
Walker-Smith, Edith (author's grand-daughter) 236, 243
Walker-Smith, Elizabeth ('Liz', author's wife) 65, 76, 88, 111, 113, 117, 121, 126-28, 130, 131, 137-39, 244, 263, 271
Walker-Smith, Hugh (author's uncle) 36
Walker-Smith, James (author's son) 21, 111, 138, 172, 188, 236, 243, 260, 269

Walker-Smith, John (author's grandfather) 2, 15, 80, 81
Walker-Smith, Laura (author's daughter) 126, 127, 118, 138, 236, 238, 242, 260, 268
Walker-Smith, Louise (author's daughter) 46, 112, 117, 126-29, 136, 138, 154, 236, 260, 266
Walker-Smith, Suki 236, 243
Walsh, Dermot 9
Walsh, Helen & Bob 93, 132
Warren, Ted (author's cousin) 10
Warren, Tom (Uncle Tom) 4, 32
Weijers, Dr 94, 96
Weir, Sue 276
Wellcome Trust Centre 117, 168, 179, 273, 274, 277, 278
Wershil, Barry 152
Wharton, Brian, 107, 133, 140 141
Wheeler, Lou 127
Whitlam, Gough 181, 252
William, Prince 262, 264
Williams, Capt. 54, 60
Williams, Christopher 147, 148, 151, 228, 229
Williams, Archbishop Rowan 269, 270
Winning, Kate 158
Wollman, David 66, 78, 109, 268
Wollstonecraft, 5, 7, 11, 17, 23, 27, 52, 260, 266
Wood, Prof. Chris 122, 123, 125, 129, 131, 133, 135, 140, 149, 167, 204
Wood, Don 72, 81, 108
Wood-Walker, Bob 101
Wright, David 77, 101
Wright, Sir Nicholas 232
Wright, Vanessa 113, 204
Wyndham, Norman 40, 87
Yap, Boh-Gee 193
York 81, 162, 163, 198, 207, 275
Young, Winifred 133, 159
Yu, John 52, 53, 71, 89, 93, 94, 97, 107, 108, 111, 112, 118-20, 194, 261, 270
Zilbauer, Matt 182
Zimbabwe (Rhodesia) 97, 101, 247, 255-57
Zoppi, Giuseppe 97
Zuckerman, Prof. Arie 143, 177, 198, 201-07, 214
Zurich 90-109, 119, 121, 148, 175, 184, 192, 267